AF835835

Handbook of Pediatric Infection Prevention and Control

Handbook of Pediatric Infection Prevention and Control

Edited by **KRISTINA A. BRYANT AND JUDITH A. GUZMAN-COTTRILL**

OXFORD
UNIVERSITY PRESS

OXFORD
UNIVERSITY PRESS

Oxford University Press is a department of the University of Oxford. It furthers the University's objective of excellence in research, scholarship, and education by publishing worldwide. Oxford is a registered trade mark of Oxford University Press in the UK and certain other countries.

Published in the United States of America by Oxford University Press
198 Madison Avenue, New York, NY 10016, United States of America.

Library of Congress Cataloging-in-Publication Data
Names: Bryant, Kristina A. (Kristina Angel), editor. | Guzman-Cottrill, Judith A., editor.
Title: Handbook of pediatric infection prevention and control /
edited by Kristina A. Bryant, Judith A. Guzman-Cottrill.
Description: New York, NY : Oxford University Press, [2019] |
Includes bibliographical references and index.
Identifiers: LCCN 2018039055 | ISBN 9780190697174 (pbk. : alk. paper)
Subjects: | MESH: Infection Control—methods | Hospitals, Pediatric—organization & administration | Hospital Units—organization & administration
Classification: LCC RJ101 | NLM WX 167 | DDC 362.1989200068—dc23
LC record available at https://lccn.loc.gov/2018039055

9 8 7 6 5 4 3 2 1

Printed by Webcom, Inc., Canada

To my parents, Leo and Nancy K, and Hannah, Jeff and Dean (KAB)

To my parents, Virgilio and Flordelis, and Jerod, Miles, and Ruby (JGC)

CONTENTS

CONTRIBUTORS

Susan Coffin, MD, MPH
Clinical Director, Division of Infectious Diseases
Children's Hospital of Philadelphia
Philadelphia, Pennsylvania

Donna Fisher, MD
Chief, Division of Pediatric Infectious Diseases
Baystate Children's Hospital
Springfield, Massachusetts
Medical Director, Hospital Epidemiology and Infection Control
Associate Professor of Pediatrics
University of Massachusetts School of Medicine
Amherst, Massachusetts

Jane M. Gould, MD
Medical Epidemiologist
Healthcare-Associated Infections/ Antimicrobial Resistance Program
Division of Disease Control
Philadelphia, Pennsylvania
Public Health Physician Consultant
Pennsylvania Department of Health
Harrisburg, Pennsylvania

Galit Holzmann-Pazgal, MD
Associate Director of Infection Prevention
Texas Children's Hospital—West Campus
Houston, Texas

Michele D. Honeycutt, MNSc, RN, CIC, FAPIC
Director of Infection Prevention
Arkansas Children's Hospital
Little Rock, Arkansas

Olivia Jackson, RN
Infection Control Coordinator
Elizabeth Seton Pediatrics Center
Yonkers, New York

Candace Johnson, MD
Assistant Professor of Pediatrics
Division of Pediatric Infectious Diseases
Columbia University Irving Medical Center
New York, New York

Manjiree V. Karandikar, MD, MBS
Assistant Professor, Division of Pediatric Infectious Diseases and Global Health
UCSF Benioff Children's Hospital
San Francisco, California

Grace M. Lee, MD, MPH
Professor of Pediatrics
Stanford University School of Medicine
Palo Alto, California

Karen Lehan, MD
Resident Physician
Department of Pediatrics
University of Texas at Austin Dell Medical School
Austin, Texas

W. Matthew Linam, MD, MS
Medical Director of Quality Improvement for Pediatric Infectious Diseases
Medical Director for the Vascular Access Team
Associate Professor, Pediatric Infectious Diseases
Emory University School of Medicine and Children's Healthcare of Atlanta
Atlanta, Georgia

Preeti Mehrotra, MD, MPH
Attending Physician
Division of Infectious Diseases
Beth Israel Deaconess Medical Center
Boston, Massachusetts

William Middlesworth, MD
Associate Professor of Surgery
Department of Surgery
Columbia University Irving Medical Center
New York, New York

Meghan Murray, RN, MPH
Doctoral Candidate
Graduate Partnership Program Fellow
National Institutes of Health
Columbia University School of Nursing
New York, New York

Natalie Neu, MD, MPH
Associate Professor of Pediatrics
Division of Infectious Diseases
Department of Pediatrics
Columbia University Irving Medical Center
New York, New York

Ann-Christine Nyquist, MD, MSPH
Medical Director, Infection Prevention and Control
Children's Hospital Colorado
Professor, Pediatrics—Infectious Diseases and Epidemiology
University of Colorado School of Medicine
Aurora, Colorado

Jared Olson, PharmD, BCCPS
Infectious Diseases Pharmacist
Department of Pharmacy
Primary Children's Hospital
Salt Lake City, Utah

Gholabamas Amin Ostovar, MD
Clinical Assistant Professor
College of Medicine
University of Arizona
Phoenix, Arizona
Department of Infection Prevention and Control
Maricopa Integrated Health System
Phoenix, Arizona

Sarah Turner Pietruszka, MD
Resident Physician
Department of Obstetrics and Gynecology
Wake Forest Baptist Health
Winston Salem, North Carolina

Claudette Poole, MD
Assistant Professor of Pediatrics
Division of Pediatric Infectious Diseases
University of Alabama at Birmingham
Birmingham, Alabama

Caroline Quach, MD, MSc, FRCPC, FSHEA
Professor, Departments of Microbiology, Infectious Disease and Immunology, and Pediatrics
University of Montreal
Medical Lead, Infection Prevention and Control
CHU Sainte-Justine
Pediatric Medical Director
OPTILAB Montreal-CHUM
Montreal, Quebec
Canada

Lorry G. Rubin, MD
Chief of Infectious Diseases
Division of Infectious Diseases, Department of Pediatrics
Steven and Alexandra Cohen Children's Medical Center of New York
Northwell Health
New Hyde Park, New York
Department of Pediatrics
Donald and Barbara Zucker School of Medicine at Hofstra/Northwell
Hempstead, New York

Lisa Saiman, MD, MPH
Professor of Pediatrics
Department of Pediatrics
Columbia University Irving Medical Center
Department of Infection Prevention and Control
New York—Presbyterian Hospital
New York, New York

Thomas J. Sandora, MD, MPH
Associate Professor of Pediatrics
Harvard Medical School
Division of Infectious Diseases
Boston Children's Hospital
Boston, Massachusetts

Aqsa Shakoor, MD
Resident Physician
Department of Surgery
Columbia University Irving Medical Center
New York, New York

Andi L. Shane, MD, MPH, MSc
Associate Professor, Infectious Diseases and Global Health
Marcus Professor, Hospital Epidemiology and Infection Control
Emory University School of Medicine
Atlanta, Georgia

Emily A. Thorell, MD, MSCI
Associate Professor, Pediatric Infectious Diseases
University of Utah School of Medicine
Director, Antimicrobial Stewardship Program and Associate Hospital Epidemiologist
Primary Children's Hospital
Salt Lake City, Utah

Meera Varman, MD
Professor, Pediatrics
Pediatric Infectious Diseases Section
Creighton University School of Medicine
Omaha, Nebraska

Vini Vijayan, MD
Assistant Professor, Pediatrics
Pediatric Infectious Diseases Section
University of Arkansas for Medical Sciences
Little Rock, Arkansas

INTRODUCTION

KRISTINA A. BRYANT AND JUDITH A. GUZMAN-COTTRILL

Children are not just small adults. For generations, pediatricians have been well aware of this fact. Some of these differences are obvious, such as weight-based medication dosing. However, when considering healthcare-associated infection prevention strategies, the differences may not be so obvious. For example, it is well established that clinicians should avoid using the femoral vein for central venous access, because femoral catheters have a higher risk of central line–associated bloodstream infection (CLABSI). This is rated a Category IA recommendation by the Centers for Disease Control and Prevention (CDC) . . . for adults. In children, however, the femoral vein has not been identified as an independent CLABSI risk factor and continues to be a suggested insertion site. Similarly, routine care and maintenance of adult catheter dressings include once-weekly dressing changes. Quite the opposite, the standard of care in the neonatal intensive care unit (NICU) setting is to only change the occlusive dressing if it becomes wet or soiled.

In the fields of healthcare epidemiology and infection prevention, evidence to guide pediatric practice has been lacking for quite some time. However, in the past few decades, more pediatric clinicians, researchers, epidemiologists, and infection preventionists have been contributing to this important field. This textbook discusses topics that pediatric providers must tackle in many settings: ambulatory clinics, emergency departments, community hospitals, and freestanding university children's hospitals. Each chapter opens with a clinical scenario (perhaps you have dealt with a few of these scenarios in real life), and follows with questions that are frequently raised when a solution is sought. We hope each chapter provides practical guidance and solutions to the problems we face daily.

We would like to acknowledge the leadership of the Pediatric Infectious Diseases Society (PIDS), who supported this book's development. PIDS is the world's largest organization of professionals dedicated to the treatment, control, and eradication of infectious diseases affecting children. From fellowship training to continuing medical education, research, regulatory issues, and guideline development, PIDS members are the core professionals advocating for the improved health of children with infectious diseases both nationally and around the world, participating in critical public health and medical professional advisory committees that determine the treatment and prevention of infectious diseases, immunization practices in children, and the education of pediatricians. For more information, visit http://www.pids.org.

We also offer our sincere thanks to the members of the Pediatric Leadership Council steering committee of the Society for Healthcare Epidemiology of America (SHEA) for their many contributions to this book, including thoughtful editorial review. We would like to acknowledge Dr. Jane Gould, who initially realized the need for this book as a resource. As a professional society, SHEA improves public health by establishing infection prevention measures and supporting antibiotic stewardship among healthcare providers. Since its founding in 1980, SHEA has helped define best practices in healthcare epidemiology worldwide.

Finally, we are compelled to provide a disclaimer. For a number of infection prevention issues in pediatrics, we do not have evidence-based guidelines to shape our practice. In daily practice, we often reach out to our friends and colleagues and ask, "How do you deal with this or that situation at your facility?" We hope this book fills a need for those who don't necessarily have the email addresses of experts in the field. We have to acknowledge however that there is often more than one "right" approach, especially in the absence of robust data. The recommendation in this book reflect the experiences of the authors and are in no way intended as mandates.

1 | Pathogens Spread via Respiratory Route

CLAUDETTE POOLE AND ANN-CHRISTINE NYQUIST

Background

Respiratory infections in children are one of the most common reasons for evaluation by healthcare personnel (HCP) in all healthcare settings. Lower respiratory tract infections (LRTI) are among the most common reasons for pediatric hospitalizations, and a common cause is viruses.[1–3] These infections pose significant challenges for infection prevention and contribute to the burden of HAIs. This is especially true in less-resourced communities.[4]

The full scope of the disease burden of respiratory infections was not fully appreciated prior to the routine use of molecular diagnostics employing polymerase chain reactions (PCR) to detect the presence of viral nucleic acids. Over the last several years, more and more investigators have started describing the burden of healthcare-associated respiratory viral infections using PCR and multiplexed testing. A recent study conducted at two large children's hospitals found the incidence rate of laboratory-confirmed hospital-acquired viral respiratory tract infection was 1.29 per 1,000 patient days, which was higher than the published rates of healthcare-associated bloodstream infections during the same time period of 0.51–0.87 per 1,000 patient days.[5] It is now estimated that HAI due to viruses contributes to around 29% of all HAI in children, which is roughly equivalent to central line-associated bloodstream infections (CLABSI), surgical site infections (SSI), and catheter-associated urinary tract infections (CAUTI) combined.

Clinical Scenario

The neonatal intensive care unit (NICU) nurse manager calls you to report a chicken pox exposure. Yesterday the four-year-old brother of twin patients was visiting his siblings' bedside in the NICU for approximately 20 minutes. Last night the sibling developed mild nasal congestion, cough, and a high fever. This morning the sibling woke up with a vesicular rash and has been diagnosed with chicken pox by his pediatrician.

Questions

How should the diagnosis of chicken pox be confirmed in the ill brother? Which patients should be placed in isolation precautions, and for how long? What options for post-exposure prophylaxis exist, and what measures should be considered for patients, visitors, or employees?

Key Challenges

The burden of respiratory pathogen transmission is particularly pronounced in facilities that care for children, for several reasons:

- The most common reason for hospitalization in previously healthy children is respiratory illness, which is largely due to viruses.[2]
- Younger children are efficient spreaders of these pathogens due to developmentally appropriate behaviors, including mouthing, thumb and finger sucking, drooling, and not being able to cover their mouths when coughing or blowing their noses.
- Family members, who may be less aware about disease transmission, provide direct hands-on care for their children while hospitalized, and then move freely throughout the hospital.
- Hospitalized children may congregate in shared areas.
- Many studies have demonstrated that young children can be asymptomatically infected with respiratory viruses or have only mild symptoms, making it difficult to identify patients to place on appropriate isolation precautions.[6,7]
- Many vaccine-preventable infections are spread via the respiratory route, such as measles (airborne transmission) and pertussis or whooping cough (droplet transmission), making younger children who have not received their vaccines particularly vulnerable.

- Some pathogens spread via the respiratory route may cause very mild symptoms or be completely asymptomatic in immune-competent hosts but can cause severe and sometimes fatal disease in certain vulnerable populations with compromised immune systems, including, but not limited to, premature neonates, patients with chronic lung disease, or post-transplant patients.[8–10]

Outbreaks of respiratory pathogens in pediatric healthcare settings, including pertussis, respiratory syncytial virus (RSV), influenza viruses, parainfluenza virus, human metapneumovirus, adenovirus, measles, and varicella, are well described in the literature.[11-19] Sources of infection include patients, visitors, and HCPs. This chapter will discuss some of the common and less common pathogens spread via the respiratory route, with suggestions for effective prevention strategies based on either best evidence or best practice. To compound the challenges of implementing effective infection prevention strategies, there is a lack of pediatric-specific research, a lack of national pediatric-specific quality measures, and the implementation of infection prevention practices that have been validated only in adult populations.[20]

Challenges in the NICU Setting

Routine screening for respiratory tract viruses in the NICU is not standard practice. Nevertheless, multiple studies have demonstrated that these pathogens are involved in disease outbreaks within the NICU, are prevalent, and are related to negative outcomes. A retrospective study querying an international database of reported outbreaks in hospitals identified 44 NICU outbreaks, with over half secondary to respiratory viral infections with a subsequent case fatality rate of 13%.[21]

In one study of premature infants, the prevalence of viral respiratory infections was 50% during the birth hospitalization. Infected babies had significantly longer hospital stays, more days of ventilation, and a higher rate of bronchopulmonary dysplasia compared to a matched cohort of babies who did not acquire a viral respiratory tract infection. No reliable clinical predictors of the presence of a respiratory virus were found.[22] A similarly designed study, conducted in Spain, found that only 9% of the babies acquired a respiratory virus.[23] Study authors postulated that the low incidence of acquisition of respiratory viruses was due to strict adherence to infection control practices, although these practices were not described. In a third study, the use of a viral respiratory panel test (either direct fluorescent antigen or PCR) at the time of a clinical sepsis evaluation performed on neonates during their birth hospitalization identified a viral respiratory tract infection in 6–10% of the evaluations done. In the same cohort, 10–15% of evaluations identified central venous catheter-associated bloodstream infections.[24-25] Collectively, these studies suggest that, before the availability of sensitive molecular testing, the ability to diagnose healthcare-associated viral infections was lacking, and until more extensive epidemiological studies are performed in different patient populations, the true prevalence of these infections will remain unknown.

Challenges in Post-Transplant Patients

Acquisition of a respiratory virus in the pre- or post-transplant period is associated with an increase in severe disease and death.[26,27] Multiple viruses, including RSV, parainfluenza, influenza, and human metapneumovirus, progress from upper respiratory tract infections to LRTIs in this patient population, with an attendant high mortality rate. Other than influenza, for which the initiation of antiviral therapy within 48 hours of symptoms was associated with a reduction in mortality, there are no effective therapies for most of the other viruses, and prevention of infection is therefore paramount.[28-30]

Challenges in Respiratory Virus Surveillance

Implementation of effective prevention strategies starts with effective surveillance. The Centers for Disease Control and Prevention (CDC) define an HAI as a localized or systemic condition resulting from an adverse reaction to the presence of an infectious agent(s) or its toxin(s).[31] There must be no evidence that the infection was present or incubating at the time of admission to the acute care setting, which is difficult to ascertain for many respiratory pathogens. It is important to note that these surveillance definitions may differ from clinical definitions. Determining the true prevalence of healthcare-associated respiratory infections is challenging for a number of reasons:

1. The incubation time of respiratory viruses varies.
2. Some viruses incubating at admission will manifest more than three days later.
3. Not all children with viral symptoms are tested.

4. Viral infections can present non-specific symptoms in certain groups of patients (e.g., NICU patients).
5. Sensitive PCR tests identify presence of viral nucleic acid for prolonged periods, which may not represent infectious virus.[32]

Suggested Approaches

Transmission and Syndromic-Based Precautions

A sound understanding of pathogen transmission is required in order to address approaches for prevention. For many respiratory pathogens, especially emerging pathogens such as Middle Eastern Respiratory Syndrome (MERS) and Severe Acute Respiratory Syndrome (SARS), knowledge and evidence regarding transmission may be lacking. As a foundation for understanding the transmission of infectious agents, the 2007 Guideline from the Healthcare Infection Control Practices Advisory Committee describes three elements: a source (reservoir) of infectious agents, a susceptible host with a portal of entry receptive to the agent, and a mode of transmission for the agent.[33] These guidelines propose using standard precautions for all, plus the implementation of empiric transmission-based precautions determined by clinical syndromes and associated symptoms (see Table 1.1). This is to minimize the spread of pathogens before the diagnosis is made.

Identifying Susceptible Hosts

Groups of patients who may be more vulnerable to pathogens include term and preterm infants; children with congenital or acquired immune deficiency; medically complex children with heart disease, lung disease, and neurodevelopmental delays; and technology-dependent children such as those with tracheostomies.

Healthcare personnel (HCP) are also at risk for the development of healthcare-associated respiratory infection. Those in the pediatric setting have a higher likelihood of exposure to vaccine-preventable illnesses such as pertussis, measles, and varicella (chicken pox). Additionally, the pregnant healthcare worker may be at risk of exposure to cytomegalovirus (CMV) and parvovirus (Fifth disease), both common childhood illnesses spread via the respiratory route that can have serious sequelae for the developing fetus.

TABLE 1.1 Examples of Suggested Empiric Precautions Based on Clinical Syndromes/Conditions Related to Pathogens Spread via the Respiratory Route, in Addition to Standard Precautions, Pending Confirmation of Diagnosis

CLINICAL SYNDROME OR CONDITION	POTENTIAL PATHOGENS	INITIAL EMPIRIC PRECAUTIONS
Meningitis		
	Neisseria meningitidis	Droplet Precautions (until 24 hours after initiation of effective antimicrobial therapy)
	Enteroviruses	Contact Precautions
Exanthems		
Petechial and/or purpura with fever (general)	*Neisseria meningitidis*	Droplet Precautions (until 24 hours after initiation of effective antimicrobial therapy)
Vesicular	Varicella-zoster (chickenpox or zoster in immunocompromised host)	Airborne plus Contact Precautions
	Herpes simplex virus, localized zoster in an immunocompetent host	Contact Precautions
Maculopapular with cough, coryza, and fever	Rubeola (measles) virus	Airborne Precautions
Respiratory tract only		
Cough/fever/pulmonary infiltrate with risk factors for *Mycobacterium tuberculosis*	*M. tuberculosis*	Airborne Precautions
Cough/fever/pulmonary infiltrate in a patient with a history of recent travel to countries with active transmission of severe acute respiratory syndrome virus (SARS-CoV), Middle Eastern Respiratory Virus (MERS), or avian influenza	*M. tuberculosis*, SARS-CoV, MERS, avian influenza	Airborne plus Contact Precautions plus eye protection
Bronchiolitis and pneumonia, in infants and young children	Respiratory syncytial virus, parainfluenza virus, adenovirus, influenza virus, human metapneumovirus	Contact plus Droplet Precautions. Can modify if pathogen identified

Finally, family members of patients and other visitors may be exposed to respiratory pathogens. Healthcare facilities can take steps to minimize these risks by educating visitors about infection prevention practices such as hand hygiene and isolation precautions (see Chapter 8).

Immunizations and Post-Exposure Prophylaxis for Specific Pathogens

Influenza

Seasonal influenza is transmitted by droplet spread. Patients are contagious for 24 hours before the onset of symptoms. Viral shedding in nasal secretions decreases within seven days, but shedding can be prolonged in young infants and immunodeficient patients for up to 10 days or longer. The incubation period is usually one to four days, with a mean of two days.[34,35]

Isolation of the Hospitalized Patient

Droplet precautions are indicated for the duration of illness. Many pediatric centers will also follow contact precautions in hospitalized patients with influenza. Patients who have a prolonged hospital stay, usually greater than a week, should be without symptoms and have a documented negative influenza test, preferably PCR, before removing droplet precautions.[36]

All HCPs should get an annual influenza vaccine.[37-39] Multiple studies have demonstrated a significant decrease in healthcare-associated influenza, especially in high-risk patient populations where HCP were mandated to receive the influenza vaccine, resulting in improved vaccination coverage.[40]

Recommended Post-Exposure Interventions

Post-exposure prophylaxis with oseltamivir (see Table 1.2) should be considered for children with significant exposure to family members or other close contacts if they are in certain high-risk categories:

1. Children at high risk of complications from influenza in whom vaccination is contraindicated;
2. Infants between three and six months of age (too young to be immunized);
3. Infants less than three months—chemoprophylaxis is not recommended due to the lack of available safety and efficacy data in this age group unless the situation is judged critical.[41]

TABLE 1.2 Oseltamivir Post-Exposure Prophylaxis Dosing

AGE	TREATMENT DOSE (FIVE DAYS)	PROPHYLAXIS DOSE (FOURTEEN DAYS)[A]
Preterm < 38 weeks postmenstrual age[b]	1 mg/kg/dose twice a day	Not recommended for infants younger than 3 months of age unless situation judged critical (limited data)
Preterm 38–40 weeks postmenstrual age[b]	1.5 mg/kg/dose twice a day	
Preterm > 40 weeks postmenstrual age through 8 months chronological age[b]	3 mg/kg/dose twice a day	
Birth–3 months[c]	3 mg/kg/dose twice a day	Not recommended for infants younger than 3 months of age unless situation judged critical (limited data)
Children 3 months to <9 months	3 mg/kg/dose twice a day	3 mg/kg/dose once daily
9–11 months[d]	3.5 mg/kg/dose twice a day	3.5 mg/kg/dose once daily
Children 1–12 years old and weighing:		
≤15 kg	30 mg/dose twice a day	30 mg once daily
> 15–23 kg	45 mg/dose twice a day	45 mg once daily
>23–40 kg	60 mg/dose twice a day	60 mg once daily
>40 kg	75 mg/dose twice a day	75 mg once daily
Children ≥ 13 years of age, and adults	75 mg/dose twice a day	75 mg once daily

[a] Duration of chemoprophylaxis in the outpatient setting is typically for seven to ten days (as recommended by the CDC and the American Academy of Pediatrics Committee on Infectious Diseases (Red Book 2018–2021) respectively). For control of outbreaks in institutional settings (e.g. long-term care facilities for elderly persons and children) and hospitals, CDC recommends antiviral chemoprophylaxis for a minimum of 2 weeks, and continuing up to 1 week after the last known case was identified. Antiviral chemoprophylaxis is recommended for all residents, including those who have received influenza vaccination.

[b] Current weight-based dosing recommendations are not appropriate for premature infants. Premature infants might have slower clearance of oral oseltamivir because of immature renal function, and doses recommended for full-term infants might lead to very high drug concentrations in this age group. CDC recommends dosing as also recommended by the American Academy of Pediatrics Committee on Infectious Diseases (Red Book 2018–2021): limited data from the National Institute of Allergy and Infectious Diseases Collaborative Antiviral Study Group provide the basis for dosing preterm infants using their postmenstrual age (gestational age + chronological age).

[c] Oral oseltamivir is approved by the FDA for treatment of acute uncomplicated influenza within 2 days of illness onset with twice-daily dosing in persons 14 days and older, and for chemoprophylaxis with once-daily dosing in persons 1 year and older. Although not part of the FDA-approved indications, use of oral oseltamivir for treatment of influenza in infants less than 14 days old, and for chemoprophylaxis in infants 3 months to 1 year of age, is recommended by the CDC and the American Academy of Pediatrics Committee on Infectious Diseases (Red Book 2018).

[d] The FDA-approved oral oseltamivir treatment dose for infants 14 days and older and less than 1 year old is 3 mg/kg twice daily, and provides oseltamivir exposure in children similar to that achieved by the approved dose of 75 mg orally twice daily for adults, as shown in two studies of oseltamivir pharmacokinetics in children (Kimberlin, 2013 [CASG 114], EU study WP22849, FDA Clinical Pharmacology Review). The American Academy of Pediatrics has recommended an oseltamivir treatment dose of 3.5 mg/kg orally twice daily for infants aged 9-11 months, on the basis of data which indicated that a higher dose of 3.5 mg/kg was needed to achieve the protocol-defined targeted exposure for this cohort as defined in the CASG 114 study (Kimberlin, 2013). It is unknown whether this higher dose will improve efficacy or prevent the development of antiviral resistance. However, there is no evidence that the 3.5 mg/kg dose is harmful or causes more adverse events to infants in this age group.

Pertussis

Bordetella pertussis (whooping cough) is a Gram-negative pleomorphic bacillus, with humans being the only known hosts. Pertussis is transmitted by droplet spread. Infected people are most contagious during the initial catarrhal stage through the third week of the paroxysmal stage. Factors affecting the length of communicability include age, immunization status, and appropriate antimicrobial therapy.[42]

Definitions of Exposure

Exposure is deemed to occur when there has been direct unmasked face-to-face (within 3 feet) contact with a contagious patient or direct contact with the secretions of the patient.[34]

Isolation of the Hospitalized Patient

Patients should remain in droplet precautions until five days after initiation of appropriate antimicrobial therapy. Many hospitals will continue droplet isolation for the duration of hospitalization due to persistent symptoms of cough. If patients have not received appropriate antibiotics, they should be placed in droplet isolation until three weeks after the onset of cough.[33]

Recommended Post-Exposure Interventions

Post-exposure prophylaxis is indicated regardless of pertussis immunization status. The antimicrobials and dosages recommended for post-exposure prophylaxis are the same as for treatment of pertussis and include azithromycin, erythromycin, clarithromycin, and trimethoprim-sulfamethoxazole.[43]

HCPs who develop a respiratory illness within 21 days of exposure to pertussis or develop symptoms consistent with pertussis should be excluded from work for at least the first five days of the recommended antimicrobial therapy (see Table 1.3). HCPs unable to take the recommended antimicrobial therapy should be excluded from work for 21 days from the onset of cough.[34,43]

Measles

Person-to-person transmission of measles is by airborne and droplet spread. The incubation period is generally 8–12 days from exposure to onset of symptoms. Measles is a notifiable disease, and once confirmed, it should be reported immediately to the local and state health departments.[44]

TABLE 1.3 Recommended Antimicrobial Therapy and Post-Exposure Prophylaxis for Pertussis in Infants, Children, Adolescents, and Adults[a]

	RECOMMENDED DRUGS		ALTERNATIVE	
AGE	AZITHROMYCIN	ERYTHROMYCIN	CLARITHROMYCIN	TMP-SMX
Younger than 1 mo.	10 mg/kg/day as a single dose daily for 5 days[b,c]	40 mg/kg/day in 4 divided doses for 14 days	Not recommended	Contraindicated at younger than 2 mos. of age
1 through 5 mos.	See above	See above	15 mg/kg per day in 2 divided doses for 7 days	2 mos. of age or older: TMP, 8 mg/kg/day; SMX, 40 mg/kg/day in 2 doses for 14 days
6 mos. or older, and children	10 mg/kg as a single dose on day 1 (maximum 500 mg), then 5 mg/kg/day as a single dose on days 2 through 5 (maximum 250 mg/day)[b,d]	40 mg/kg/day in 4 divided doses for 7–14 days (maximum 1–2 g/day)	15 mg/kg/day in 2 divided doses for 7 days (maximum 1 g/day)	See above
Adolescents and adults	500 mg as a single dose on day 1, then 250 mg as a single dose on days 2 through 5[b,d]	2 g/day in 4 divided doses for 7–14 days	1 g/day in 2 divided doses for 7 days	TMP, 320 mg/day; SMX, 1600 mg/day in 2 divided doses for 14 days

TMP, trimethoprim; SMX, sulfamethoxazole.

[a] Centers for Disease Control and Prevention. Recommended antimicrobial agents for the treatment and postexposure prophylaxis of pertussis: 2005 CDC guidelines. *MMWR Recomm Rep*. 2005;54(RR-14):1–16.

[b] Azithromycin should be used with caution in people with prolonged QT interval and certain proarrhythmic conditions.

[c] Preferred macrolide for this age because of the risk of idiopathic hypertrophic pyloric stenosis associated with erythromycin.

[d] A 3-day course of azithromycin for post-exposure prophylaxis or treatment has not been validated and is not recommended.

Definitions of Exposure

An exposed individual is anyone who has been in the room with a patient with measles who is not immune and not wearing appropriate personal protective equipment (PPE), such as a fit-tested N-95 mask or Powered Air Purifying Respirator (PAPR). Measles virus can remain infectious in the air for up to two hours after an infectious person leaves the area.[34]

Evidence of Immunity to Measles

1. History of two doses of measles vaccine more than six weeks prior to the exposure. In the United States, the first dose of measles vaccination is usually given at 12–15 months of age, followed by a second dose at 4–6 years of age;
2. Laboratory evidence of immunity (positive IgG serology);
3. Laboratory confirmation of past disease (positive serology, positive viral culture, or PCR for measles)[44]

Isolation of the Hospitalized Patient

A patient with confirmed or suspected measles should be placed on airborne precautions until four days after the appearance of the rash in otherwise healthy children, and for the duration of the illness in immunocompromised patients. Patients who are susceptible to measles and who have been exposed should be placed on airborne precautions from day 5 after the exposure until 21 days from the last exposure (or 28 days from the last exposure if the susceptible person has received immunoglobulin prophylaxis).[33]

Table 1.4 describes recommended interventions post-exposure to measles.

Varicella-Zoster Virus

Primary varicella infection (chicken pox) and disseminated zoster in immunocompromised hosts are spread by airborne and contact routes. The contagious period extends from up to 48 hours before the appearance of rash until all skin lesions are crusted over, usually about five days in normal hosts. The incubation period for chicken pox is 10–21 days (median 14 days) but can be up to 28 days if varicella-zoster immunoglobulin (VariZIG) or intravenous immune globulin (IGIV) is given.

An immunocompetent person with zoster (shingles) involving a dermatomal rash can transmit the infection to a susceptible person by direct contact. Infectious virus is released from the skin vesicles onto the susceptible person's hands, with subsequent transfer to the mucous

TABLE 1.4 Measles Post-Exposure Interventions[71]

MEASLES VACCINATION RECOMMENDED FOR:	IMMUNE GLOBULIN RECOMMENDED FOR:	IMMUNE GLOBULIN DOSING
All exposed persons ≥ 6 months of age who have not been vaccinated, or have only received one vaccine and have no contraindications to vaccination. Measles vaccine should be given to susceptible individuals within 72 hours of measles exposure.	1. Pregnant women without evidence of immunity 2. Severely immunocompromised patients regardless of immunologic or vaccination status 3. Patients with a primary immunodeficiency 4. Bone marrow transplant patients until at least 12 months after finishing all immunosuppressive therapy, or longer if developed graft-vs-host disease 5. Patients with acute lymphocytic leukemia within and until 6 months after completion of immunosuppressive chemotherapy 6. Patients with HIV who have a CD4 count < 15% for all ages or < 200 lymphocytes/mm^3 for children older than 5 years 7. Infants < 12 months of age whose mothers received biological response modifiers during pregnancy Immune globulin should be administered within 6 days of exposure	1. IGIM 0.50mL/ kg (maximum dose volume 15 mL) 2. IGIV 400 mg/kg

membranes of the eyes or mouth. Prevention of transmission requires adequately covering the rash to avoid contact.[33]

Definitions of Exposure

HCPs who have face-to-face or direct patient contact without appropriate PPE (gown, gloves, and N-95 mask or PAPR) are considered exposed. Patients who share the same patient room or bathroom, or have face-to-face or direct contact, are considered exposed.

Isolation of the Hospitalized Patient

1. Chicken pox or disseminated zoster:
   Airborne and contact isolation until all lesions are crusted (typically 5 days for an immunocompetent host, significantly longer for immunocompromised hosts);
2. Breakthrough chicken pox in previously vaccinated child:
   Airborne and contact isolation until no new lesions are occurring (i.e., all skin lesions do not have to all be resolved);
3. Immunocompetent person with zoster (shingles) involving a dermatomal rash: Contact isolation until all lesions are crusted;
4. For exposed patients without evidence of immunity to varicella:
   Airborne and contact isolation from eight days after first exposure to the index patient until 21 days after last exposure to the index patient (extend to 28 days if VariZIG or IGIV has been given).[33,34]

Hospital Exposure Considerations

See Figure 1.1.

Identify all persons involved in the exposure and determine their evidence of immunity:

Varicella: A significant hospital exposure would be considered all those in the same room or adjacent beds in a large ward or those who had face-face contact with a person with varicella or disseminated herpes zoster.

Dermatomal Zoster: A significant hospital exposure would be considered if direct contact occurred between the susceptible person and the uncovered rash of the person with zoster, or intimate contact such as hugging or kissing before the person adequately covered the rash to prevent transmission.

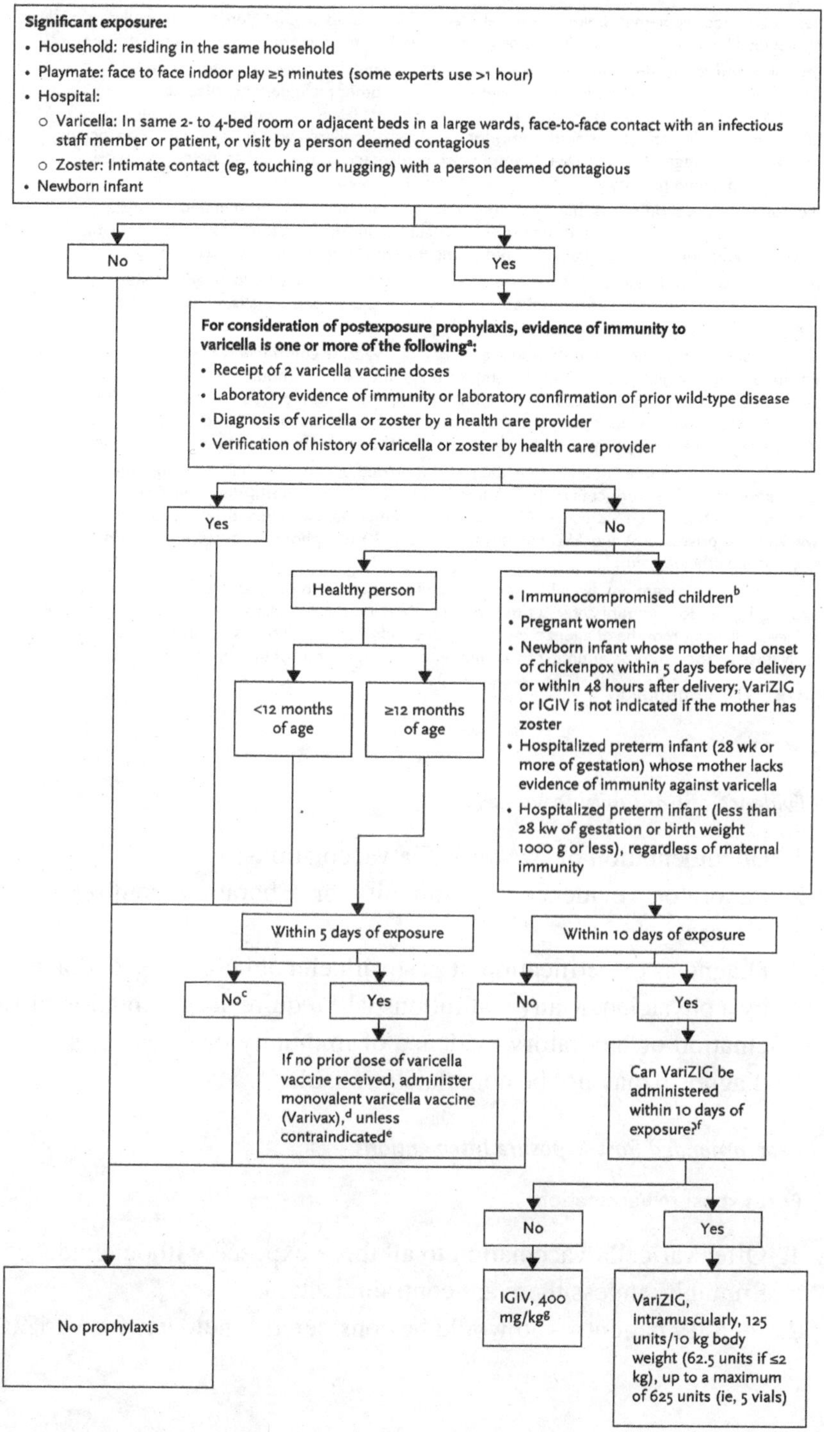

FIGURE 1.1 Varicella exposure algorithm.

Reproduced with permission from *AAP Red Book 2015*.[34]

a. People who receive hematopoietic stem cell transplants should be considered nonimmune regardless of previous history of varicella disease or varicella vaccination in themselves or in their donors.

b. Immunocompromised children include those with congenital or acquired T-lymphocyte immunodeficiency, including leukemia, lymphoma, and other malignant neoplasms affecting the bone marrow or lymphatic system; children receiving immunosuppressive therapy, including ≥2 mg/kg/day of systemic prednisone (or its equivalent) for ≥14 days; all children with human immunodeficiency virus (HIV) infection regardless of CD4+ T-lymphocyte percentage; and all hematopoietic stem cell transplant patients regardless of pretransplant immunity status.

c. No postexposure prophylaxis, but age-appropriate vaccination still recommended for protection against subsequent exposures. If the exposure occurred during an outbreak, 2-dose vaccination is recommended for preschool-aged children younger than 4 years for outbreak control.

d. If 1 prior dose of varicella vaccine has been received, a second dose should be administered at ≥4 years of age. If the exposure occurred during an outbreak, a second dose is recommended for preschool-aged children younger than 4 years for outbreak control.

e. Contraindications include patients who are allergic to a vaccine component, or who are immunocompromised (see above footnote), or pregnant. Caution should be used in patients receiving salicylates. Vaccine may not be as effective if patient has recently received Immune Globulin Intravenous, whole blood, or plasma transfusions, and for this reason, it is recommended that varicella vaccine be withheld for 3 to 11 months, depending on the dose, after administration of these products.

f. Varicella Zoster Immune Globulin (VariZIG) was approved by the US Food and Drug Administration in December 2012. The product is manufactured by Cangene Corporation (Winnipeg, Canada) and distributed in the United States by FFF Enterprises (Temecula, California; 800-843-7477; **www.fffenterprises.com**) and ASD Healthcare (Frisco, TX) (telephone, 800-746-6273; online at **www.asdhealthcare.com**).

g. If VariZIG and IGIV are not available, some experts recommend prophylaxis with oral acyclovir (20 mg/kg per dose administered 4 times per day, with a maximum daily dose of 3200 mg) or oral valacyclovir (if >3 months of age; 20 mg/kg per dose administered 3 times per day, with a maximum daily dose of 3000 mg) beginning 7 to 10 days after exposure and continuing for 7 days.

FIGURE 1.1 Continued

Evidence of Immunity to Varicella

1. Documentation of two varicella vaccinations;
2. Laboratory evidence of immunity or laboratory confirmation of disease;
3. Diagnosis or verification of past varicella or herpes zoster diagnosed by a physician. Many institutions will require documentation of vaccination or laboratory evidence of immunity or disease, as clinical diagnosis may not be completely reliable.[45]

Recommended Post-Exposure Interventions

Post-Exposure Vaccination

1. Offer varicella vaccination to all those exposed without evidence of immunity unless there are contraindications.
2. Identify patients who would be considered candidates for VariZIG.

Three factors need to be met to consider administering VariZIG:

a. A significant exposure occurred;
b. The exposed person has no evidence of immunity;
c. The exposed person has a high risk for developing severe disseminated disease.

Table 1.5 describes antiviral and immune globulin dosing. VariZIG should be administered to appropriate candidates within 10 days of exposure. If VariZIG is unavailable, IGIV is an appropriate alternative. If both VariZIG and IGIV are unavailable, prophylaxis with a seven-day course of acyclovir or valacyclovir can be considered, starting 7–10 days after exposure.[46]

Mycobacterium tuberculosis

Children less than 10 years old infected with *Mycobacterium tuberculosis* are rarely contagious. The usual source of infection for children is an adult household contact who quite frequently may accompany the child into the hospital. For infection control purposes, the child being evaluated for tuberculosis (TB) should be initially placed in airborne isolation until the adults accompanying the child have been screened and the household contact source identified. For continued isolation precautions, whether the child has contagious disease needs to be considered. All cases of suspected or confirmed TB should be reported to the local health department's TB control program.

TABLE 1.5 Antiviral and Immune Globulin Dosing

Acyclovir (IV)	Valacyclovir (PO)
20mg/kg/dose given 4 times a day with a maximum daily dose of 3200 mg	20mg/kg/dose given 3 times a daily, max daily dosing of 3000mg
VariZIG (IM)	**IGIV (IV)**
< 2kg 62.5 units (0.5 vial) 2.1 kg–10 kg 125 units (1 vial) 10.1 kg–20kg 250 units (2 vials) 20.1 kg–30 kg 375 units (3 vials) 30.1 kg–40 kg 500 units (4 vials) > 40 kg 625 units (5 vials)	400mg/kg

1. Only adults who have been screened and cleared should be allowed to visit the child. Many hospitals only allow parents or guardians to visit after screening and clearance for contagious TB.
2. Household contacts accompanying the child should be managed with TB precautions until they have been screened and either determined to be clear of pulmonary TB. If the contact is determined to have active pulmonary TB disease, the contact should be restricted from hospital entry until he/she has initiated appropriate therapy *and* has three consecutive acid-fast bacilli (AFB)–negative sputum smears collected at least eight hours apart. Household contacts should wear a surgical mask upon entry to the hospital until they are in a negative-pressure room with their child, and they should avoid visiting common areas of the hospital until they have been cleared of active TB. Close collaboration with local public health officials is strongly advised when determining TB clearance for household contacts.

Children with the following disease states are potentially contagious and require continued airborne precautions:

1. Cavitary lung disease;
2. Extensive lung involvement;
3. AFB-positive sputum;
4. Laryngeal involvement;
5. Neonates and infants with congenital TB undergoing endotracheal intubation, or other oropharyngeal procedures that may result in aerosolization of respiratory secretions.

In these circumstances, the hospitalized child should remain on airborne-isolation precautions until effective therapy has been administered and/or:

1. If patient was initially AFB-smear-positive—have three daily consecutive negative sputum smears.
2. If extensive pulmonary disease/cavitary lung disease—until coughing has abated.

In addition to placing the patient in an airborne-isolation room, all health-care personnel and visitors entering the room should wear a personally "fit tested" and "sealed" N95-particulate respirator or PAPR.[47,48] OSHA requires annual fit testing.

Children with extrapulmonary TB or pulmonary disease without cough and who have negative-sputum AFB smears, in addition to their adult companions who have been cleared of having contagious pulmonary TB, do not require continuation of airborne precautions.[34]

Recommended Post-Exposure Interventions

HCPs who have been exposed to a child, or, more frequently, to their adult companion with confirmed contagious TB, should undergo screening for *M. tuberculosis* infection. An exposure would be sharing an airspace with the infected individual without the use of a N95-particulate respirator or PAPR, or where the contagious individual has not been appropriately wearing a surgical mask while in transit. Exposure can occur for laboratory personnel by handling potentially infected material without the appropriate protective equipment. Recommended screening is the tuberculin skin test (TST) or gamma interferon release assay (IGRA) in HCPs with prior recorded negative TB screening tests. If testing remains negative, a TST or IGRA should be repeated in 8–10 weeks' time. In HCPs with a documented prior positive TST or IGRA, a symptom questionnaire should be completed. HCPs with a positive TST or IGRA, or with a positive symptom questionnaire, should then have a chest radiograph to evaluate for pulmonary *M. tuberculosis* disease and consideration of treatment of either latent infection or disease. Employees found to have pulmonary disease should be excluded from work until they have initiated treatment and have three documented negative sputum smears for AFB that have been obtained between 8 and 12 hours apart, and at least one has been obtained as an early morning specimen.[47]

M. tuberculosis exposure in certain high-risk groups should warrant consideration of initiating preventative isoniazid treatment. Examples of this would be a significant exposure in a nursery, NICU, or bone marrow transplant unit. If an adult who has spent a significant amount of time in one of these types of units is subsequently found to have contagious *M. tuberculosis*, the infants or immunocompromised children who have shared an airspace with the contagious adult are at high risk of developing *M. tuberculosis* disease. A tiered, ring approach starts with screening household contacts of the contagious healthcare worker by TST or IGRA, usually performed by the local health department's TB control program. Only if household contacts of the HCP are found to be infected should the patients with the highest likelihood of exposure be evaluated, and if any of those are found to be infected, the remoter contacts should also be evaluated.

Exposed vulnerable patients such as children younger than four years and immunocompromised patients should first be evaluated for *M. tuberculosis* disease, in addition to the placement of a TST. If disease is initially excluded, treatment for presumptive latent TB infection (LTBI) should be initiated (even if an initial TST is negative) for 8–10 weeks, followed by a repeat TST. Although each situation warrants an independent assessment, this tiered approach has been recommended to limit unnecessary screening and treatment while identifying those most at risk.[49]

Special Considerations for Pregnant and Breastfeeding Healthcare Personnel

Cytomegalovirus

Cytomegalovirus (CMV) is a ubiquitous virus, and most people will acquire infection during their lifetime. CMV infection may be an asymptomatic infection, or it may result in a mild infectious mononucleosis type of infection in immune-competent hosts. It is the most common congenital infection, although 70% of infections are asymptomatic. Ten percent result in severe symptomatology, including fetal loss, severe intrauterine growth retardation (IUGR), microcephaly, retinitis, profound neurodevelopmental delay, and sensorineural hearing loss. Between 15% and 30% of congenitally infected infants who appear asymptomatic at birth will go on to develop sensorineural hearing loss over the next five or six years.[50-53]

The highest prevalence of CMV acquisition is among toddlers. Horizontal transmission is common among babies and toddlers who attend daycare,[54] and infected babies and toddlers will asymptomatically shed large quantities of virus in their saliva and urine.[52] Multiple studies have demonstrated that women who work in daycare centers are at increased risk of acquiring CMV infection compared to the general population.[55] In contrast, pediatric nurses have the same risk of infection and seroconversion rates as the general population.[56] This disparity is most likely related to care practices, with pediatric nurses adhering to hand hygiene and the use of barrier precautions when handling bodily fluids.

Some healthcare institutions have infection control policies that restrict pregnant HCPs from taking care of patients known to be infected with CMV. This policy is fundamentally flawed, not evidence-based, and may result in unnecessary anxiety or in a false sense of security. Studies have demonstrated that infants and toddlers infected with CMV can shed large quantities of virus in both their saliva and their urine for many months, and most of these children are without symptoms.[57] Several studies have demonstrated that adherence to strict hand hygiene procedures when taking care of babies and toddlers, in conjunction with refraining from kissing, effectively prevents transmission.[58,59] With adherence to these practices, the seroconversion rates of pediatric and obstetric nurses are the same as the general population (around 1–2% per year).[60–63] Standard precautions are sufficient for the care of CMV-infected infants and children.

Parvovirus

Parvovirus B19 is another ubiquitous virus, with seroprevalence rates of 5–10% in young children, 50% in young adults, and 90% in the elderly. Infection may result in asymptomatic infection, mild upper respiratory tract infection, or classic erythema infectiosum (Fifth disease) of childhood. Other, less-common presentations include polyarthropathy syndrome or petechial, papular-purpuric-gloves-and-socks syndrome. More serious syndromes include hydrops fetalis/congenital anemia when the fetus is infected during the first 20 weeks of pregnancy, transient aplastic crisis in patients with hemaglobinopathies, and chronic anemia/pure red cell aplasia in immunocompromised hosts.[35]

Parvovirus is shed in respiratory secretions and is spread via the contact and droplet routes. Patients are contagious before the development of rash in erythema infectiosum or joint complaints in polyarthropathy syndrome, and are no longer contagious once the classic symptoms of rash or joint pain develop. Therefore, standard precautions are recommended for most patients with parvovirus infection. Infants with hydrops are not contagious.[64]

In contrast, immunocompromised patients, or those with aplastic crises, generally remain contagious after the development of symptoms and should be placed on contact and droplet precautions. Most experts recommend that pregnant HCPs should avoid caring for immunocompromised patients with chronic Parvovirus B19 infection or patients with aplastic crisis.[34,64]

Zoster in the Breastfeeding Mother

Direct contact with the rash is required to transmit viral infection to a susceptible host. A term newborn should not be removed from the mother in the event she develops zoster, as the infant has passive immunity to zoster from transplacental maternal antibodies. Increased precautions should be considered in preterm infants as they are likely to lack adequate maternal antibodies, whose transfer occurs later in gestation.

Transmission can be prevented by covering the rash and using standard precautions. A mother should continue to breastfeed her newborn infant, provided that the rash is adequately covered. If the rash involves a breast, she should avoid feeding her infant on the affected breast, but may continue to feed her infant on the unaffected side. HCPs with zoster can continue to work, provided the rash can remain adequately covered. HCPs with facial lesions should be restricted from patient care in high-risk groups who are vulnerable to varicella infection, until all the lesions have crusted over.

Influenza in the Mothers of Neonates

Expectant mothers should be offered the inactivated influenza vaccine during each pregnancy to provide passive immunity to their newborn infants.[65] In the event a mother with a newborn infant becomes ill with influenza, the mother should be started on antiviral medications, but her infant should not be removed from her. Breastfeeding should continue, with efforts at strict hand hygiene and the mother wearing a surgical mask while handling her baby, for the duration of symptoms.[66,67] She and the baby should not have access to the general nursery.

If the baby is being cared for in the nursery or the NICU, the mother should wear a surgical mask on entry into the unit, perform hand hygiene, and use contact precautions when handling her baby. She should continue to either offer expressed breast milk, or nurse her infant.

Protection of the Healthcare Personnel and Minimizing Contribution to Healthcare-Associated Infections

Infectious diseases are an occupational hazard for HCPs; individuals working within healthcare settings may also serve as the source of HAIs. There are three basic interventions HCPs can take to minimize these risks. These include:

1. Maintaining strict adherence to universal precautions, as well as recommended additional precautions based on risk of exposure to patients and their secretions. This would include proper training on effective hand hygiene techniques, as well as the appropriate use of PPE;
2. Refraining from presenting to work when sick with a potentially contagious illness;
3. Remaining up-to-date with recommended vaccinations.

HCP are defined by the CDC as including physicians, nurses, emergency medical personnel, dental professionals and students, medical and nursing students, laboratory technicians, pharmacists, hospital volunteers, and administrative staff.

In 2010, the American Academy of Pediatrics issued an initial policy statement, "Recommendation for Mandatory Influenza Immunization of All Health Care Personnel," which they reaffirmed in 2015.[39] A growing body of evidence shows that high influenza vaccination rates among HCPs decrease HAIs due to influenza.[68,69] Additionally, data support that high immunization rates in healthcare settings can only be achieved through mandatory programs. The Advisory Committee on Immunization Practices (ACIP) began recommending influenza vaccinations in the 1980s,[70] but it only has been steadily improving in recent years, reaching 75% during the 2013–2014 season. Coverage in HCPs who reported mandatory vaccination requirements approached 98% and was significantly higher in healthcare facilities that offered free on-site vaccinations over multiple days.[71]

Emerging Respiratory Viruses (MERS and SARS)

Over the past decade, there have been several outbreaks of novel strains of coronaviruses: notably, severe acute respiratory syndrome (SARS) and Middle Eastern respiratory syndrome (MERS). These outbreaks involved high transmission rates to HCPs and high mortality rates.[72,73] Critical lessons learned from these outbreaks to prevent transmission of these types of respiratory pathogens in healthcare settings include the need for organizational leadership, the presence of clear administrative policies, and an adequate infrastructure to successfully implement effective infection control practices, such as environmental and engineering controls, administrative controls, safer work practices, and PPE. The CDC has published comprehensive guidelines for infection control in healthcare facilities for both SARS and MERS.[74,75]

The basic principles follow.

Minimize Chance of Exposures

This focuses on prompt identification and isolation. These should include both symptom and travel screening when scheduling appointments or upon arrival to a healthcare facility. Signage should raise awareness and educate regarding hand hygiene and cough etiquette. Facilities should provide supplies to perform hand hygiene, tissues, face masks, and receptacles for disposal. Patients identified as high risk should be placed in a private room immediately, and placed in an airborne isolation room as soon as possible.

Ensure Adherence to Standard, Contact, and Airborne Precautions

All HCPs should be adequately educated on the proper use of PPE. HCPs must wear a respirator that is at least as protective as a fit-tested, National Institute for Occupational Safety and Health (NIOSH)-certified disposable N95 face mask. Face shields or goggles must be worn for any aerosol-generating procedures such as intubation or suctioning.

Limit Visitor Access and Movement Within the Facility; Monitor and Manage Ill and Exposed Healthcare Personnel

Currently the recommendation is for HCPs to report any respiratory or febrile illness that occurs within 14 days of exposure to either of these viruses. They should be promptly evaluated and excluded from working. Asymptomatic HCPs who have had an unprotected exposure to a patient with confirmed MERS-related coronavirus should be excluded from work for 14 days; and to confirmed SARS, for 10 days after the date of the last high-risk exposure, to monitor for the onset of illness.

Approach to the Clinical Scenario

Given the seriousness of the exposure outlined earlier in the chapter, the diagnosis of varicella should be confirmed with laboratory tests. Varicella direct stain, culture, or PCR of the lesions can be used. Varicella IgM serology is not a reliable method for routine confirmation of varicella, although a positive result indicates current or recent varicella zoster virus.

All patients in the adjacent beds in the same room of the infants of the ill brother would be considered exposed. All these patients, in addition to the infant siblings, should be placed in airborne isolation eight days after first exposure to the index patient until 21 days after the last exposure, unless the patient was given immunoglobulin, which extends their period of isolation to 28 days after last exposure.

Healthcare facilities should employ a standardized approach to defining exposures and the need for post-exposure prophylaxis. A typical process is outlined below:

1. HCP, patients, and visitors who have had close face-to-face contact with the contagious sibling should be contacted to ascertain their

immunity to varicella and to determine options for those without immunity. Occupational Health should be notified to confirm that all healthcare staff have documented immunity to varicella.

2. Varicella vaccination should be given within 72 hours and up to 120 hours after exposure if the person is not immune to varicella and there are no contraindications for vaccination. This should then be followed by a second dose of vaccine at the age-appropriate interval after the first dose. This would be the most appropriate first step for all otherwise-healthy exposed employees, visitors, and patients.
3. All those exposed should be evaluated to determine whether VariZIG is indicated (Figure 1.1). VariZIG should ideally be administered within 96 hours, but it may still be beneficial if administered within 10 days of exposure. If VariZIG is unavailable, administer IGIV instead.
4. Oral acyclovir or oral valacyclovir can be administered beginning 7–10 days after exposure and continued for seven days for both immunocompromised patients and adults without evidence of immunity when vaccination is contraindicated, as well as in otherwise-healthy children. However, in immunocompromised people, VariZIG or IVIG is preferred (see #3 above).

Unresolved Issues

Respiratory Virus Healthcare-Associated Infection Surveillance

Knowledge of the incubation period of respiratory pathogens is essential in the investigation, control, and classification of infections as healthcare-associated versus community-associated. Definitions for HAI viral respiratory infections are not standardized, and institutions may use slightly different criteria to define the minimum duration of hospitalization before the onset of symptoms to classify an infection as healthcare-associated. This makes benchmarking difficult. In general, standardized definitions require the presence of symptoms compatible with viral respiratory infection and virus detection. Quach et al. noted substantial but different healthcare-associated viral infection rates in two children's hospitals, providing a roadmap for future work to further define healthcare-associated viral respiratory infections and to evaluate best practices for preventing such infections.[5]

References

1. U.S. Department of Health and Human Services, Health Resources and Services Administration, Maternal and Child Health Bureau. *Child Health USA 2012*. Rockville, Maryland: U.S. Department of Health and Human Services, Maternal and Child Health Bureau; 2013.
2. Jain S, Williams DJ, Arnold SR, et al. Community-acquired pneumonia requiring hospitalization among U.S. children. *N Engl J Med*. 2015;372:835–845.
3. Jain S, Self WH, Wunderink RG, et al. Community-acquired pneumonia requiring hospitalization. *N Engl J Med*. 2015;373:2382.
4. Lonngren C, Morrow BM, Haynes S, Yusri T, Vyas H, Argent AC. North–South divide: distribution and outcome of respiratory viral infections in paediatric intensive care units in Cape Town (South Africa) and Nottingham (United Kingdom). *J Paediatr Child Health*. 2014;50:208–215.
5. Quach C, Shah R, Rubin LG. Burden of healthcare-associated viral respiratory infections in children's hospitals. *J Pediatric Infect Dis Soc*. 2018;7:18–24.
6. Raymond J, Aujard Y. Nosocomial infections in pediatric patients: a European, multicenter prospective study. European Study Group. *Infect Control Hosp Epidemiol*. 2000;21:260–263.
7. Campins M, Vaque J, Rossello J, et al. 1993. Nosocomial infections in pediatric patients: a prevalence study in Spanish hospitals. EPINE Working Group. *Am J Infect Control*. 2016;21:58–63.
8. Miller EK, Bugna J, Libster R, et al. Human rhinoviruses in severe respiratory disease in very low birth weight infants. *Pediatrics*. 2012;129:e60–e67.
9. Henrickson KJ, Hoover S, Kehl KS, Hua W. National disease burden of respiratory viruses detected in children by polymerase chain reaction. *Pediatr Infect Dis J*. 2004;23:S11–S18.
10. Hall CB, Powell KR, MacDonald NE, et al. Respiratory syncytial viral infection in children with compromised immune function. *N Engl J Med*. 1986;315:77–81.
11. Langley JM, Hanakowski M. Variation in risk for nosocomial chickenpox after inadvertent exposure. *J Hosp Infect*. 2000;44:224–226.
12. Atkinson WL, Markowitz LE, Adams NC, Seastrom GR. Transmission of measles in medical settings—United States, 1985–1989. *Am J Med*. 1991;91:320S–324S.
13. Hatherill M, Levin M, Lawrenson J, Hsiao NY, Reynolds L, Argent A. Evolution of an adenovirus outbreak in a multidisciplinary children's hospital. *J Paediatr Child Health*. 2004;40:449–454.
14. Moisiuk SE, Robson D, Klass L, et al. Outbreak of parainfluenza virus type 3 in an intermediate care neonatal nursery. *Pediatr Infect Dis J*. 1998;17:49–53.
15. Hall CB. Nosocomial respiratory syncytial virus infections: the "Cold War" has not ended. *Clin Infect Dis*. 2000;31:590–596.
16. Maltezou HC, Drancourt M. Nosocomial influenza in children. *J Hosp Infect*. 2003;55:83–91.
17. Christie CD, Glover AM, Willke MJ, Marx ML, Reising SF, Hutchinson NM. Containment of pertussis in the regional pediatric hospital during the Greater Cincinnati epidemic of 1993. *Infect Control Hosp Epidemiol*. 1995;16:556–563.

18. Valenti WM, Pincus PH, Messner MK. Nosocomial pertussis: possible spread by a hospital visitor. *Am J Dis Child.* 1980;134:520–521.
19. Outbreaks of pertussis associated with hospitals—Kentucky, Pennsylvania, and Oregon, 2003. *MMWR.* 2005;54:67–71.
20. Foster CB, Sabella C. Health care-associated infections in children. *JAMA.* 2011;305:1480–1481.
21. Civardi E, Tzialla C, Baldanti F, Strocchio L, Manzoni P, Stronati M. Viral outbreaks in neonatal intensive care units: what we do not know. *Am J Infect Control.* 2013;41:854–856.
22. Bennett NJ, Tabarani CM, Bartholoma NM, et al. Unrecognized viral respiratory tract infections in premature infants during their birth hospitalization: a prospective surveillance study in two neonatal intensive care units. *J Pediatr.* 2012;161:814–818.
23. Gonzalez-Carrasco E, Calvo C, Garcia-Garcia ML, et al. [Viral respiratory tract infections in the Neonatal Intensive Care Unit]. *An Pediatr (Barc).* 2015;82:242–246.
24. Ronchi A, Michelow IC, Chapin KC, et al. Viral respiratory tract infections in the neonatal intensive care unit: the VIRIoN-I study. *J Pediatr.* 2014;165:690–696.
25. Kidszun A, Hansmann A, Winter J, et al. Detection of respiratory viral infections in neonates treated for suspicion of nosocomial bacterial sepsis: a feasibility study. *Pediatr Infect Dis J.* 2014;33:102–104.
26. Hutspardol S, Essa M, Richardson S, et al. Significant transplantation-related mortality from respiratory virus infections within the first one hundred days in children after hematopoietic stem cell transplantation. *Biol Blood Marrow Transplant.* 2015;21:1802–1807.
27. Campbell AP, Guthrie KA, Englund JA, et al. Clinical outcomes associated with respiratory virus detection before allogeneic hematopoietic stem cell transplant. *Clin Infect Dis.* 2015;61:192–202.
28. Shah DP, Shah PK, Azzi JM, El Chaer F, Chemaly RF. Human metapneumovirus infections in hematopoietic cell transplant recipients and hematologic malignancy patients: a systematic review. *Cancer Lett.* 2016;379:100–106.
29. Kmeid J, Vanichanan J, Shah DP, et al. Outcomes of influenza infections in hematopoietic cell transplant recipients: application of an immunodeficiency scoring index. *Biol Blood Marrow Transplant.* 2016;22:542–548.
30. Shah DP, Shah PK, Azzi JM, Chemaly RF. Parainfluenza virus infections in hematopoietic cell transplant recipients and hematologic malignancy patients: a systematic review. *Cancer Lett.* 2016;370:358–364.
31. Horan TC, Andrus M, Dudeck MA. CDC/NHSN surveillance definition of health care-associated infection and criteria for specific types of infections in the acute care setting. *Am J Infect Control.* 2008;36:309–332.
32. Self WH, Williams DJ, Zhu Y, et al. Respiratory viral detection in children and adults: comparing asymptomatic controls and patients with community-acquired pneumonia. *J Infect Dis.* 2016;213:584–591.
33. Siegel JD, Rhinehart E, Jackson M, Chiarello L. Guideline for isolation precautions: preventing transmission of infectious agents in health care settings. *Am J Infect Control.* 2007;35:S65–S164.
34. Kimberlin DWB, MT, Jackson MA, Long SS, eds. *Red Book: 2015 report of the Committee on Infectious Diseases.* Elk Grove Village, IL: American Academy of Pediatrics; 2015:1151.

35. Uyeki TM, "Influenza viruses." In: Cherry JD, Demmler-Harrison GJ, Kaplan SL, Steinbach WJ, Hotez PJ, eds. *Feigin and Cherry's textbook of pediatric infectious diseases 7th edition*, Vol. 2. Philadelphia, PA: Saunders Elsevier; 2014:2326–2359.
36. Centers for Disease Control and Prevention National Center for Immunization and Respiratory Diseass. Influenza (flu) prevention strategies for seasonal influenza in healthcare settings. Guidelines and recommendations. https://www.cdc.gov/flu/professionals/infectioncontrol/healthcaresettings.htm
37. Bernstein HH, Starke JR, American Academy of Pediatrics. Committee on Infectious Diseases. Policy statement—recommendation for mandatory influenza immunization of all health care personnel. *Pediatrics*. 2010;126:809–815.
38. Committee on Infectious Diseases. Recommendations for prevention and control of influenza in children, 2016–2017. *Pediatrics.*2016;138:e20162527.
39. Committee on Infectious DiseasesInfluenza immunization for all health care personnel: keep it mandatory. *Pediatrics.* 2015;136:809–818.
40. Frenzel E, Chemaly RF, Ariza-Heredia E, et al. Association of increased influenza vaccination in health care workers with a reduction in nosocomial influenza infections in cancer patients. *Am J Infect Control*. 2016;44:1016–1021.
41. Fiore AE, Fry A, Shay D, et al. Antiviral agents for the treatment and chemoprophylaxis of influenza—recommendations of the Advisory Committee on Immunization Practices (ACIP). *MMWR Recomm Rep*. 2011;60:1–24.
42. Cherry JD, Heininger U. "Pertussis and other Bordetella infections." In: Cherry JD, Demmler-Harrison GJ, Kaplan SL, Steinbach WJ, Hotez PJ, eds. *Feigin and Cherry's textbook of pediatric infectious diseases 7th edition*, Vol. 2. Philadelphia, PA: Saunders Elsevier; 2014:1616–1639.
43. Tiwari T, Murphy TV, Moran J, CDC National Immunization Program. Recommended antimicrobial agents for the treatment and postexposure prophylaxis of pertussis: 2005 CDC guidelines. *MMWR Recomm Rep*. 2005;54:1–16.
44. McLean HQ, Fiebelkorn AP, Temte JL, Wallace GS, CDC. Prevention of measles, rubella, congenital rubella syndrome, and mumps, 2013: summary recommendations of the Advisory Committee on Immunization Practices (ACIP). *MMWR Recomm Rep*. 2013;62:1–34.
45. Centers for Disease Control and Prevention National Center for Immunization and Respiratory Diseases (NCIRD) Division of Viral Diseases. Assessing immunity to varicella. https://www.cdc.gov/chickenpox/hcp/immunity.html.
46. Centers for Disease Control and Prevention. Updated recommendations for use of VariZIG—United States, 2013. *MMWR*. 2013;62:574–576.
47. Jensen PA, Lambert LA, Iademarco MF, Ridzon R, CDC. Guidelines for preventing the transmission of *Mycobacterium tuberculosis* in health-care settings, 2005. *MMWR Recomm Rep*. 2005;54: 1–141.
48. National Tuberculosis Controllers Association, CDC. Guidelines for the investigation of contacts of persons with infectious tuberculosis. Recommendations from the National Tuberculosis Controllers Association and CDC. *MMWR Recomm Rep*. 2005;54:1–47.
49. Cruz AT, Starke JR. A current review of infection control for childhood tuberculosis. *Tuberculosis (Edinb)*. 2011;91(Suppl 1):S11–S15.

50. Fowler KB, McCollister FP, Dahle AJ, Boppana S, Britt WJ, Pass RF. Progressive and fluctuating sensorineural hearing loss in children with asymptomatic congenital cytomegalovirus infection. *J Pediatr*. 1997;130:624–630.
51. Fowler KB, Boppana SB. Congenital cytomegalovirus (CMV) infection and hearing deficit. *J Clin Virol*. 2006;35:226–231.
52. Boppana SB, Fowler KB. Persistence in the population: epidemiology and transmission. In: Arvin A, Campadelli-Fiume G, Mocarski E, et al. (eds.). *Human herpes viruses: biology, therapy, and immunoprophylaxis*. New York, NY: Cambridge University Press; 2007: 795–813.
53. Rosenthal LS, Fowler KB, Boppana SB, et al. Cytomegalovirus shedding and delayed sensorineural hearing loss: results from longitudinal follow-up of children with congenital infection. *Pediatr Infect Dis J*. 2009;28:515–520.
54. Pass RF, Hutto SC, Reynolds DW, Polhill RB. Increased frequency of cytomegalovirus infection in children in group day care. *Pediatrics*. 1984;74:121–126.
55. Adler SP. Cytomegalovirus and child day care. Evidence for an increased infection rate among day-care workers. *N Engl J Med*. 1989;321:1290–1296.
56. Hyde TB, Schmid DS, Cannon MJ. Cytomegalovirus seroconversion rates and risk factors: implications for congenital CMV. *Rev Med Virol*. 2010;20:311–326.
57. Murph JR, Bale JF, Jr. The natural history of acquired cytomegalovirus infection among children in group day care. *Am J Dis Child*. 1988;142:843–846.
58. Adler SP, Finney JW, Manganello AM, Best AM. Prevention of child-to-mother transmission of cytomegalovirus by changing behaviors: a randomized controlled trial. *Pediatr Infect Dis J*. 1996;15:240–246.
59. Adler SP, Finney JW, Manganello AM, Best AM. Prevention of child-to-mother transmission of cytomegalovirus among pregnant women. *J Pediatr*. 2004;145:485–491.
60. Hatherley LI. Is primary cytomegalovirus infection an occupational hazard for obstetric nurses? A serological study. *Infect Control*. 1986;7:452–455.
61. Dworsky ME, Welch K, Cassady G, Stagno S. Occupational risk for primary cytomegalovirus infection among pediatric health-care workers. *N Engl J Med*. 1983;309:950–953.
62. Yow MD, Lakeman AD, Stagno S, Reynolds RB, Plavidal FJ. Use of restriction enzymes to investigate the source of a primary cytomegalovirus infection in a pediatric nurse. *Pediatrics*. 1982;70:713–716.
63. Bolyard EA, Tablan OC, Williams WW, Pearson ML, Shapiro CN, Deitchmann SD. Guideline for infection control in healthcare personnel, 1998. Hospital Infection Control Practices Advisory Committee. *Infect Control Hosp Epidemiol*. 1998;19:407–463.
64. Centers for Disease Control and Prevention. Risks associated with human parvovirus B19 infection. *MMWR*. 1989;38:81–88, 93–97.
65. Centers for Disease Control and Prevention National Center for Immunization and Respiratory Diseases. Guidelines for vaccinating pregnant women. https://www.cdc.gov/vaccines/pregnancy/hcp/guidelines.html. Accessed November 6, 2018.
66. Sendelbach DM, Sanchez PJ. Varicella, influenza: not necessary to separate mother and infant. *Pediatrics*. 2012;130:e464; author reply 65–66.
67. Cantey JB, Bascik SL, Heyne NG, et al. Prevention of mother-to-infant transmission of influenza during the postpartum period. *Am J Perinatol*. 2013;30:233–240.

68. Frenzel E, Chemaly RF, Ariza-Heredia E, et al. Association of increased influenza vaccination in health care workers with a reduction in nosocomial influenza infections in cancer patients. *Am J Infect Control* 2016;44:1016–1021.
69. Ahmed F, Lindley MC, Allred N, Weinbaum CM, Grohskopf L. Effect of influenza vaccination of healthcare personnel on morbidity and mortality among patients: systematic review and grading of evidence. *Clin Infect Dis*. 2014;58:50–57.
70. Centers for Disease Control and Prevention. Prevention and control of influenza. *MMWR*. 1984;33:253–260, 65–66.
71. Black CL, Yue X, Ball SW, et al. Influenza vaccination coverage among health care personnel—United States, 2013–14 influenza season. *MMWR*. 2014;63:805–811.
72. Loeb M, McGeer A, Henry B, et al. SARS among critical care nurses, Toronto. *Emerg Infect Dis*. 2004;10:251–255.
73. Ho PL, Tang XP, Seto WH. SARS: hospital infection control and admission strategies. *Respirology*. 2003;8(Suppl):S41–S45.
74. National Center for Immunization and Respiratory Diseases (NCIRD) Division of Viral Diseases. Severe acute respiratory syndrome (SARS) III. Infection control in healthcare facilities; supplement 1: Infection control in healthcare, home, and community settings. Public health guidance for community-level preparedness and response to severe acute respiratory syndrome (SARS). https://www.cdc.gov/sars/guidance/i-infection/downloads/I-infection-full.pdf. Accessed November 6, 2018.
75. National Center for Immunization and Respiratory Diseases (NCIRD), Division of Viral Diseases. Middle East respiratory syndrome (MERS) interim infection prevention and control recommendations for hospitalized patients with Middle East respiratory syndrome coronavirus (MERS-CoV). https://www.cdc.gov/coronavirus/mers/infection-prevention-control.html. Accessed November 6, 2018.

2 | Device-Associated Infections (Outside of the Neonatal Intensive Care Unit)

MANJIREE V. KARANDIKAR, GRACE M. LEE,
GALIT HOLZMANN-PAZGAL, AND SUSAN COFFIN

THE STRATEGIES USED TO PREVENT device-associated infections in children can vary, depending on many patient-specific factors, including the child's age and physical location when receiving inpatient pediatric care. This chapter provides guidance for preventing device-associated infections outside of the neonatal intensive care unit (NICU) setting. (Refer to Chapter 3 for NICU-specific recommendations.)

Ventilator-Associated Events (VAE)

Manjiree V. Karandikar and Grace M. Lee

Background

Ventilator-associated pneumonia (VAP) is the second-most-common hospital-acquired infection in pediatric and neonatal intensive care units (ICUs).[1,2] Pediatric VAP has been associated with increased duration of mechanical ventilation and increased hospital length of stay. While attributable mortality to VAP in pediatric patients is not well studied, mortality rates in patients with VAP are estimated to be as high as 10–20%.[2] VAP is also associated with increased healthcare costs. A single-center study in pediatric ICU patients estimated the direct cost of VAP during an admission to be $30,931 (95% confidence interval [CI], $18,349 to $82,638).[2]

Surveillance for VAP in Pediatric Patients

Surveillance data from the National Healthcare Safety Network (NHSN) suggest that the incidence of VAP is trending down. Between 2008 and

2012, VAP incidence in pediatric ICU (PICU) patients decreased from 1.9 to 0.7 per 1000 ventilator days.[3] Along similar lines, VAP incidence from neonatal ICU (NICU) patients decreased from 1.6 to 0.6 per 1000 ventilator days from 2008 to 2012.[3] More recent data from NHSN from 2013 suggest the incidence of VAP in children ranges from 0.4 to 0.7 per 1000 ventilator days, and comprises approximately 10% of all pediatric device–related infections reported to NHSN.[4]

Despite overall improvements in pediatric VAP rates, national surveillance for VAP has been challenging, particularly in neonates and children, due to the subjective nature of diagnosing VAP based on chest radiograph (CXR) findings, lack of specificity of clinical signs and symptoms, and paucity of literature regarding sensitivity of diagnostic testing.[2] As a consequence, the utility of VAP surveillance has come under scrutiny.[5–7] Clinical and radiographic findings have limited sensitivity for detecting pneumonia and often do not correlate with histological findings upon autopsy.[5,8] Neonates and children may also have progression of underlying disease that meets surveillance criteria for VAP, despite alternative known causes. The reliance on non-specific clinical signs or symptoms and subjective interpretations of radiographic findings increases the chance of inter-rater variability in reporting.[5–7] Additionally, the focus on VAP alone for surveillance provides an incomplete picture, as it does not consider alternative etiologies for deterioration while receiving mechanical ventilation, including many non-infectious etiologies that may also be preventable.[5] Given concerns about both the validity and reliability of diagnosing VAP using existing definitions, particularly in an era of public reporting and pay-for-performance, the Centers for Disease Control and Prevention (CDC) replaced VAP surveillance criteria in adult populations with a broader definition, termed *ventilator-associated events* (VAE), in 2013.

Clinical Scenario

During patient rounds in the PICU, a critical care physician states that he is treating two ventilated patients for bacterial pneumonia. He asks about changes in the CDC definition of VAP, and if this terminology should be used for his patients. He then asks what preventative measures can be taken to prevent VAE in the PICU.

Questions

Do these patients meet criteria for pediatric VAP? How does pediatric VAP differ from pediatric VAE? Why is pediatric VAE different from adult

VAE? Are there pediatric-specific interventions that can be implemented in the inpatient setting to prevent VAE?

Key Challenges and Suggested Approaches

Applying adult VAE definitions to children

The adult definition of VAE encompasses three nested definitions[6]:

1. Criteria for the broadest definition, *ventilator-associated condition (VAC)*, are met by worsening oxygenation while on mechanical ventilation after a period of improvement or stability, based on changes in daily minimum positive end expiratory pressure (PEEP) by 3 or more, or daily minimum fraction of inspired oxygen (FiO_2) by 0.2 or more.
2. Patients with VAC events who also have abnormal temperature or white blood cell (WBC) count and are started on antibiotics for at least four calendar days within two days of the increase in PEEP or FiO_2 meet criteria for *infection-related ventilator-associated complications (IVAC)*.
3. Patients with IVAC with concomitant potentially pathogenic organisms detected via culture or alternative respiratory diagnostic testing meet surveillance definitions for *possible VAP (PVAP)*.

The challenge in applying the adult VAE criteria to pediatric populations lies in the inherent difference between underlying physiology and ventilation strategies used in neonatal and pediatric populations compared to adults. For example, the use of mean airway pressure (MAP) as a criterion may better reflect underlying changes in lung compliance and oxygenation in neonatal and pediatric patients, rather than PEEP.[9] Furthermore, the adult definition of VAE excludes patients receiving high-frequency ventilation, a common ventilation modality used in critically ill neonatal and pediatric populations. Exclusion of high-frequency ventilation in children would limit the impact of a PEEP-based VAE definition on improvement efforts.

With regard to IVAC, definitions of abnormal WBC count may differ for neonates and children, compared to adults. Temperature abnormalities may also be masked when applying the adult VAE definition to NICU settings, due to external active thermoregulation of premature infants. Early work suggests that criteria for abnormal temperature and WBC in neonates and children offer little discriminatory capacity for identifying infectious causes of VAC, while adding surveillance burden.[10] In addition, criteria for antibiotic use associated with IVAC may differ for neonates and young infants, since dosing intervals may differ from adults'.

Suggested Approaches

Redefine Ventilator-Associated Events in Children

An adaptation of the adult VAE definition has been recently described for use in neonates and children. Like the adult definition for VAE, pediatric VAE also consists of three nested definitions (Figure 2.1).[10] The broadest category, termed *pediatric VAC*, is defined as an increase in the daily minimum MAP by ≥4 cm H_2O, or an increase in the daily minimum FiO_2 by ≥0.25 for two or more days following at least two days of stable or decreasing daily minimum MAP or FiO_2.[9] This MAP-based definition includes patients receiving high-frequency ventilation. Patients with VAC with new antimicrobial use are classified as "*pediatric VAE with antimicrobial use*," or *AVAC*. Because temperature and WBC count criteria were not found to be useful in discriminating IVAC episodes in neonates and children, these criteria were removed, and the definition was renamed to describe whether or not antimicrobials were administered for four or more calendar days.[10] While AVAC does not distinguish between infectious and non-infectious etiologies, it nevertheless offers useful information that may be relevant for antimicrobial stewardship efforts. Positive diagnostic tests for respiratory infection among pediatric AVAC cases meet criteria for pediatric *possible VAP (PVAP)*. Like AVAC, pediatric PVAP may have limited utility for public reporting or determining pay-for-performance; however, it may offer opportunities for internal quality-improvement

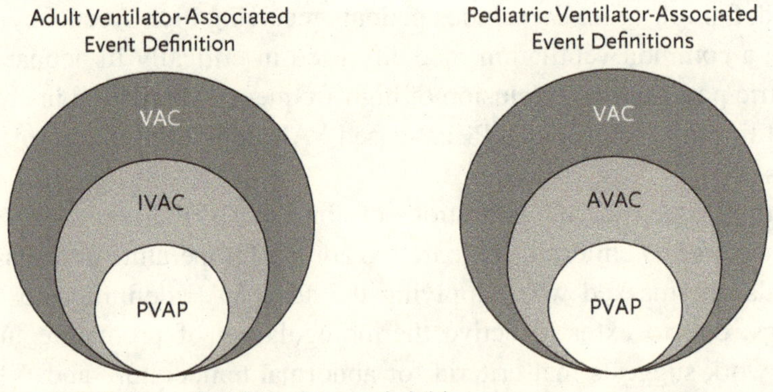

FIGURE 2.1 Definition of VAE in adults and children.

efforts. Key differences between adult and pediatric VAE definitions are described in Table 2.1.

Pediatric VAP vs. Pediatric VAE

Pediatric data comparing traditional VAP definitions with VAE are limited. One study compared pediatric VAE with NHSN-defined VAP events during the same period by requiring onset within +/– one week. Poor overlap was found between pediatric VAE definitions and the pediatric VAP surveillance definition, ranging from 6% for pediatric VAC to 16% for pediatric PVAP.[10] In a retrospective single-center study in Greece, application of the adult VAE criteria to a pediatric population also showed poor concordance between the two definitions.[11] Limited overlap has also been described for adult VAP and adult VAE definitions.[5] This may in part be due to poor sensitivity of the VAP definitions for diagnosing pneumonia, as well as to the inclusion of additional non-infectious etiologies for deterioration caught by application of VAC criteria.

With regard to outcomes, the majority of studies in adult and pediatric populations suggest that patients with VAC are at higher risk for in-hospital mortality, prolonged hospitalizations, and prolonged mechanical ventilation than control patients without VAE.[7,9,11,12] This is in contrast to studies focused on outcomes attributable to pediatric VAP compared to similarly ill children without VAP, where little impact has been observed on mortality or duration of ventilation.[13]

Key Challenges in Prevention

Several prospective cohort studies have identified a few factors independently shown to be associated with the development of pediatric VAP, including the presence of a genetic syndrome, postsurgical admission, prior antibiotic therapy, use of narcotic medications, presence of enteral feeds, reintubation, and transport out of the ICU.[2] In NICU patients, low birthweight may be a risk factor for the development of VAP, although low birthweight is also a risk factor for longer duration of mechanical ventilation. Prior bloodstream infection has been identified as a risk factor for VAP.[2] While data are limited with regard to their efficacy, VAP prevention efforts have typically focused on maintaining oral hygiene, head-of-bed elevation, and minimizing disruption of the circuit.[2,14]

As we adopt pediatric VAE definitions for use in national surveillance, we will need to identify and implement key interventions to reduce the

TABLE 2.1 Comparison of Adult and Pediatric VAE Definitions

	ADULT VAE	PEDIATRIC VAE
Definition of *Ventilator-Associated Condition (VAC)*: Baseline period of stability or improvement on the ventilator for ≥2 calendar days followed by at least one of the following, sustained for ≥2 calendar days:		
	Increase in daily minimum **PEEP** values of **≥ 3 cm H_2O** over the daily minimum PEEP of the first day in the baseline period; *And/Or:* Increase in daily minimum FiO_2 of **≥0.20 (20 points)** over the daily minimum FiO_2 of the first day in the baseline period.	Increase in daily minimum **MAP** values of **≥4 cm H_2O** over the daily minimum MAP of the first day in the baseline period; *And/Or:* Increase in daily minimum FiO_2 of **≥0.25 (25 points)** over the daily minimum FiO_2 of the first day in the baseline period.
Definition of *Infection-related Ventilator Associated Complication (IVAC)*: On or after calendar day 3 of mechanical ventilation and within 2 calendar days before or after the onset of worsening oxygenation, the patient meets the following criteria to the right		
	Temperature >38°C or <36°C, OR WBC count ≥12,000 cells/mm3 or ≤4,000 cells/mm3; ***And*** **A new antimicrobial agent started and continued for ≥4 calendar days.**	Not Applicable
Definition of *Pediatric VAC with antimicrobial use (AVAC)*: On or after calendar day 3 of mechanical ventilation and within 2 calendar days before or after the onset of worsening oxygenation, the patient meets the criteria at right		
	Not Applicable	**A new antimicrobial agent started and continued for ≥4 calendar days.**

Definition of *Possible Ventilator-Associated Pneumonia (PVAP)*: On or after calendar day 3 of mechanical ventilation and within 2 calendar days before or after the onset of worsening oxygenation:		
	Criteria met per current CDC NHSN Adult VAE guidelines: concurrent purulent pulmonary secretions and a positive quantitative or semi-quantitative culture for a potentially pathogenic organism. * Patients can also qualify for probable pneumonia on the basis of histological changes or positive laboratory tests for *Legionella sp.* and selected respiratory viruses.	Criteria met per current CDC NHSN Adult VAE guidelines.
Qualified ventilation modes	Patients are included in surveillance if they are receiving a conventional mode of ventilation through a tracheostomy or by endotracheal intubation. Patients are **EXCLUDED** from VAE surveillance during periods of time when they are receiving high-frequency ventilation, Patients are **EXCLUDED** from VAE surveillance if they are receiving extracorporeal life support (extracorporeal membrane oxygenation).	Patients are included in surveillance if they are receiving a conventional mode of ventilation through a tracheostomy or by endotracheal intubation. Patients are **INCLUDED** in VAE surveillance during periods of time when they are receiving high-frequency ventilation. Patients are **EXCLUDED** from VAE surveillance if they are receiving extracorporeal life support (extracorporeal membrane oxygenation).

* *Purulence* is defined as ≥25 neutrophils and ≤10 epithelial cells per low-power field on Gram stain of an endotracheal aspirate or bronchoalveolar lavage specimen.

risk of VAE. In order to pursue these interventions, however, we will need a robust understanding of risk factors and infectious and non-infectious etiologies of pediatric VAE in a wide range of U.S. hospitals, particularly given the limited overlap between pediatric VAE and VAP.

Suggested Approaches to Prevention

Current work to identify potential risk factors for VAE in the pediatric population is ongoing. Risk factors for pediatric VAE are likely to vary by ICU type (i.e., PICU, cardiac intensive care unit [CICU], NICU). In PICU/CICU settings, preliminary data suggest that use of neuromuscular blockade and positive fluid balance are associated with greater risk of pediatric VAE, while recent sedative weaning or interruption is protective.[10,15] For comparison, potential risk factors identified in adults include mandatory modes of mechanical ventilation, excess fluid balance, and exposures to paralytics, sedatives, and opioid analgesics.[7] We also anticipate that etiologies of pediatric VAE will vary by ICU type.[10,15] In PICU/CICU settings, the majority have been due to non-infectious causes, such as pulmonary edema, atelectasis, acute respiratory distress syndrome (ARDS), recent surgical procedures, and sepsis; however, pneumonia remains a significant challenge for prevention. Findings are similar in adult populations, where common etiologies include respiratory infections (25–40% of cases), fluid overload (20–40% of cases), atelectasis (10–15% of cases), and ARDS (10–20% of cases).[7]

Based on these preliminary data, a VAE bundle for pediatric populations is in development, focusing on key intervention strategies against the most preventable conditions associated with VAC events (Figure 2.2).

Suggested Components of VAE Prevention

1. Minimize the need for intubation, and optimize infection prevention practices during intubation procedure.
2. Optimize care processes while on the ventilator to minimize the duration of ventilation and risk for infection.
3. Schedule weaning and extubation-readiness assessments.
4. Minimize the need for re-intubation.

Some suggested components for prevention are similar to the current Institute of Healthcare Improvement VAP bundle, consisting of head-of-bed elevation, oral hygiene, scheduled weaning and extubation-readiness

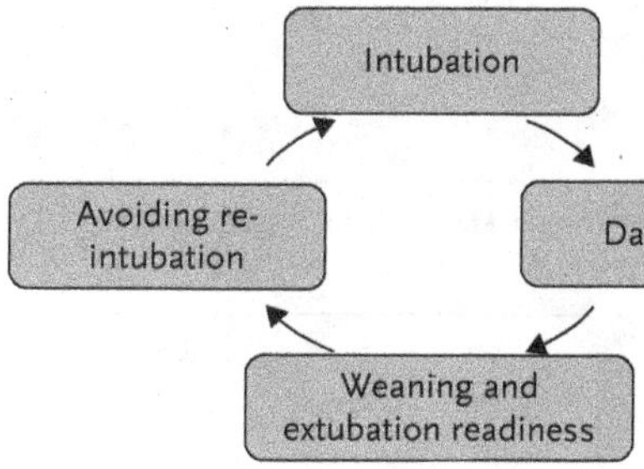

FIGURE 2.2 Targeting stages of ventilation for pediatric VAE prevention.[13]

assessments, hand hygiene, and secretion management.[14] Additional components of VAE prevention in children may include scheduled assessment and management of pain and sedation, early mobility, assessment and management of goal-directed fluid balance, and optimizing ventilator management strategies to reduce atelectrauma, barotrauma, and volutrauma.[17] For comparison, six interventions have been proposed to combat VAE in adults, including minimizing sedation, enhancing the performance of daily paired spontaneous awakening trials and spontaneous breathing trials, mobilizing patients, conservative fluid management, low tidal volume ventilation, and restrictive thresholds for blood transfusion.[17]

Approach to the Clinical Scenario

To meet criteria for VAE, the patients described in the clinical scenario must have had a period of stability or improvement on the ventilator for at least two calendar days, defined as stable or decreasing daily minimum MAP or FiO_2 values. The daily minimum is the lower value of FiO_2 or MAP during a calendar day that is maintained for at least one hour.

Step 1: Determine whether the patient experienced a VAC

After a period of stability or improvement, a patient will qualify for a VAC if they meet one of the following criteria sustained **over 2 calendar days**.

1. Increase in daily minimum FiO_2 of **≥0.25 (25 points)** over the daily minimum FiO_2 in the baseline period
2. Increase in the daily minimum MAP value of **≥4 cm $H_2$0** over the daily minimum MAP in the baseline period

For examples, see Table 2.2.

TABLE 2.2 Definition of VAC

MECHANICAL VENTILATION DAY	DAILY MINIMUM MAP	DAILY MINIMUM FIO_2	VAE
1	12	0.4	
2	11	0.4	
3	10	0.4	
4	14	0.4	VAC criteria met
5	15	0.5	
6	15	0.4	

Step 2: Determine if the patient meets criteria for AVAC

If on or after calendar day 3 of mechanical ventilation, and within two calendar days before or after the onset of worsening oxygenation, the patient is started on a new antimicrobial for a duration of four or more calendar days, the patient meets the definition for AVAC. A list of acceptable antimicrobials can be found in the CDC NHSN VAE guidelines.[6]

Step 3: Determine if the patient meets criteria for PVAP

The patient meets criteria for PVAP if on or after calendar day 3 of mechanical ventilation, and within two calendar days before or after the onset of worsening oxygenation, the patient has evidence of recent antimicrobial use *and* concurrent purulent pulmonary secretions, and a positive quantitative or semi-quantitative culture for a potentially pathogenic organism. *Purulence* is defined as ≥25 neutrophils and ≤10 epithelial cells per low-power field on Gram stain of an endotracheal aspirate or bronchoalveolar lavage specimen. Patients can also qualify for probable pneumonia on the basis of histological changes or positive laboratory tests for *Legionella* species and selected respiratory viruses as defined by CDC NHSN criteria.[6]

Unresolved Issues

These new pediatric VAE surveillance definitions provide opportunities to broaden our efforts for prevention, by shifting the focus from pneumonia to a definition that includes both infectious and non-infectious etiologies. In addition, the transition from subjective criteria to objective, readily measurable criteria allows for improved inter-rater reliability among providers and between hospitals. Patients who experience a VAE episode are at higher risk for morbidity and mortality, and identifying associated key risk factors is the first step in prevention and improved outcomes.

In an era where antimicrobial stewardship is becoming an increasing priority, VAE surveillance may identify potential stewardship program targets by enhancing our understanding of the indications for and duration of antibiotic use in this population of patients. However, specifics regarding surveillance of antimicrobial use in patients with AVAC with concomitant renal failure or in neonatal populations, where antibiotic dosing may differ from adults', have yet to be elucidated. Since pediatric patients may also have fewer invasive diagnostic tests, it remains unclear how variations in clinical practice will affect rates of PVAP in the pediatric population.

Additional efforts to define and characterize pediatric VAE are ongoing, and additional issues surrounding the subtleties of applying VAE to the pediatric population will soon become apparent with implementation of this new surveillance definition. Patients transitioned from conventional mechanical ventilation to high-frequency ventilation are likely to meet criteria for pediatric VAE, which may be appropriate, as use of high-frequency ventilation is more common in patients with acute or subacute deterioration. As extracorporeal membrane oxygenation (ECMO) patients are excluded from the pediatric definition of VAE, the impact on pediatric VAE surveillance remains to be determined. In conditions where hyperoxia is part of clinical management—for example, in patients with pulmonary hypertension—the impact on VAE surveillance also remains unclear, as these patients may be more likely to meet criteria for pediatric VAE, despite the higher FiO_2 threshold used in children. An additional component specific to pediatrics is the management of postsurgical patients after complex revisions in their underlying anatomy, such as postsurgical cardiac patients with structural heart defects. These issues highlight the need for ongoing efforts to assess preventability, while also challenging our current paradigms for prevention.

Central Line–Associated Bloodstream Infections (CLABSI)

Galit Holzmann-Pazgal

Background

Like adults in the ICU, pediatric patients in the PICU are at increased risk for central line–associated bloodstream infection (CLABSI) due to frequent use of central vascular catheters (CVC), the presence of multiple CVC, the emergency nature of line insertions, frequent and repeated access of CVC, and prolonged duration of catheter use. Per NHSN data published in 2015, mean PICU CLABSI rates ranged from 0.3 to 1.3 per 1000 line days, depending on the patient population (medical, surgical, or cardiovascular (CV). CLABSI rates in pediatric patients outside the PICU on medical wards are surprisingly high as well, with a mean rate of 1.1/1000 reported to NHSN. Pediatric oncology patients with long-term CVC have even higher rates of CLABSI, at 2.1–2.4/1000 line days.[18] A multicenter study of U.S. hospitals from 2008 to 2011 found that a pediatric CLABSI was associated with a mean attributable cost of $55,646 and attributable length of stay (LOS) of 19 days.[19]

Clinical Scenario

Despite reportedly high compliance with central-line insertion and maintenance bundles, rates of CLABSI in the PICU have not decreased for the last two years and remain higher than rates reported by "benchmark" hospitals. The medical director of the unit has asked about additional interventions to reduce CLABSI.

Questions

What are the standard components of a central line insertion bundle, to ensure standardization of best practices when a new CVC is placed? What "bundle" exists for care and maintenance of CVCs to further minimize risk of CLABSI?

Key Challenges

Device utilization and duration of catheterization are important risk factors for CLABSI. Pediatric ICUs have some of the highest device-utilization rates (DUR) reported to NHSN, with a mean of 0.72 (median 0.75) devices/patient days in CV PICU.[18] Additional risk factors for CLABSI in pediatric patients, similar to adults', include microbial colonization at catheter insertion site or hub, immunocompromised status, and inadequate CVC care. Unlike in adults, the femoral insertion site has not been clearly associated with an increased infection risk.[20,21]

Additional pediatric data regarding risk factors for CLABSI in the PICU include arterial catheterization, ECMO, and presence of genetic abnormalities.[22] Independent risk factors for pediatric CLABSI in peripherally inserted central catheters (PICCs) in patients outside the PICU include catheter duration >21 days, parenteral nutrition as the indication for central line, prior PICC-associated CLABSI, PICU exposure during hospitalization, and presence of an underlying metabolic condition. Other risk factors outside the PICU include younger age, presence of underlying malignancy, and PICC placement in a lower extremity.[23] A single-center pediatric cardiac ICU study found the following independent risk factors: non-elective admission, presence of non-cardiac comorbidities, initial low absolute neutrophil count, substantial blood product exposure, use of hydrocortisone, and CVC in place for at least seven days.[24]

CVC insertion and maintenance bundles have become the centerpiece of CLABSI prevention and has been shown to be effective when implemented reliably.[25,26]Additional interventions, including chlorhexidine bathing, antiseptic-containing hubs/connectors, antibiotic-impregnated catheters, antiseptic dressings, and catheter lock therapy, may also play a role in pediatric CLABSI prevention in certain populations or when CLABSIs continue to occur despite consistent maximal adherence to insertion and maintenance bundle hygiene.

Suggested Approaches

Perform active surveillance for CLABSI

- Utilize consistent definitions for CLABSI (such as the CDC's NHSN definitions) and benchmark to insure consistency and reliability.
- Perform surveillance in both the ICU and non ICU setting.
- Educate healthcare providers CLABSI rates in their units to increase awareness and promote a culture of safety and about CLABSI prevention.
- Maintain adequate nurse to patient ratios (at least 1:2 in ICU) and minimize floating/visiting nurses who may not be as aware of unit policies.[20,21]
- Maintain adequate staffing of infection preventionists so as to maintain surveillance and educational activities.[20]
- Utilize ultrasound guidance to facilitate insertion accuracy.[21]

Utilize Insertion Bundles

Insertion bundles are an essential component of CLABSI prevention in pediatrics. Use of insertion checklists has demonstrated success in decreasing CLABSI rates (Handout 2.1). An example checklist for a CLABSI-prevention maintenance bundle has been developed by the CDC and is available here: https://www.cdc.gov/HAI/pdfs/bsi/checklist-for-CLABSI.pdf. Checklists stress the use of aseptic technique for line placement, using and empowering an observer to "stop the line" if there is a breach in aseptic technique, and stressing hand hygiene. Use of an insertion kit or cart containing all necessary supplies is recommended.

Unique CVC insertion issues in pediatrics

While the general principles for insertion of CVC in children mirror those in adults, there are some important differences.

Femoral insertion site While insertion checklists used in adult ICUs will specifically discourage use of the femoral site, no definitive data support an increased risk of CLABSI in pediatric patients with a femoral insertion site. In fact, femoral vein insertion site was linked with a relatively lower risk of thrombotic complications.[27] One pediatric study did find that patients with femoral PICC lines inserted for prolonged antimicrobial therapy did have a twofold increase in overall complications.[28] Additional data have demonstrated that subcutaneous tunneling of CVC in the femoral site of PICU patients significantly decreased the rate of CVC colonization.[29] In general, there is no specific recommendation to avoid the femoral insertion site in younger pediatric patients when prolonged duration of catheterization is not anticipated. However, insertion site care must be meticulous, particularly in diapered children.

Chlorhexidine Skin Disinfection An alcoholic chlorhexidine product is recommended for skin antisepsis for line insertion.[20,21] The use of chlorhexidine in infants under two months of age has historically been controversial in pediatrics. More recently, the manufacturer contraindication statement for this age group has been modified to "Use with caution" rather than the previous "Do not use" statement. A survey of U.S. pediatric institutions indicated that more than 50% of pediatric centers do use chlorhexidine in patients under two months of age, including neonates, with varying restrictions.[30]

Utilize Maintenance Bundles

Maintenance bundles for the ongoing care of CVC have also been shown to be effective in preventing CLABSI. An example checklist for CLABSI

HANDOUT 2.1 Sample Insertion Checklist

Instructions: Assisting nurse is to audit practices related to insertion technique for all central venous catheters and return to unit director or designee.

Did the Provider/Staff Attending:	Please circle answer		Comments
Wash hands using soap or hand sanitizer prior to start? (ask if unsure).	Yes	No	
Prep the insertion site with chlorhexidine for 30 seconds on a dry site or 2 minutes on a moist site?	Yes	No	
Wear a head cover, mask, sterile gown, and sterile gloves during entire procedure?	Yes	No	
Drape the patient from head to toe?	Yes	No	
Was sterile field maintained during the procedure?	Yes	No	
Was Biopatch placed at the insertion site? (Biopatch restriction per unit policy)	Yes	No	
Was dressing labeled with insertion date and dressing date?	Yes	No	
Did the Assisting Physician/Nurse:			
Wash hands using soap or hand sanitizer prior to start? (ask if unsure).	Yes	No	
Wear a head cover, mask, gown, and gloves?	Yes	No	

Unit: ____________________

Physician: ____________________

Insertion Date/Time: ____________________

Person completing audit: ____________________

Reason for insertion:

☐ Emergent ☐ Elective

☐ Initial insertion ☐ Other

☐ Re-wire ☐ Surgery

Site: ☐ Right ☐ Left

☐ IJ ☐ EJ ☐ SC ☐ FEM ☐ PIC ☐ UVC/UAC

Other ____________________

Other Comments: ____________________

prevention maintenance bundle has been developed by the CDC, and is available here: https://www.cdc.gov/HAI/pdfs/bsi/checklist-for-CLABSI.pdf. Daily review and physician documentation of central-line necessity, and prompt removal of unnecessary central lines in order to decrease duration of catheterization, are important components of CVC maintenance. CVC hubs should be disinfected immediately prior to access for at least 5 seconds, using either an alcohol/chlorhexidine preparation or 70% sterile alcohol, then allowed to dry prior to access.[20]

Disinfection should occur before every single access (including routine flushing), and disinfectant allowed to dry prior to access. Tubing changes for infusions other than blood products or lipids should take place every 96 hours. Tubing for blood and lipid formulations should be changed within 24 hours of infusion initiation.[21]

Dressing changes should be performed at least every seven days, or sooner if the dressing is soiled or not intact. Gauze dressings should be changed at least every two days, or sooner if needed.[20,21]

Utilization of disinfecting caps to cover needleless connectors has also demonstrated a benefit in decreasing CLABSI in several studies.[31–33]

Unique maintenance issues in pediatrics

Non-tunneled/Unsutured CVC An exception to dressing-change frequency in pediatrics relates to selected patients in which a non-tunneled CVC may become dislodged with dressing changes. This is often the case in very young or neonatal patients, as lines are not sutured in place and can move when manipulated. For this reason, it is reasonable to change dressings less frequently in this population as long as dressings remain intact, clean, and dry.[20]

Antimicrobial/Antiseptic-impregnated catheters Additional CLABSI prevention approaches include the use of antimicrobial catheters. These can be used in pediatrics in certain patients if CLABSI rates remain high despite implementation of insertion and maintenance bundles.[34–36] However, these catheters are often not available in the smaller sizes necessary in neonates or smaller patients.

Chlorhexidine Dressings In 2017, the CDC's Healthcare Infection Control Practices Advisory Committee (HICPAC) reviewed the existing literature specific to the use of chlorhexidine-impregnated dressings for prevention of intravascular catheter-related infections.[37] Based on this review, chlorhexidine dressings over catheter insertion sites are recommended for adults over 18 years of age. In addition, no recommendation could be made about the use of chlorhexidine-impregnated dressings to protect the site of short-term, non-tunneled CVCs for pediatric patients less than 18 years old and non-premature neonates, due to the lack of sufficient evidence from published, high-quality studies about efficacy and safety in this age group.

Daily Chlorhexidine Bathing In addition to chlorhexidine patches, daily chlorhexidine bathing in children over two months old utilizing chlorhexidine wipes is recommended and has been demonstrated to decrease the incidence of hospital-acquired bacteremia and CLABSI in pediatric patients by at least 34%.[38] No serious adverse events occurred. Blood concentrations of chlorhexidine in pediatric patients over two months of age receiving daily bathing with the chlorhexidine wipes were measured, and only 15% had measurable chlorhexidine levels above the limit of detection. No trend of chlorhexidine accumulation was noted with repeated bathing exposure.[39] (For additional discussion about the use of chlorhexidine in young and premature infants, please also refer to Chapter 3.)

Special pediatric populations (Immunocompromised and intestinal failure patients)

Lock therapy: CVC lock therapy can be utilized to prevent CLABSI in certain populations with long-term CVC. Data demonstrate that *ethanol* lock therapy is effective in significantly reducing the incidence of CLABSI in pediatric patients with intestinal failure receiving long-term total parenteral nutrition (TPN) as well as pediatric oncology patients.[40–43]

Taurolidine lock therapy has also been shown to be effective in significantly decreasing the incidence of CLABSI in both pediatric oncology patients and patients receiving home TPN due to intestinal failure.[44,45] Taurolidine is not available in the United States.

Antibiotic lock therapy has also been utilized effectively to prevent CLABSI in pediatric oncology, intestinal failure, and hemodialysis patients with long-term CVC access. Vancomycin is the most frequently utilized antimicrobial agent in these studies.[21] Use of antibiotic lock therapy must be balanced with the potential for emergence of antimicrobial resistance with this therapy.

Approach to the Clinical Scenario

The clinical scenario asks about additional interventions to reduce CLABSI when rates remain higher than reported by "benchmark" hospitals despite reportedly high compliance with central line insertion and maintenance bundles. To recap, the usual components of a CVC insertion bundle are:

- Perform hand hygiene before insertion.
- Adhere to aseptic technique.
- Use maximal sterile barrier precautions (i.e., mask, cap, gown, sterile gloves, and sterile full body drape).
- Choose the best insertion site to minimize infections and noninfectious complications based on individual patient characteristics.
- Prepare the insertion site with >0.5% chlorhexidine with alcohol.
- Place a sterile gauze dressing or a sterile, transparent, semipermeable dressing over the insertion site.
- For patients 18 years of age or older, use a chlorhexidine impregnated dressing with an FDA-cleared label that specifies a clinical indication for reducing CLABSI for short-term non-tunneled catheters, unless the facility is demonstrating success at preventing CLABSI with baseline prevention practices.

A CVC maintenance bundle typically includes the following components:

- Comply with hand hygiene requirements.
- Bathe patients over two months of age with a chlorhexidine preparation on a daily basis.
- Scrub the access port or hub with friction immediately prior to each use with an appropriate antiseptic (chlorhexidine, povidone iodine, an iodophor, or 70% alcohol).
- Use only sterile devices to access catheters.
- Immediately replace dressings that are wet, soiled, or dislodged.
- Perform routine dressing changes using aseptic technique with clean or sterile gloves.
- Change gauze dressings at least every two days or semipermeable dressings at least every seven days.
- For patients 18 years of age or older, use a chlorhexidine-impregnated dressing with an FDA-cleared label that specifies a clinical indication for reducing CLABSI for short-term non-tunneled catheters, unless the facility is demonstrating success at preventing CLABSI with baseline prevention practices.

- Change administrations sets for continuous infusions no more frequently than every 4 days, but at least every 7 days.
- If blood or blood products or fat emulsions are administered change tubing every 24 hours.

Unresolved Issues

Specific CLABSI prevention strategies do not exist for certain pediatric populations. The incidence of CLABSI in patients receiving ECMO therapy has increased, based on data from several pediatric studies. In one unit, CLABSI rates for PICU patients on ECMO were tenfold higher than for non-ECMO patients.[46] Infection rates as high as 24.9 CLABSI/1000 ECMO days have been noted, and CLABSI is the most common infectious bacterial complication for pediatric ECMO patients.[47,48] Major risk factors for CLABSI on ECMO include duration of bypass, and cardiothoracic patients with post-operative open chests while on ECMO.[47–50] Potential interventions to decrease CLABSI rates on ECMO have been proposed in several small single-center intervention studies, but there are no definitive trials or guidelines to support particular interventions beyond those previously recommended for general CLABSI prevention.

Patients with short bowel syndrome and intestinal failure requiring chronic TPN are another challenging population. These children have higher risk of CLABSI due to numerous factors, including an altered intestinal microbiome, longstanding CVC use, impaired immunity, and impaired gut absorption.[21] Effective preventive measures such as ethanol locks have been reported, but the indications for use are not yet established.[20]

Catheter-Associated Urinary Tract Infections (CAUTI)

Susan Coffin

Background

Catheter-associated urinary tract infections (CAUTI) are the third-most-common HAIs experienced by hospitalized children. In addition, they can cause secondary bloodstream infections in patients who develop urosepsis. Rigorous epidemiological analysis has demonstrated that hospitalized children who develop a CAUTI experience, on average, a 2.4-day prolonged hospitalization and an excess average cost of $7200.[51, 52]

The microbiology of CAUTI in hospitalized children is similar to that reported for community-onset UTIs; enteric organisms such as *Klebsiella* and *Escherichia coli* predominate. Additional pathogens that have been frequently reported include *Pseudomonas, Enterococcus,* and *Enterobacter.*[51,53] When compared to a community-onset UTI, however, there is a greater risk that a healthcare-associated CAUTI will be caused by a resistant organism.

Risk factors for pediatric CAUTI[53,54] include:

- Duration of catheterization
- Being on contact precautions
- Prior catheterization
- Congenital syndrome
- Structural or functional urinary tract abnormality.

Clinical Scenario

Despite an aggressive campaign to decrease CAUTI, rates in a PICU have not decreased for the last two years and remain higher than rates reported by "benchmark" hospitals. The medical director of the unit has asked about additional interventions to reduce CAUTI, specifically asking about prevention bundles, which have been similarly used in CLABSI prevention.

Question

What are the typical components of a CAUTI prevention bundle?

Key Challenges

Prevention of CAUTI in children presents unique challenges.

Paucity of data

Despite the significant burden these infections pose to children, our understanding of the most effective strategies to prevent CAUTI in children is somewhat limited due to the paucity of pediatric studies. However, indirect evidence from adult studies has been used by pediatric investigators to develop pediatric CAUTI prevention bundles. Several single-center studies report the successful reduction of pediatric CAUTI after implementation of a CAUTI prevention bundle that was adapted from evidence-based adult prevention bundles.[51,55]

Different disease processes might require different approaches to infection prevention

Congenital abnormalities of the genitourinary tract are relatively common among hospitalized children on a surgical service. Although maintaining a closed drainage system is a key element of adult CAUTI prevention bundles, pediatric urologists have argued that there are specific clinical scenarios that require an open drainage system. These include recent complex surgical repair or reconstruction of congenital abnormalities of the urogenital system. In addition, some urologists and neonatologists believe that it is important to maintain a low-pressure urinary drainage system in premature infants who require urinary catheterization. We do not have sufficient data to determine whether there are specific patients who would benefit more from an open drainage system despite an increased risk of CAUTI.

Lack of pediatric-specific resources

Not all preventive resources are available for small children. For example, appropriately sized condom catheters are not available for young boys who need accurate measurement of urinary output. To minimize the risk of reflux of urine from a catheter back into the bladder, some institutions have included "direct drainage of urine into collecting system" in their CAUTI prevention bundle, to prevent urine reflux (from tubing that connects the catheter to the collecting system) back into the bladder. However, the small size of some children makes redundant loops of tubing inevitable, and this increases the risk of reflux of urine from the collecting system backwards into the bladder. Lastly, urinary catheter insertion kits have been a commonly recommended strategy to prevent adult CAUTI. However, fewer vendors produce pediatric urinary catheter insertion kits.

Surveillance challenges

New tools to support electronic surveillance for CAUTI have been developed. However, investigators have noted that inaccurate documentation can introduce errors in CAUTI surveillance. For example, electronic medical record (EMR) documentation may erroneously indicate that a patient has an indwelling urinary catheter when a patient is actually receiving intermittent catheterization.[56]

Suggested Approaches

Determine the indication for insertion of urinary catheter

Placement of a urinary catheter should be avoided whenever possible. Pediatric providers should consider the use of in-and-out catheterization as an alternative to an 2indwelling urinary catheter for young boys who cannot use a condom catheter, if they are continent and cooperative. Recommended preapproved indications for insertion of an indwelling urinary catheter include:

- Peri-operative use for selected surgical procedures
- Continuous monitoring of urine output in the critically ill patient
- Management of acute urinary retention and urinary obstruction
- Assistance in pressure ulcer healing for incontinent patients
- At patient/family request to improve comfort, or for comfort during end-of-life care
- For patients with abnormal GU systems
- To promote continuous bladder emptying and/or to prevent caustic harm during certain chemotherapy protocols.

These indications should also be used for a daily assessment of catheter necessity. Patients who no longer meet these indications should have their catheters removed promptly.

Prevention bundles

Prevention bundles have been derived from adult, evidence-based bundles. Elements that have been included in published reports of pediatric CAUTI prevention bundles include[51,55]:

- Simulation training of catheter insertion using male and female mannequins.
- Place urinary catheter only for preapproved indications.
- Conduct a daily assessment of catheter necessity.
- Maintain aseptic technique for catheter insertion.
- Use insertion checklist to monitor insertion technique.

- Keep urinary collection system closed and below the level of the bladder.
- Use a secural device to stabilize catheter.
- Empty urinary collection system when two-thirds full or every 8 hours (whichever is sooner).
- Do not routinely change indwelling urinary catheters or collection systems.
- Perform meatal/perineal care at least once per day and whenever soiled.

Insertion Checklists

Several institutions have developed urinary catheter insertion checklists. These lists provide a detailed, step-by-step approach to guide catheter insertion:

- Obtain catheter insertion kit or gather all necessary equipment.
- Perform hand hygiene and don non-sterile, procedure gloves.
- Cleanse meatal/perineal area with sterile water and gauze.
- Remove procedure gloves, perform hand hygiene, don sterile gloves.
- Cover legs, lower abdomen, and buttocks with sterile drapes.
- Swab urethral meatus 3x with sterile betadine and allow to air dry.
- Insert catheter to the Y bifurcation; if first attempt at catheter insertion fails, obtain new sterile catheter.
- Inflate catheter balloon with sterile water.
- Apply secural device to anchor catheter to patient's lower leg.
- Connect catheter to urinary drainage system.
- Position urinary collection system below level of the bladder.

Additional practices that can be considered, particularly if CAUTI rates remain elevated, include:

- Episodic audits of patients with urinary catheters to ensure:
  - o Indication for catheterization is present
  - o Catheter is secured and below the level of the bladder
  - o Urinary collection system is no more than two-thirds full.
- Nurse-driven protocols for catheter removal when the indication for urinary catheterization is resolved
- Use of bladder scanners to assess urinary retention.

Approach to the Clinical Scenario

In the hospital described in the clinical scenario, CAUTI rates in a PICU have not decreased for the last two years and remain higher than rates reported by "benchmark" hospitals despite an aggressive campaign to decrease them. The medical director of the unit asked about additional interventions to reduce CAUTI, specifically asking about prevention bundles, which have been similarly used in CLABSI prevention.

As previously reviewed, potential components of a prevention bundle may include:

- Simulation training of catheter insertion using male and female mannequins.
- Place urinary catheter only for preapproved indications.
- Conduct a daily assessment of catheter necessity.
- Maintain aseptic technique for catheter insertion.
- Use insertion checklist to monitor insertion technique.
- Keep urinary collection system closed and below the level of the bladder.
- Use a secural device to stabilize catheter.
- Empty urinary collection system when two-thirds full or every 8 hours (whichever is sooner).
- Do not routinely change indwelling urinary catheters or collection systems.
- Perform meatal/perineal care at least once per day and whenever soiled.

Unresolved Issues

Several unresolved issues in CAUTI prevention include the use of antiseptic solution versus sterile saline for meatal cleaning before catheterization, and antibiotic prophylaxis at catheter removal to prevent UTI. In addition, specific recommendations are needed for high-risk patients such as those with neurogenic bladder or abnormal genitourinary anatomy. Currently, pediatric data are lacking, therefore general recommendations are not available.

References

1. Centers for Disease Control and Prevention, National Healthcare Safety Network (NHSN). *Pneumonia (ventilator-associated [VAP] and non-ventilator-associated pneumonia [PNEU]) event*. 2016. Accessed June 10, 2016.

2. Foglia E, Meier MD, Elward A. Ventilator-associated pneumonia in neonatal and pediatric intensive care unit patients. *Clin Microbiol Rev.* 2007;20(3):409–425.
3. Patrick SW, Kawai AT, Kleinman K, et al. Health care–associated infections among critically ill children in the US, 2007–2012. *Pediatrics.* 2014;134(4):705–712.
4. Dudeck M, Edwards J, Allen-Bridson K, et al. National Healthcare Safety Network report, data summary for 2013, device-associated module. *Am J Infect Control.* 2015;43(3):206–221.
5. Klompas M. Ventilator-associated conditions versus ventilator-associated pneumonia: different by design. *Curr Infect Dis Rep.* 2014;16(10):430.
6. Centers for Disease Control and Prevention, National Healthcare Safety Network (NHSN). *Ventilator-associated events.* 2016. https://www.cdc.gov/nhsn/pdfs/validation/2016/pcsmanual_2016.pdf. Accessed June 10, 2016.
7. Corcoros NM, Klompas M. Ventilator-associated events and their prevention. *Infect Dis Clin North Am.* 2016;30(4):887–908.
8. Tejerina E, Esteban A, Fernandez-Segoviano P, et al. Accuracy of clinical definitions of ventilator-associated pneumonia: comparison with autopsy findings. *J Crit Care.* 2010;25(1):62–68.
9. Corcoros NM, Kleinman K, Priebe GP, et al. Ventilator associated events in neonates and children—a new paradigm. *Crit Care Med.* 2016;44(1):14–22.
10. Corcoros NM, Priebe GP, Logan LK, et al. A pediatric approach to ventilator-associated event surveillance. *Infect Control Hosp Epidemiol.* 2017;38(3): 327–333.
11. Iosifidis E, Chochliourou E, Violaki A, et al. Evaluation of the new Centers for Disease Control and Prevention ventilator-associated event module and criteria in critically ill children in Greece. *Infect Control Hosp Epidemiol.* 2016;37(10):1162–1166.
12. Cirulis M, Hamele M, Stockmann C, Bennett T, Bratton S. Comparison of the new adult ventilator-associated event criteria to the Centers for Disease Control and Prevention pediatric ventilator-associated pneumonia definition (PNU2) in a population of pediatric traumatic brain injury patients. *Pediatr Crit Care Med.* 2016;17(2):157–164.
13. Klompas M, Branson R, Eichenwald EC, et al. Strategies to prevent ventilator-associated pneumonia in acute care hospitals. *Infect Control Hosp Epidemiol.* 2014;35(Suppl 2):S133–S154.
14. Curley MA, Schwalenstocker JK, Deshpande, CC, et al. Tailoring the Institute for Health Care Improvement 100,000 Lives Campaign to pediatric settings: the example of ventilator-associated pneumonia. *Pediatr Clin N Am.* 2006;53(6):1231–1251.
15. Corcoros NM, Gray JE, Priebe GP, et al. Identifying factors associated with pediatric ventilator-associated conditions in six U.S Hospitals. *Crit Care Med.* 2015;43(12 Suppl):77.
16. Cocoros N, Gray J, Priebe G, et al. Identifying factors associated with pediatric ventilator-associated conditions in 6 U.S. hospitals. *Crit Care Med.* 2015;43:77.
17. Klompas M. Potential strategies to prevent ventilator-associated events. *Am J Respir Crit Care Med.* 2015;192(12):1420–1430.
18. Dudeck MA, Edwards JR, Allen-Bridson K, et al. National Healthcare Safety Network report, data summary for 2013, device-associated module. *Am J Infect Control.* 2015;43:206–221.

19. Goudie A, Dynan L, Brady PW, Rettiganti M, Attributable cost and length of stay for central line–associated bloodstream infections. *Pediatrics*. 2014;133:e1525–e1532.
20. Marschall J, Mermel LA, Fakih M, et al. Strategies to prevent central line-associated bloodstream infections in acute care hospitals: 2014 update. *Infect Control Hosp Epidemiol.* 2014;35:753–771.
21. O'Grady NP, Alexander M, Burns LA, et al. Guidelines for prevention of intravascular catheter-related infections. *Am J Infect Control.* 2011;39:S1–S34.
22. Smith MJ. Catheter-related bloodstream infections in children. *Am J Infect Control.* 2008;36:S173.e1–S173.e3.
23. Advani S, Reich NG, Sengupta A, Gosey L, Milstone AM. Central line–associated bloodstream infection in hospitalized children with peripherally inserted central venous catheters: extending risk analyses outside the intensive care unit. *Clin Infect Dis.* 2011;52:1108–1115.
24. Costello, JM, Graham DA, Morrow DF. Risk factors for central line-associated bloodstream infection in a pediatric cardiac intensive care unit. *Pediatric Critical Care Medicine.* 2009;10(4):453–459.
25. Edwards JD, Herzig C, Liu H, et al. Central line–associated blood stream infections in pediatric ICUs: longitudinal trends and compliance with bundle strategies. *Am J Infect Control.* 2015;43;489–493.
26. Li L, Fortin E, Tremblay C, Ngenda-Muadi M, Quach C. Central line–associated bloodstream infections in Quebec intensive care units: results from the Provincial Healthcare-Associated Infections Surveillance Program (SPIN). *Infect Control Hosp Epidemiol.* 2016;37:1186–1194.
27. de Jonge RC, Polderman KH, Gemke RJ. Central venous catheter use in the pediatric patient: mechanical and infectious complications. *Pediatr Crit Care Med.* 2005;6:329–339.
28. Barrier A, Williams DJ, Connelly M, Creech CB. Frequency of peripherally inserted central catheter complications in children. *Pediatr Infect Dis J.* 2012;31:519–520.
29. Nahum EN, Levy I, Katz J, et al. Efficacy of subcutaneous tunneling for prevention of bacterial colonization of femoral central venous catheters in critically ill children. *Pediatr Infect Dis J.* 2002;21:1000–1004.
30. Tamma PD, Aucott SW, Milstone AM. Chlorhexidine use in the neonatal intensive care unit: results from a national survey. *Infect Control Hosp Epidemiol.* 2010;31:846–849.
31. Menyhay SZ, Maki DG. Preventing central venous catheter-associated bloodstream infections: development of an antiseptic barrier cap for needleless connectors. *Am J Infect Control.* 2008;36:S174e1–S175e5.
32. Sweet MA, Cumpston A, Briggs F, Craig M, Hamadani M. Impact of alcohol-impregnated port protectors and needleless neutral pressure connectors on central line–associated bloodstream infections and contamination of blood cultures in an inpatient oncology unit. *Am J Infect Control.* 2012;40:931–934.
33. Wright MO, Tropp J, Schora DM, et al. Continuous passive disinfection of catheter hubs prevents contamination and bloodstream infection. *Am J Infect Control.* 2013;41:33–38.
34. Bhutta A, Gilliam C, Honeycutt M, et al. Reduction of bloodstream infections associated with catheters in paediatric intensive care unit: stepwise approach. *BMJ.* 2007;334:362–365.

35. Chelliah A, Heydon KH, Zaoutis TE, et al. Observational trial of antibiotic coated central venous catheters in critically ill pediatric patients. *Pediatr Infect Dis J.* 2007;26:816–820.
36. Weber JM, Sheridan RL, Fagan S, Ryan CM, Pasternack MS, Tompkins RG. Incidence of catheter-associated bloodstream infection after introduction of minocycline and rifampin antimicrobial-coated catheters in a pediatric burn population. *J Burn Care Res.* 2012;33:539–543.
37. Centers for Disease Control and Prevention. 2017 Recommendations on use of chlorhexidine-impregnated dressings for prevention of intravascular catheter-related infections: An update to the 2011 guidelines for the prevention of intravascular catheter-related infections from the Centers for Disease Control and Prevention. Centers for Disease Control and Prevention, National Center for Emerging and Zoonotic Infectious Diseases, Division of Healthcare Quality and Promotion. Available at: https://www.cdc.gov/infectioncontrol/guidelines/pdf/bsi/c-i-dressings-H.pdf. Accessed date October 26, 2018.
38. Milstone AM, Elward A, Song X, et al. Daily chlorhexidine bathing to reduce bacteraemia in critically ill children: a multicenter, cluster-randomised crossover trial. *Lancet.* 2013 Mar 30;381(9872):1099–1106. doi:10.1016/S0140-6736(12)61687-0
39. Lee A, Harlan R, Breaud AR, et al. Blood concentrations of chlorhexidine in hospitalized children undergoing daily chlorhexidine bathing. *Infect Control Hosp Epidemiol.* 2011;32:395–397.
40. Maiefski M, Rupp ME, Hermsen ED. Ethanol lock technique: review of the literature. *Infect Control Hosp Epidemiol.* 2009;30:1096–1108.
41. Schoot RA, van Ommen CH, Stijnen T, et al. Prevention of central venous catheter-associated bloodstream infections in paediatric oncology patients using 70% ethanol locks: a randomized controlled multi-centre trial. *Eur J Cancer.* 2015;51:2031–2038.
42. Ardura MI, Lewis J, Tansmore JL, Harp PL, Dienhart MC, Balint JP. Central catheter-associated bloodstream infection reduction with ethanol lock prophylaxis in pediatric intestinal failure. *JAMA Pediatr.* 2015;169:324–331.
43. Oliveira C, Nasr A, Brindle M, Wales PW. Ethanol locks to prevent catheter-related bloodstream infections in parenteral nutrition: a meta-analysis. *Pediatrics.* 2012;129:318–329.
44. Handrup MM, Moller JK, Schroder H. Central venous catheters and catheter locks in children with cancer: a prospective randomized trial of taurolidine versus heparin. *Pediatr Blood Cancer.* 2013;60:1292–1298.
45. Chu, HP, Brind J, Tomar R, Hill S. Significant reduction in central venous catheter-related bloodstream infections in children on HPN after starting treatment with taurolidine line lock. *JPGN.* 2012;55:403–407.
46. Odetola FO, Moler FW, Dechert RE, VanDerElzen K, Chenoweth C. Nosocomial catheter-related bloodstream infections in a pediatric intensive care unit: risk and rates associated with various intravascular technologies. *Pediatr Crit Care Med.* 2003;4:432–436.
47. Brown KL, Ridout DA, Shaw M, et al. Healthcare-associated infection in pediatric patients on extracorporeal life support: the role of multidisciplinary surveillance. *Pediatr Crit Care Med.* 2006;7:546–550.
48. O'Neill JM, Schutze GE, Heulitt MJ, Simpson PM, Taylor BJ. Nosocomial infections during extracorporeal membrane oxygenation. *Intens Care Med.* 2001;27:1247–1253.

49. Kaczala GW, Paulus SC, Al-Dajani N, et al. Bloodstream infections in pediatric ECLS: usefulness of daily blood culture monitoring and predictive value of biological markers. The British Columbia experience. *Pediatr Surg Int*. 2009;25:169–173.
50. Steiner, CK, Stewart DL, Bond SJ, Hornung CA, McKay VJ. Predictors of acquiring a nosocomial bloodstream infection on extracorporeal membrane oxygenation. *J Pediatr Surg*. 2001;36:487–492.
51. Davis KF, Coebaugh AM, Eithum BL, et al. Reducing catheter-associated urinary tract infections: a quality improvement initiative. *Pediatrics*. 2014;134:e857.
52. Lo E, Nicolle LE, Coffin SE, et al. Strategies to prevent catheter-associated urinary tract infections in acute care hospitals: 2014 update. *Infect Control Hosp Epidemiol*. 2014;35(S2):S32–S47.
53. Kabbani, MS, Ismail, SR, Fatima, A, Shafi, R, Idris, JA, Mehmood, A, Singh, RA, Elbarabry, M, Hijazi, O, Hussein, MA. Urinary tract infection in children after cardiac surgery: Incidence, causes, risk factors and outcomes in a single-center study. *J Infect Pub Health*. 2016 (advance access).
54. Lee, NG, Marchalik D, Lipsky A, Rushton G, Pohl HG, Song X. Risk factors for catheter-associated urinary tract infections in a pediatric institution. *J Urol*. 2015;195:1306–1311.
55. Duzkaya, DS, Bozkurt, G, Uysal, G, Yakut, T. The Effects of Bundles on Catheter-Associated Urinary Tract Infections in the Pediatric Intensive Care Unit. *Clin Nurse Specialist*. Nov/Dec, 2016:341–346.
56. Sen AI, Balzer K, Mangino D, et al. Electronic surveillance for catheter-associated urinary tract infections at a university-affiliated children's hospital. *Am J Infect Control*. 2016;44:599–601.

3 | Device-Associated Infections in the Neonatal Intensive Care Unit (NICU)

CAROLINE QUACH

Background

Infants, especially preterm, in neonatal intensive care units (NICU) are especially susceptible to healthcare-associated infections (HAI), given their immature immune system, the acuity of care needed, and the frequency of invasive procedures performed.[1–3] Moreover, HAIs have major impacts on premature infant outcomes. HAIs in the NICU have been associated with a twofold increase in the risk of death.[4,5] Even bacteria usually considered as commensals, such as coagulase-negative staphylococci, had a reported mortality of 1.6% when causing bloodstream infections.[6] Bloodstream infections caused by Gram-negative bacilli (e.g., Enterobacteriaceae) have been associated with a 10.5% mortality rate in the absence of a drug-resistant organism, while in the presence of a multidrug-resistant organism, the mortality rate has been as high as 28.6%.[7] Postnatal sepsis, occurring in infants born before 30 weeks of gestation, doubles the risk of cerebral palsy at two years of age,[8] and coagulase-negative staphylococcal bloodstream infections have been associated with a 5.6-fold increase in the risk of cerebral palsy at 18–24 months of age.[8,9]

Infection prevention and control interventions and recommendations in the NICU should therefore aim to decrease HAIs in general, and device-associated infections in particular, given the adverse outcomes associated with HAIs in this age group. Neonates differ from older infants and children in many ways, including their immature immune system, immature skin, and their developing, but not yet formed, microbiota. Unlike in older children, infants' microbiota has not reached maturity and is therefore, in theory, more amenable to change; the impact of these modifications is yet to be determined. In light of this uncertainty, the precaution principle should be applied, weighing potential risks against benefits, when an intervention to prevent an infection is implemented.

Clinical Scenario

You are working with your staff neonatologists in creating a Best Practice Guideline to prevent central line–associated bloodstream infections (CLABSIs) in the NICU setting. One of the physicians is concerned about the safety of chlorhexidine gluconate (CHG)–containing skin antiseptics for premature neonates. She is concerned that CHG will cause skin irritation in infants with very low birthweight (VLBW) (those weighing <1500 grams at birth).

Question

What infection prevention strategies are safe and effective to prevent device-associated infections in the NICU setting?

Key Challenges

The neonatal microbiome and its evolution over time creates unique challenges for infection prevention.

Microbiota Evolution in Infants

"Microbiota" is the sum of all microbial life, including bacteria, fungi, archaea, and viruses, living in and on the human body, and is influenced by what/whom we have encountered. The adult microbiota consists of tenfold more cells than those of human origin, with the vast majority residing in the gastrointestinal (GI) tract.[10] While in utero, infants are considered to reside in a sterile or nearly sterile environment.[11] The fetal intestine is therefore sterile.[12] Having a greater number of bifidobacteria, a lower number of *Escherichia coli* (and other Enterobacteriaceae), and *Clostridioides difficile* with a greater bacterial diversity has been considered a "beneficial" profile[13]—less likely to be associated with necrotizing enterocolitis (NEC)[14–16] and late-onset sepsis.[17] Acquisition of one's microbiota starts at birth and is influenced by various factors, including the maternal GI and cervical flora, mode of delivery, environment, feeding mode, and administration of antimicrobials. Time since birth has a major influence on the composition of an infant's microbiota.

Mode of Delivery

Fecal colonization is delayed in infants born by cesarean section, with lower numbers of *Bacteroides fragilis*[18] and a different bacterial composition than that of infants born by vaginal delivery.[19] Vaginally delivered infants acquire bacterial communities resembling their own mother's vaginal microbiota, whereas infants born by cesarean section harbor bacterial communities more similar to those found on the skin surface (*Staphylococci, Corynebacterium*, and *Propionibacterium spp.*).[20]

Feeding Mode

The GI microbiota of a healthy 31-week premature infant on fortified breast milk was shown to be dominated initially with *E. coli* and replaced, over the second to third week of life, by *S. anginosus* and *C. butyricum* (anaerobes), illustrating a switch to a fermentation-based metabolism.[21] Feeding mode (breastmilk vs. formula) also influences the GI microbiota.[22] Penders et al. analyzed fecal samples collected at four weeks of age in a large Dutch birth cohort (1,032 infants). The following factors were independently associated with a "better" microbiota: vaginal delivery, exclusive breast-feeding, absence of hospitalization, absence of prematurity, and having older siblings.[13]

Exposure to Antimicrobials

The impact of antimicrobial administration (ampicillin and gentamicin) on NICU infants' microbiota has been studied. Serial stool samples were collected from infants admitted to a level III NICU in the United States during their first three weeks of life ($n = 74$). Only 18% had not received antibiotics. The predominant bacterial genera during the first week of life varied according to antimicrobial status: in infants who had not received antimicrobials, *Staphylococcus* (41%), *Enterococcus* (26%), and *Enterobacter* (19%) dominated, compared to a predominance of *Enterococcus* (34%) and *Clostridium* (33%) in infants who had received intense antimicrobial courses, defined as those lasting from five to seven days. In the third week of life, infants who had not received antimicrobials harbored a majority of *Enterobacter* (36%), *Enterococcus* (17%), *Clostridia* (17%), *Veillonella* (16%), and *Escherichia* (11%), compared to a predominance of *Enterobacter* (47%) and *Enterococcus* (35%) in infants who had received intense antimicrobial courses. This highlights the marked decrease in bacterial diversity and a higher relative abundance of *Enterobacter* associated with the administration of ampicillin and gentamicin in the first week of life.[23]

Prematurity

The GI microbiota is different in preterm neonates from that of healthy, full-term neonates, with the preterm GI microbiota having less biodiversity.[24,25] In one study of preterm NICU infants,[26] *Ureaplasma* was the dominant species in the first week of life in gastroesophageal specimens, but *Staphylococci* were the predominant bacteria overall. By the fourth week of life, Gram-negative bacteria increased and accounted for 50% of the total organisms. The GI microbiota of extremely low birthweight infants (those weighting <750 grams at birth) who received prolonged antimicrobial therapy, total parenteral nutrition, delayed oral feeding, and intubation showed a lower bacterial diversity.[27] It is, however, likely that antibiotic use and the lack of breast milk exposure influenced GI microbiota development more than prematurity itself.

Microbiota of the Hospital Environment

Built hospital environments also have microbiota. These are complex ecosystems that are composed of all microbial life that exists indoors, and include human pathogens and commensals (colonizers) that interact with each other but also with their environment.[28] In a survey of a hospital environment using non–culture-based methods, the composition of airborne bacterial communities differed between outdoor air, mechanically ventilated rooms, and window-ventilated rooms, with highest diversity in outdoor air. The relative abundance of bacteria closely related to human pathogens was higher indoors than outdoors and was found to be higher in rooms with lower airflow rates and lower relative humidity. Architectural characteristics of a hospital—in particular, ventilation—affect the environmental microbiota.[28]

The NICU environment has been shown to have an impact on neonates' microbiota, with microorganisms identified on NICU surfaces before being found in infants' guts.[10] The most probable reservoir for GI-colonizing microbiota is tubing (e.g., nasogastric feeding tube), infants' incubators, and sinks, but healthcare workers' hands showed variable amounts of potential fecal colonizers.[11] A survey of the environment of two level-III NICUs in San Diego using culture-independent methods found species of *Enterobacter, Neisseria, Pseudomonas, Streptococcus*, and *Staphylococcus* in abundance in both NICUs,[29] emphasizing the importance of proper environmental cleaning, in particular of high-touch areas.

Gastrointestinal Microbiota in Infants, and Health Outcomes

Various factors influence infants' microbiota development, but how many of those changes actually impact infants' overall health? Several studies suggest that changes in microbiota may be associated with adverse health outcomes. In a nested case–control study of premature infants who developed late-onset sepsis, the mean gestational age of cases and controls was 27 weeks, with an average postnatal age at sepsis onset of 25 days. The authors detected a higher proportion of organisms in the *Firmicutes* phylum (i.e., *Staphylococci*) in the stools of infants with late-onset sepsis, two weeks before diagnosis. However, the authors did not find any difference in bacterial diversity at the time or near the time of sepsis onset. Bifidobacteria (anaerobes) counts were lower in cases with late-onset sepsis at all time-points, compared to controls. It was rather a distortion in the normal microbiota composition and not an enrichment of potential pathogens that seemed associated with late-onset sepsis in this patient population.[17] As for necrotizing enterocolitis (NEC), Wang et al.[16] studied 10 preterm infants with, and 10 without, NEC. The microbiota analysis revealed that patients with NEC had even less bacterial diversity than premature infants without NEC, with an increase in abundance of Gammaproteobacteria (i.e., Enterobacteriaceae), but a decrease in other bacterial species. NEC could thus be associated with a severe lack of bacterial diversity, which could allow a single dominant microorganism to take over following widespread use of antimicrobials.[16] A small case control study performed to look at the microbiota in infants with NEC did not find a difference in bacterial diversity between cases and controls at the time of NEC diagnosis. However, in the week prior to the diagnosis of NEC, the authors found an increase in Enterobacteriaceae and *S. epidermidis.*[14] Another case–control study of premature infants evaluated whether early microbial community could be predictive of later NEC. The authors reported that a lower microbial diversity in the first week of life and the absence of *Propionebacterium* were associated with NEC onset. Interestingly, in infants who developed early-onset NEC, the predominant microbial community (>98%) between days 4–9 of life was the Firmicutes (mainly *Staphylococcus* and *Enterococcus*). This predominantly Gram-positive signature was not shared by any of the infants in the control group. For later-onset NEC cases, the predominant microbial community between days 10 and 16 of life that preceded NEC onset included a Gram-negative Proteobacteria signature—specifically, Enterobacteriaceae, of which the dominant genera were *Enterobacter* and *Escherichia.*[15]

Evolution of Skin Microbiota

The composition of the microbial skin communities evolves over the first year of life, along with skin maturation.[30] This change in composition is associated with an increasing diversity with age. Early on, the main colonizing organism is coagulase-negative *Staphylococci*—this predominance is seen until infants reach four to six months of age. Moreover, the composition of the infant skin microbiota—like in adults—appears to vary by anatomical site. The cutaneous microbiota may be acquired from the environment (mother, nurses and other healthcare workers), but it is also likely to be influenced by the GI microbiota, which in turn has been shown to be impacted by systemic antimicrobial utilization, among other things.[23]

With these data in hand, infection prevention and control in the NICU should aim to decrease HAIs, while limiting the impact on neonates' microbiota, as the short-term and long-term outcomes of microbiota modifications in early life are not yet clear.

Suggested Approaches

Central Line–Associated Bloodstream Infections

The most important identified risk factor for bloodstream infections in the NICU has been the use of central venous catheters (CVC), or central lines. In the province of Quebec (Canada), mandatory year-round participation in CLABSI surveillance for all intensive care units (ICU) has been ongoing since 2007.[31,32] Although decrease in CLABSI incidence rates over time has been seen for adult ICUs and level-II/III NICUs, pooled mean rates have remained higher in the NICU: 4.20/1000 CVC-days, compared to 1.04/1000 CVC-days in adult teaching ICUs between 2007 and 2014, inclusively.[31] In the United States, the National Healthcare Safety Network (NHSN) showed that, for NICU level-III, pooled mean CLABSI rates ranged from 0.7/1000 CVC-days (birthweight >2500 g) to 2.1/1000 CVC-days (birthweight 750 g or less), compared to CLABSI rates in adult medical major teaching ICUs of 1.2/1000 CVC-days.[3]

Several reasons may explain higher NICU CLABSI rates in extremely low birthweight infants. Translocation from the neonates' immature GI tract, including *Staphylococci*, may be a source of bloodstream infections not preventable by CVC insertion and maintenance bundles.[33] Evidence for CVC insertion and maintenance bundles in these populations is less robust[2] than in adult settings, thus leading to greater heterogeneity in bundle elements for children compared to adults.[34–36] Moreover, neonates tend to have much longer CVC dwell times, emphasizing the importance of maintenance bundle adherence,[37,38] and premature infants' skin may be more likely to be damaged and a point of entry for bloodstream infections.[33] Successful strategies include incorporating elements based on facility-specific challenges, involving parents in prevention efforts, and holding regular meetings with stakeholders to discuss outcomes and directions.[39–41] Finally, if, despite compliance with the basic suggested preventive measures, CLABSI rates remain high, additional interventions are suggested, as described next.

Bundles—Basic Preventive Measures

Based on current research, the use of central line bundles is critical in the prevention of HAIs in the NICU (see Table 3.1 for insertion and maintenance bundle recommendations). Studies have shown that standardized CVC care with checklists for monitoring adherence to insertion and maintenance bundles have helped to decrease CLABSI rates in the NICU.[2,36]

CVC Insertion

The Centers for Disease Control and Prevention (CDC) recommends the use of a standardized central line insertion checklist applied by a dedicated and trained team. The catheter type should be selected before the procedure is initiated and should have the minimum number of ports and lumens necessary for care. Maximum sterile barrier precautions should be used: the infant should be covered with sterile drapes, and healthcare workers within the sterile perimeter should wear a mask, sterile gown, and sterile gloves. The skin at the insertion site should be disinfected. Although CHG has not been approved for use in infants less than two months of age,[42] experience shows that it may be used safely, leading the US Food and Drug Administration (FDA) to change the CHG (2%) and isopropyl alcohol (70%) product label to state: "Use with care in premature infants or infants under two months of age. These products may cause irritation or chemical burns." In some institutions, CHG-based products are used for all neonates requiring CVC insertion. Other centers with extremely premature infants (<28 weeks of gestational age) will use

TABLE 3.1 CVC Bundles: Insertion and Maintenance

INSERTION BUNDLE	MAINTENANCE BUNDLE
a) Establish a central line kit, cart, tray, or box before procedure.	a) Daily evaluate catheter site for signs of infection, to assess dressing integrity, and catheter necessity (removal when no longer necessary).
b) Perform proper hand hygiene before and after manipulating catheter site or inserting central line.	b) Perform proper hand hygiene before and after accessing catheter or before and after dressing change.
c) Maximal barrier precautions for providers and patients (including sterile gown, sterile gloves, surgical mask, hat, sterile drape).	c) Develop and use standardized tubing setup, kit, and items needed for dressing change (define package contents for providers).
d) Insertion training for all providers or dedicated teams, and insertion checklist to complete during/after procedure.	d) Standardized recommended catheter site care (i.e., CDC recommends gauze change every 2 days or clear dressing change every 7 days unless soiled, damp, or loose).
e) Disinfect skin with appropriate antiseptic before catheter insertion—15–60 seconds, 30–60 seconds to air dry or until fully dried.	e) Dressing change and skin disinfection when dressing is soiled, damp, or loose.
f) No iodine for skin preparation or for insertion site disinfection.	f) Maintain sterile techniques with catheter hub/cap/tubing care, access, or change (i.e., "scrub the hub").
g) Use sterile transparent semipermeable dressing or sterile gauze to cover catheter insertion site.	g) Prepackaged cap change kit/cart/ location including masks and sterile gloves (all individuals involved in dressing change are required to wear both mask and sterile gloves).

2% aqueous CHG, but will advocate that, once the skin is dried, CHG should be rinsed off the skin with sterile water to prevent burns. Table 3.2, Box 3.1, and Table 3.3 detail practices in one hospital. Guidelines recommend scrubbing the insertion site for at least 30 seconds, then allowing it to dry fully.[2,43–45] However, premature neonates' skin is fragile; therefore, vigorous scrubbing should be avoided. There are no evidence-based optimal catheter sites for CVC insertion in neonatal patients, unlike in the adult population, but the jugular and femoral veins are the most commonly used in neonates.[45]

TABLE 3.2 Product Use for Skin Disinfection Prior to CVC Insertion

BIRTHWEIGHT	GESTATIONAL AGE	CHRONOLOGICAL AGE	CHG FOR CVC INSERTION AND DRESSING CHANGE
≤1000 g	≤28 weeks	<28 days	2% aqueous CHG
≤1000 g	≤28 weeks	≥28 days	0.5% CHG in 70% alcohol
≤1000 g	29–35 weeks	≥28 days	0.5% CHG in 70% alcohol
>1000 g	29–35 weeks	All ages	0.5% CHG in 70% alcohol
>1000 g	>35 weeks	All ages	0.5% CHG in 70% alcohol

CHG: Chlorhexidine gluconate

CVC Maintenance

CVC maintenance is essential in the prevention of CLABSIs, in particular in the NICU, given the long CVC dwell time. The CDC recommends that hubs should be scrubbed with 70% alcohol/2% chlorhexidine for at least five seconds and allowed to completely air dry before the CVC is accessed.[46] Tubing-change techniques should be sterile: use sterile gloves and a mask with a sterile barrier under the central line.[44] Some centers have opted for clean tubing-change techniques, which have included gloves with sterile gauze barriers under the central line. However, clean tubing change was found to be less effective in the prevention of CLABSI than a sterile technique.[44] A recent report described a quality improvement project in NICUs: "SLUG Bug" (Standardized Line Care Under Guideline Recommendations) aimed to identify element(s) of the CVC maintenance bundle that were actually effective at reducing the incidence of CLABSIs. The bundle elements that significantly reduced CLABSI rates in the NICU were the use of sterile technique for tubing changes (defined by institution ward policy, but that included at least hand hygiene, use of sterile gloves and mask, with use of sterile barrier under the catheter), in addition with hub-care compliance monitoring (monitoring being implemented using the institution policy).[44] Sterile tubing change alone decreased CLABSI rates by 0.51/1000 CVC days on average, while adding hub-care compliance monitoring was associated with an average decrease in CLABSI rates of 1.25/1000 CVC days, for both elements together.

Dressing change is also a critical part of the maintenance bundle. The designated team should define the frequency of the dressing change, depending on the specific central line (Broviac, peripherally inserted central catheter [PICC], subclavian, jugular, femoral, etc.). Recommendations have been to change the dressing weekly or as needed, if the dressing

BOX 3.1 PROCEDURE FOR SKIN ANTISEPSIS

Instructions

Before Procedure

1. Perform skin assessment including skin maturity.
2. Depending on the characteristics of the patient and the procedure to be performed, choose the appropriate *solution* AND *product* (single-use swabs or single-use swab sticks) for skin antisepsis.
3. Disinfect skin by applying the right antiseptic solution to sufficient skin area.

   If using **2% aqueous Chlorhexidine Gluconate (CHG) solution**:

   - Apply antiseptic to the skin. Swab gently.
   - Allow to dry for 2 minutes before beginning procedure.
   - Do not blow on or wave hand over the site to speed drying.
   - After 2 minutes, remove any excess solution with a sterile gauze.
   - **For neonates <26 weeks gestation and who are <48 hours old,** after 2 minutes of exposure, *rinse the skin with sterile water* and allow to dry before applying the dressing.

   If using **0.5% CHG in 70% alcohol solution** or **2% CHG in 70% alcohol solution**:

   - Apply antiseptic to the skin.
   - Allow antiseptic to dry completely before beginning the procedure. A minimum of 30 seconds is required for these products to act.
   - Do not blow on or wave hand over the site to speed drying.
   - Take care not to allow the solution to pool under the infant or child. If a spill occurs, change the linen as soon as possible. Do not leave the infant or child lying on the wet linen.
4. Perform procedure as per pertaining protocol.

After Procedure

5. Clean the skin with water anywhere the antiseptic may have pooled. Check sheets under the neonate and change them if antiseptic solution may have spilled onto them.
6. Document procedure, including use and type of antiseptic solution, response of patient, and skin integrity pre-/post-procedure in the progress notes.

TABLE 3.3 Skin Antiseptic Products Selection

BIRTHWEIGHT AND GESTATIONAL AGE	ACTUAL AGE	CORRECTED AGE	PRODUCT
Extremely premature			
<1000 g **OR** <28 weeks	<4 weeks		**2% aqueous CHG**
<1000 g **OR** <28 weeks	≥4 weeks	<4 weeks	**0.5% CHG in 70% alcohol**
Premature			
≥1000 g **AND** ≥28 weeks	≥4 weeks	<4 weeks	**0.5% CHG in 70% alcohol**
Term newborn			
	<4 weeks		**0.5% CHG in 70% alcohol**
Age 4 weeks or more			
Extremely premature Premature		≥4 weeks (≥44 weeks post-conception)	**2% CHG in 70% alcohol**
Term	≥4 weeks		
Older child			

becomes soiled, damp, or loose. Some centers have aimed to decrease dressing changes to a minimum, especially when the transparent dressing is used to stabilize the CVC in extremely premature infants. In these particular cases, the dressing is only changed if soiled, damp, or loose, or after two to four weeks when skin has matured, or when a stabilization device has been installed.[47] The CVC insertion site should be assessed daily, with documentation of date and time of each dressing change. If signs of infection appear, the CVC should ideally be removed after discussion with the NICU team, and a root-cause analysis performed to understand how to improve practices.

Chlorhexidine Gluconate Bathing

When, despite the implementation of insertion and maintenance CVC bundles, CLABSI incidence rates remain high, CHG bathing with a CHG-impregnated cloth may be added.[48] Based on previously published studies, CHG bathing has been part of CLABSI prevention protocols in most settings outside of the NICU, as CHG-impregnated cloths are not formally approved for use in infants less than two months of age.[49] Studies that support the use of CHG bathing have shown that CHG is effective in preventing healthcare-associated infections and bloodstream infections in ICU settings. In adult ICUs, CHG bathing was associated with a 50% reduction in CLABSI rates.[50–52] In the pediatric population, a randomized controlled trial found a decrease in primary bloodstream infections in pediatric ICUs (PICUs) and a 48% reduction in CLABSI rates.[53] Similarly, CHG use in the NICU setting was shown to decrease CLABSI rates more than 65%, without adverse events.[54]

Concerns about CHG bathing include the potential for systemic absorption. CHG has been detected in the blood of some preterm and term infants after whole-body washing, mainly when specimens were procured by capillary technique, probably representing topical contamination.[55] CHG used for skin antisepsis prior to CVC placement for neonates weighing 1500 g or more, seven days of age or older, was not associated with dermatitis. In that study, of the 48 enrolled infants, seven (14.6%) had detectable CHG concentrations ranging from 13 to 100 μg/L.[56] A study of preterm neonates (median gestational age 28 2/7 weeks), who had one limb washed with a 2% CHG-impregnated cloth before PICC placement, showed that half had a detectable CHG concentration, with levels ranging from 1.6 to 206 μg/L; no infant developed dermatitis.[57] In children aged over three months, CHG blood level was detected after daily bathing in fewer than 10% of children enrolled (mean concentration 57 μg/L), with no evidence of accumulation.[58] Despite extensive use and evidence that some absorption occurs, CHG has not been associated with any documented neurological adverse event, at all blood levels reported in studies, except when instilled directly in the middle ear.[55] A survey of 44 American and 13 Canadian freestanding children's hospital done in 2012 showed that 10% of NICUs were already using CHG baths.[59] Moreover, in 2012, the FDA changed the CHG-impregnated cloth label to state that these could be "use(d) with care in premature infants or infants under two months of age."[49]

At the Montreal Children's Hospital, to limit the potential impact of CHG on the developing skin microbiota, routine CHG bathing has been implemented only for infants with a CVC. Infants with a birth weight of >1000 g are bathed with a 2% CHG-impregnated cloth, using two cloths per infant, according to the bathing schedule described in Table 3.4. Infants with a birthweight of 1000 g or less are bathed with sterile water until day 10 of life, then with a mild soap until day of life 28, after which time, 2% CHG-impregnated cloths are used, but only if a CVC is still present (Table 3.4). CHG washing every other day is probably the optimal schedule, as

TABLE 3.4 Bathing Schedule by Birthweight and Age

BIRTHWEIGHT	GESTATIONAL AGE	CHRONOLOGICAL AGE	BATHING FREQUENCY	PRODUCT USED
≤1000 g	≤28 weeks	0–10 days	Twice a week	Sterile water
≤1000 g	≤28 weeks	11–28 days	Twice a week	Mild soap
≤1000 g	≤28 weeks	≥28 days	Twice a week	CHG-impregnated cloth
≤1000 g	29–35 weeks	≥28 days	Every other day	CHG-impregnated cloth
>1000 g	29–35 weeks	All ages	Every other day	CHG-impregnated cloth
>1000 g	>35 weeks	All ages	Daily	CHG-impregnated cloth

CHG: chlorhexidine gluconate

the skin bacterial burden increases back to baseline 48 hours after a CHG bathing.[60]

Additional Interventions

Chlorhexidine-impregnated sponges (e.g. Biopatch™) placed over the catheter insertion site are used, in some settings, as an adjunctive intervention to decrease the risk of CLABSI. In the adult population, use of such sponges was shown to decrease CLABSI from 1.3 to 0.40/1000 CVC-days.[61] In a multicenter collaborative study involving 29 PICUs in the United States, chlorhexidine sponge use was *not* associated with a statistically significant decrease in CLABSI rates.[36] There are no efficacy or effectiveness data for chlorhexidine sponges in the NICU setting. The survey of American and Canadian freestanding children's hospitals revealed that 46% of NICUs were using chlorhexidine sponge, with more American than Canadian settings using chlorhexidine-based products at the CVC exit site.[59] The National Health Service (NHS) recommends that, if used, chlorhexidine sponges be restricted to neonates 27 weeks of gestational age or older who are at least seven days of age, and to avoid excessive pressure over the patch, as this can cause pressure necrosis of the skin.[62]

A recent Cochrane Database systematic review was performed to determine the effectiveness of *chlorhexidine-based dressings* in the prevention of CLABSI in the NICU. Although use of such dressings decreased catheter colonization, there was no significant difference observed in major outcomes like sepsis and CLABSI, when compared to polyurethane dressing. Chlorhexidine dressings, when coupled with alcohol skin cleansing in neonates, did, however, increase markedly the risk of contact dermatitis in preterm infants[63] and should therefore not be used. In view of new data, the CDC's Healthcare Infection Control Practices Advisory Committee (HICPAC) updated, in 2017, their 2011 recommendations on the use of CHG-impregnated dressings for the prevention of intravascular catheter-related infections. They recommended against the use of CHG-impregnated dressings to protect the site of short-term, non-tunneled CVCs for premature neonates due to risk of serious adverse skin reactions. However, due to the lack of sufficient evidence, no recommendation could be made for non-premature neonates.[64]

A recent Cochrane Database systematic review studied the use *of antimicrobial-impregnated CVCs* to prevent CLABSI in the neonatal population. Only one randomized or quasi-randomized study was identified, showing that silver zeolite-impregnated umbilical venous catheters reduced CLABSI incidence in very preterm infants by almost 90%, for a number needed to treat for benefit of 6,[65] but it highlighted the lack of studies in this population. *Antibiotic locks'* effectiveness for the prevention of CLABSI in the NICU was reviewed in a meta-analysis and was shown to decrease the incidence of confirmed CLABSI by 85%. However, the effectiveness of antibiotic locks against suspected CLABSI, all CLABSIs, and mortality, when pooled as a single composite estimate, was not statistically significant.[66] The studies included in this meta-analysis, however, used different antimicrobials for locking (vancomycin, fucidic acid, and amikacin) and none presented data on the impact of antibiotic locks on antimicrobial resistance.

Ethanol locks have been shown to decrease the incidence of CLABSI. A randomized controlled trial in pediatric oncology patients showed that using 70% ethanol locks (left for two hours, then flushed with saline, every one to six weeks) decreased by almost 50% the risk of CLABSI compared with heparin locks.[67] A meta-analysis revealed that, in pediatric patients with intestinal failure, ethanol locks decreased the risk of CLABSI by 81%.[68] No randomized controlled trial was found in the neonatal population. A systematic review of ethanol lock use (all age groups) showed that, depending on the ethanol concentration, structural changes and abnormalities in catheter integrity were noted in polyurethane catheters, with elution of polymers. It also increased the risk of thrombosis compared with heparin. Systemic side effects and transaminase elevation were also reported.[69] If transaminase elevation was seen in the older age groups, one can wonder if there is a risk of unacceptably high blood alcohol concentration if ethanol locks are used in the neonatal population. A pilot study followed blood alcohol concentration in 10 patients (mean age 3.5 months, mean weight 4.5 kg) after a one-time 0.4 ml infusion of ethanol 70%. Nine of 10 patients in the study had baseline hepatic blood work within normal limits. Eight patients had undetectable five-minute blood alcohol concentrations (the remaining two patients had an alcoholemia of 0.011%), and all 10 patients were undetectable at the one-hour concentrations.[70] There are no data on the repeated use of ethanol locks in the neonatal population.

Disinfectant caps (70% isopropyl alcohol) have been used with the objective of decreasing bacterial colonization of connectors, therefore lowering the risk of CLABSI. Although no data exist in the neonatal population, a quasi-experimental study in an trauma ICU showed that its use decreased the risk of CLABSI by approximately 40%.[71] Our NICU has used alcohol disinfectant caps, but we have not evaluated their impact on CLABSI rates.

Ventilator-Associated Pneumonia (VAP) and Ventilator-Associated Events (VAE)

NICUs in the U.S. have reported ventilator-associated pneumonia (VAP) incidence rates that vary between 0.1 and 1.0/1000 ventilator-days, depending on birthweight categories.[72] However, incidence rates of VAP are difficult to interpret and difficult to use for benchmarking, since the definition requires a lot of interpretation and is not based on quantitative measures. Moreover, given the underlying medical conditions present in neonates admitted to the NICU (e.g., respiratory distress syndrome, chronic lung disease), it is often quite difficult to differentiate an acute infection from a deterioration due to the underlying process.[73,74] Using a blind-protected catheter to avoid contamination of upper respiratory microorganisms, Spanish researchers collected bronchoalveolar lavage, using samples for quantitative cultures from patients meeting the CDC definition for VAP and requiring the isolation of $>10^3$ colony-forming unit/mL for VAP diagnosis.[75] They reported a pooled VAP incidence rate of 10.9/1000 ventilator-days, much higher than what is reported by the NHSN, with a predominance of Gram-negative organisms. The only risk factor that was associated with the development of VAP was the duration of ventilation.

To improve objectivity, reliability, and efficiency, and to allow for external comparability, the CDC modified its approach to VAP surveillance in adults to include the surveillance of all complications of mechanical ventilation. The new ventilator-associated event (VAE) framework is detailed in Chapter 2. An adaptation of the adult ventilator-associated condition (VAC) definition has been proposed for the pediatric population, replacing the PEEP/FiO_2 (positive end expiratory pressure/fraction of inspired oxygen) criterion by an increase in minimum daily FiO_2 by ≥0.25, or the mean airway pressure (MAP) by ≥4.0. Using this definition, one group showed that patients with VAC in the PICU and NICU had substantially higher mortality rates and longer duration of hospitalization, ICU stay and ventilation.[74] An adaptation of the infection-related ventilator-associated complication (IVAC) definition for children and neonates is available, as criteria used to detect an infection in adults (e.g., fever) are rarely seen in premature infants.

VAP Bundles in Neonates

Currently, guidelines for the prevention of VAE are not available; we must thus rely on guidelines that were developed for the prevention of VAP. These have been recommended to prevent VAP in preterm neonates[76] (Table 3.5): (1) Avoid intubation if possible (consider noninvasive ventilation methods such as nasal continuous positive airway pressure [CPAP]); (2) minimize the duration of mechanical ventilation (limit sedation, assess readiness to extubate daily, avoid unplanned extubation and reintubation); and (3) provide regular oral care with sterile water, minimize breaks in the ventilator circuit, and change the ventilator circuit only if it is visibly soiled or malfunctioning.

The following interventions may also be considered, but their impact on VAP is unclear: (1) lateral recumbent positioning; (2) reverse Trendelenburg positioning; (3) closed/in-line suctioning.

Given the lack of data on safety and risks and the unknown impact on VAP rates in preterm neonates, the following measures are generally not recommended: (1) regular oral care with antiseptic; (2) histamine H_2-receptor antagonists; (3) prophylactic broad-spectrum antibiotics; (3) spontaneous breathing trials.

Finally, the following are not applicable to preterm neonates: (1) daily interruption of sedation; (2) prophylactic probiotics; (3) endotracheal tubes equipped with subglottic secretion drains; (4) silver-coated endotracheal tubes.

TABLE 3.5 Recommended Interventions to Prevent VAP in Premature Neonates

RECOMMENDATIONS	RATIONALE	INTERVENTION	QUALITY OF EVIDENCE
Basic practices	May lower VAP rates, minimal risk of harm; benefits likely outweigh potential risks	Use noninvasive positive pressure ventilation	High
		Minimize duration of mechanical ventilation	High
		Assess readiness to extubate daily	Low
		Manage patients without sedation when possible	Low
		Avoid unplanned extubation	Low
		Minimize breaks in ventilator circuit	Low
		Change ventilator circuit only if visibly soiled or malfunctioning	Low
Special approaches	Unknown impact on VAP rates; risk of harm minimal; reasonable to consider implementing if rates remain elevated despite basic practices	Lateral recumbent positioning	Low
		Reverse Trendelenburg positioning	Low
		Closed/in-line suctioning systems	Low

A NICU level-II/III in Egypt evaluated the impact of their prevention bundle on VAP rates.[77] The VAP definition used was: Neonatal patients mechanically ventilated ≥48 hours with new onset and persistent abnormal chest radiograph, worsening of gas exchange (i.e., desaturation, increased oxygen requirement, or increased ventilator demand); and three or more of: temperature instability with no other recognized cause; new onset of purulent sputum, change in character of sputum, increased respiratory secretions, or increased suctioning requirement; apnea, tachypnea, nasal flaring with retraction of the chest wall or grunting; wheezing, rales, or rhonchi; cough; and bradycardia (<100 beats/min) or tachycardia (>170 beats/min).

Using the following bundle—head of bed elevation 30^0–45^0, hand hygiene practice reinforcement, sterile suctioning and handling of respiratory equipment, intubation/re-intubation and endotracheal tube suction as strictly indicated by unit protocol, changing ventilator circuit if visibly soiled or mechanically malfunctioning, proper timed mouth care with normal saline and suction of oropharyngeal secretions, daily evaluation for readiness for extubation and sedation vacation for sedated patients—the authors showed a decrease in their VAP incidence rate between the pre-intervention and the post-intervention phases (six months each) with a three-month implementation phase in between. VAP rates decreased from 36.4 to 23/1000 ventilator days (RR 0.565; 95% CI 0.408, 0.782). These incidence rates are, however, much higher than what is reported in the United States.

The following elements of a VAP bundle were put in a clinical care protocol in one NICU in the U.S. and may be a useful model[78]:

1. Hand hygiene; wear gloves when manipulating equipment potentially contaminated with oral secretions;
2. Limit potential cross-contamination of the endotracheal tube used (new sterile tube for each attempt), no contact between tube and patient environment;
3. Clear secretions from oropharynx before manipulating tube or patient, using a closed suctioning system, suctioning as needed without the use of normal saline;
4. Feed the infant to avoid gastric distension and reflux;
5. Position in the midline and lateral position while mechanically ventilating as tolerated;
6. Perform oral care starting no later than 24 hours after intubation, aiming for areas of known increased bacterial colonization, using sterile water;
7. Use a separate suction canister and tubing for oral and tracheal suction: to avoid opening a closed system, change in-line suction only when soiled or otherwise indicated; clean the reusable resuscitation bag connector with alcohol after each manipulation and keep the bag and suction catheters off the patient's bed, and stored in a separate, cleaned, non-sealed plastic bag—storage bags for oral suction catheters should be changed every 24 hours. Drain ventilator condensate away from patient every two to four hours before repositioning, and change the ventilator circuit when visibly soiled.

Catheter-Associated Urinary Tract Infections

The burden associated with catheter-associated urinary tract infections (CAUTIs) is not well defined in the neonatal population. PICUs reporting to NHSN had pooled mean rates between 1.2 and 3.4/1000 catheter-days, depending on PICU type.[72] A retrospective chart review from a level-III NICU in the U.S. revealed that 1.7% of neonates admitted to the unit had a diagnosis of UTI. However, only 65 of 137 UTIs were healthcare-associated, and there were no data about device use.[79] CAUTI is part of our surveillance program in our level-III NICU,[80] with annual incidence rates varying from 0.0 to 22.2 per 1000 catheter-days, but with very low device use—probably selecting the most at-risk neonates for urinary catheter use.

Prevention Guidelines

There are no specific guidelines for the prevention of CAUTI in the neonatal population, presumably because the burden associated with CAUTI is not documented and because urinary catheters are only rarely used in the NICU—with device utilization ratios (DUR; catheter-days/patient days) of 0.1 or lower,[80] compared with DUR of 0.2 in PICUs and up to 0.7 in adult ICUs.[72] A scoping review of international guidelines or national recommendations on infection prevention and control or HAI-prevention in neonatal and pediatric populations was recently performed. Of the 10 documents included in the final review and assessed, none addressed CAUTI prevention in the neonatal population.[81] The basic practices, as recommended by Society for Healthcare Epidemiology of America (SHEA) and Infectious Disease Society of America (IDSA), should be applied to neonates[82]: these are detailed in Chapter 2.

(A) Use appropriate technique for **catheter insertion**:

1. Insert urinary catheters only when necessary for patient care, and leave in place only as long as indications remain;
2. Consider other methods for bladder management;
3. Practice hand hygiene immediately before insertion of the catheter: also before and after any manipulation of the catheter site or apparatus;
4. Insert catheters following aseptic technique and using sterile equipment;
5. Use sterile gloves, drape, and sponges; a sterile or antiseptic solution for cleaning the urethral meatus; and a sterile single-use packet of lubricant jelly for insertion;

6. Use the smallest catheter to allow proper drainage and minimize urethral trauma.

(B) Ensure appropriate **management of indwelling catheters**:

1. Properly secure indwelling catheters after insertion to prevent movement and urethral traction;
2. Maintain a sterile, continuously closed drainage system;
3. Replace the catheter and the collecting system using aseptic technique when breaks in aseptic technique, disconnection, or leakage occur;
4. For examination of fresh urine, collect a small sample by aspirating urine from the needleless sampling port with a sterile syringe/cannula adaptor after cleansing the port with disinfectant;
5. Maintain unobstructed urine flow.

The impact of these recommendations in the NICU, however, has not been assessed.

Approach to the Clinical Scenario

There are a number of infection prevention strategies to prevent device-associated infections in the NICU that are safe and effective. Specifically, there are data supporting the effectiveness of CHG-containing products for skin asepsis upon central line insertion and CHG wipes for regular body washes to decrease the risk of CLABSIs in the neonatal ICU population. Moreover, routine use of CHG-containing products in the neonatal population born at >28 weeks of gestational age and >1000 g is well tolerated. In younger infants, aqueous CHG (without alcohol) used for CVC insertion is well tolerated. In the very young and premature, one may choose to rinse off CHG, once dried, with sterile water to prevent skin burns.

Regular body washes with CHG wipes should be kept as an additional approach if basic measures (CVC insertion and maintenance bundles) have been implemented and audited with good compliance and when CLABSI rates remain high. Given the developing infant's microbiota, and given the absorption of CHG from the skin—with no clinical evidence of harm—the precautionary principle in this vulnerable population would argue that the balance of benefits should outweigh potential and theoretical risks to support implementation of this intervention. In this particular case:

- Complications and sequelae associated with CLABSI are clear in NICU patients, and CHG bathing decreases CLABSI incidence;
- Antimicrobial treatments for CLABSI will modify infants' gut microbiota, prolong the length of NICU stay, and the need for an IV access;
- CHG bathing is also likely to modify infants' skin microbiota—the duration and impact of this is unclear;
- CHG-containing products are absorbed through the skin—but animal models and clinical surveillance have not identified any clinical harm associated with detectable levels at the levels described in neonates.

CHG bathing in the NICU should thus be reserved for infants with a CVC, old enough to tolerate CHG without skin burn risk (>28 weeks of gestation, >1000 g at birth, OR >28 days of age), and in settings where the overall CLABSI incidence is high.

Unresolved Issues

Existing recommendations to decrease device-associated HAIs in the NICU have rarely been evaluated in the neonatal population. Extrapolation from pediatric or adult preventive measures is often necessary, weighing the risks and benefits of these interventions specifically for the neonatal population, in light of their developing microbiota, and keeping the precautionary principle in mind. More studies, specific to this population, are needed, and a better understanding of the short-term and long-term impacts of modifying neonates' microbiota is crucial.

Acknowledgments

I would like to thank Gaelle DeLisle for her help with elements of the literature review.

References

1. Brodie SB, Sands KE, Gray JE, et al. Occurrence of nosocomial bloodstream infections in six neonatal intensive care units. *Pediatr Infect Dis J*. 2000;**19**(1):56–65.
2. Schulman J, Stricof R, Stevens TP, et al. Statewide NICU central-line–associated bloodstream infection rates decline after bundles and checklists. *Pediatrics*. 2011;**127**(3):436–444.

3. Hocevar SN, Edwards JR, Horan TC, Morrell GC, Iwamoto M, Lessa FC. Device-associated infections among neonatal intensive care unit patients: incidence and associated pathogens reported to the National Healthcare Safety Network, 2006–2008. *Infect Control Hosp Epidemiol.* 2012;**33**(12):1200–1206.
4. Goldmann DA, Freeman J, Durbin WA, Jr. Nosocomial infection and death in a neonatal intensive care unit. *J Infect Dis.* 1983;**147**(4):635–641.
5. Auriti C, Maccallini A, Di Liso G, Di Ciommo V, Ronchetti MP, Orzalesi M. Risk factors for nosocomial infections in a neonatal intensive-care unit. *J Hosp Infect.* 2003;**53**(1):25–30.
6. Blanchard AC, Quach C, Autmizguine J. Staphylococcal infections in infants: updates and current challenges. *Clin Perinatol.* 2015;**42**:119–132.
7. Tsai MH, Chu SM, Hsu JF, et al. Risk factors and outcomes for multidrug-resistant gram-negative bacteremia in the NICU. *Pediatrics.* 2014;**133**(2):e322–329.
8. Shah DK, Doyle LW, Anderson PJ, et al. Adverse neurodevelopment in preterm infants with postnatal sepsis or necrotizing enterocolitis is mediated by white matter abnormalities on magnetic resonance imaging at term. *J Pediatr.* 2008;**153**(2):170–175.
9. Schlapbach LJ, Aebischer M, Adams M, et al. Impact of sepsis on neurodevelopmental outcome in a Swiss national cohort of extremely premature infants. *Pediatrics.* 2011;**128**(2):e348–e357.
10. Qin J, Li R, Raes J, et al. A human gut microbial gene catalogue established by metagenomic sequencing. *Nature.* 2010;**464**(7285):59–65.
11. Brooks B, Firek BA, Miller CS, et al. Microbes in the neonatal intensive care unit resemble those found in the gut of premature infants. *Microbiome.* 2014;**2**(1):1.
12. Fanaro S, Chierici R, Guerrini P, Vigi V. Intestinal microflora in early infancy: composition and development. *Acta Paediatrica.* 2003;**91**(441):48–55.
13. Penders J, Thijs C, Vink C, et al. Factors influencing the composition of the intestinal microbiota in early infancy. *Pediatrics.* 2006;**118**(2):511–521.
14. Mai V, Young CM, Ukhanova M, et al. Fecal microbiota in premature infants prior to necrotizing enterocolitis. *PLoS ONE.* 2011;**6**(6):e20647.
15. Morrow AL, Lagomarcino AJ, Schibler KR, et al. Early microbial and metabolomic signatures predict later onset of necrotizing enterocolitis in preterm infants. *Microbiome.* 2013;**1**(1):13.
16. Wang Y, Hoenig JD, Malin KJ, et al. 16S rRNA gene-based analysis of fecal microbiota from preterm infants with and without necrotizing enterocolitis. *ISME J.* 2009;**3**(8):944–954.
17. Mai V, Torrazza RM, Ukhanova M, et al. Distortions in development of intestinal microbiota associated with late onset sepsis in preterm infants. *PLoS ONE.* 2013;**8**(1):e52876.
18. Gronlund MM, Lehtonen OP, Eerola E, Kero P. Fecal microflora in healthy infants born by different methods of delivery: permanent changes in intestinal flora after cesarean delivery. *J Pediatr Gastroenterol Nutr.* 1999;**28**(1):19–25.
19. Liu D, Yu J, Li L, et al. Bacterial community structure associated with elective cesarean section versus vaginal delivery in Chinese newborns. *J Pediatr Gastroenterol Nutr.* 2015;**60**(2):240–246.

20. Dominguez-Bello MG, Costello EK, Contreras M, et al. Delivery mode shapes the acquisition and structure of the initial microbiota across multiple body habitats in newborns. *Proc Natl Acad Sci U S A.* 2010;**107**(26):11971–11975.
21. Brown CT, Sharon I, Thomas BC, Castelle CJ, Morowitz MJ, Banfield JF. Genome resolved analysis of a premature infant gut microbial community reveals a *Varibaculum cambriense* genome and a shift towards fermentation-based metabolism during the third week of life. *Microbiome.* 2013;**1**(1):30.
22. Yoshioka H, Iseki K, Fujita K. Development and differences of intestinal flora in the neonatal period in breast-fed and bottle-fed infants. *Pediatrics.* 1983;**72**(3):317–321.
23. Greenwood C, Morrow AL, Lagomarcino AJ, et al. Early empiric antibiotic use in preterm infants is associated with lower bacterial diversity and higher relative abundance of *Enterobacter*. *J Pediatr.* 2014;**165**(1):23–29.
24. Schwiertz A, Gruhl B, Lobnitz M, Michel P, Radke M, Blaut M. Development of the intestinal bacterial composition in hospitalized preterm infants in comparison with breast-fed, full-term infants. *Pediatr Res.* 2003;**54**(3):393–399.
25. Millar MR, Linton CJ, Cade A, Glancy D, Hall M, Jalal H. Application of 16S rRNA gene PCR to study bowel flora of preterm infants with and without necrotizing enterocolitis. *J Clin Microbiol.* 1996;**34**(10):2506–2510.
26. Milisavljevic V, Garg M, Vuletic I, et al. Prospective assessment of the gastroesophageal microbiome in VLBW neonates. *BMC Pediatr.* 2013;**13**:49.
27. Gewolb IH, Schwalbe RS, Taciak VL, Harrison TS, Panigrahi P. Stool microflora in extremely low birthweight infants. *ADC Fetal & Neonatal Ed.* 1999;**80**(3): F167–F173.
28. Kembel SW, Jones E, Kline J, et al. Architectural design influences the diversity and structure of the built environment microbiome. *ISME J.* 2012;**6**(8):1469–1479.
29. Hewitt KM, Mannino FL, Gonzalez A, et al. Bacterial diversity in two neonatal intensive care units (NICUs). *PLoS ONE.* 2013;**8**(1):e54703.
30. Capone KA, Dowd SE, Stamatas GN, Nikolovski J. Diversity of the human skin microbiome early in life. *J Invest Dermatol.* 2011;**131**(10):2026–2032.
31. Li L, Fortin E, Tremblay C, Ngenda-Muadi M, Quach C, for SPIN-BACC. Central-line–associated bloodstream infections in Quebec intensive care units: results from the Provincial Healthcare-Associated Infections Surveillance Program (SPIN). *Infect Control Hosp Epidemiol.* 2016;**37**(10):1186–1194.
32. Fontela PS, Platt RW, Rocher I, et al. Surveillance Provinciale des Infections Nosocomiales (SPIN) program: implementation of a mandatory surveillance program for central line–associated bloodstream infections. *Am J Infect Control.* 2011;**39**(4):329–335.
33. Dahan M, O'Donnell S, Hebert J, et al. CLABSI risk factors in the NICU: potential for prevention: a PICNIC study. *Infect Control Hosp Epidemiol.* 2016;**37**(12):1446–1452.
34. Huskins WC. Quality improvement interventions to prevent healthcare-associated infections in neonates and children. *Curr Opin Pediatr.* 2012;**24**(1):103–112.
35. Smulders CA, van Gestel JP, Bos AP. Are central line bundles and ventilator bundles effective in critically ill neonates and children? *Intensive Care Med.* 2013;**39**(8):1352–1358.
36. Miller MR, Niedner MF, Huskins WC, et al. Reducing PICU central line–associated bloodstream infections: 3-year results. *Pediatrics.* 2011;**128**(5):e1077–1083.

37. Miller MR, Griswold M, Harris JM 2nd, et al. Decreasing PICU catheter-associated bloodstream infections: NACHRI's quality transformation efforts. *Pediatrics.* 2010;**125**(2):206–213.
38. Milstone AM, Reich NG, Advani S, et al. Catheter dwell time and CLABSIs in neonates with PICCs: a multicenter cohort study. *Pediatrics.* 2013;**132**(6):e1609–1615.
39. Fisher D, Cochran KM, Provost LP, et al. Reducing central line–associated bloodstream infections in North Carolina NICUs. *Pediatrics.* 2013;**132**(6):e1664–e1671.
40. McMullan C, Propper G, Schuhmacher C, et al. A multidisciplinary approach to reduce central line–associated bloodstream infections. *Joint Commission Journal on Quality and Patient Safety/Joint Commission Resources.* 2013;**39**(2):61–69.
41. Neill S, Haithcock S, Smith PB, et al. Sustained reduction in bloodstream infections in infants at a large tertiary care neonatal intensive care unit. *Adv Neonatal Care.* 2016;**16**(1):52–59.
42. U.S. Food and Drug Administration. Chloraprep single swabstick. 2012. Available at: http://www.accessdata.fda.gov/drugsatfda_docs/appletter/2012/020832Origs030, 021555Orig1s017ltr.pdf. Accessed November 16, 2016.
43. O'Grady NP, Alexander M, Burns LA, et al. Guidelines for the prevention of intravascular catheter-related infections. *Am J Infect Control.* 2011;**39**(4 Suppl 1): S1–S34.
44. Piazza AJ, Brozanski B, Provost L, et al. SLUG Bug: quality improvement with orchestrated testing leads to NICU CLABSI reduction. *Pediatrics.* 2016;**137**(1): e20143642.
45. The Joint Commission. Preventing central line–associated bloodstream infections: useful tools, an international perspective. 2013. Available at: http://www.jointcommission.org/CLABSIToolkit. Accessed November 2, 2018.
46. Marschall J, Mermel LA, Fakih M, et al. Strategies to prevent central line–associated bloodstream infections in acute care hospitals: 2014 update. *Infect Control Hosp Epidemiol.* 2014;**35**(7):753–771.
47. Moore D, Rodrigues R, St-Martin L, Perpete C, Quach C. Infection control guidelines for insertion and care of central venous catheters—The Montreal Children's Hospital. Montreal: McGill University Health Centre; 2013.
48. O'Grady NP, Alexander M, Burns LA, et al. Guidelines for the prevention of intravascular catheter-related infections. *Clin Infect Dis.* 2011; **52**(9):e162–e193.
49. U.S. Food and Drug Administration. 2% chlorhexidine gluconate (CHG) cloth. 2012. Available at: http://www.fda.gov/Safety/MedWatch/SafetyInformation/Safety-RelatedDrugLabelingChanges/ucm307387.htm. Accessed November 16, 2016.
50. Climo MW, Yokoe DS, Warren DK, et al. Effect of daily chlorhexidine bathing on hospital-acquired infection. *N Engl J Med.* 2013;**368**(6):533–542.
51. Montecalvo MA, McKenna D, Yarrish R, et al. Chlorhexidine bathing to reduce central venous catheter–associated bloodstream infection: impact and sustainability. *Am J Med.* 2012;**125**(5):505–511.
52. Exline MC, Ali NA, Zikri N, et al. Beyond the bundle—journey of a tertiary care medical intensive care unit to zero central line–associated bloodstream infections. *Crit Care.* 2013;**17**(2):R41.
53. Milstone AM, Elward A, Song X, et al. Daily chlorhexidine bathing to reduce bacteraemia in critically ill children: a multicentre, cluster-randomised, crossover trial. *Lancet.* 2013;**381**(9872):1099–1106.

54. Quach C, Milstone AM, Perpete C, Bonenfant M, Moore DL, Perreault T. Chlorhexidine bathing in a tertiary care neonatal intensive care unit: impact on central line–associated bloodstream infections. *Infect Control Hosp Epidemiol.* 2014;**35**(2):158–163.
55. Cowen J, Ellis SH, McAinsh J. Absorption of chlorhexidine from the intact skin of newborn infants. *Arch Dis Child.* 1979;**54**(5):379–383.
56. Garland JS, Alex CP, Uhing MR, Peterside IE, Rentz A, Harris MC. Pilot trial to compare tolerance of chlorhexidine gluconate to povidone-iodine antisepsis for central venous catheter placement in neonates. *J Perinatol.* 2009;**29**(12):808–813.
57. Chapman AK, Aucott SW, Gilmore MM, Advani S, Clarke W, Milstone AM. Absorption and tolerability of aqueous chlorhexidine gluconate used for skin antisepsis prior to catheter insertion in preterm neonates. *J Perinatol.* 2013;**33**(10):768–771.
58. Lee A, Harlan R, Breaud AR, et al. Blood concentrations of chlorhexidine in hospitalized children undergoing daily chlorhexidine bathing. *Infect Control Hosp Epidemiol.* 2011;**32**(4):395–397.
59. Klieger SB, Potter-Bynoe G, Quach C, Sandora TJ, Coffin SE. Beyond the bundle: a survey of central line–associated bloodstream infection prevention practices used in US and Canadian pediatric hospitals. *Infect Control Hosp Epidemiol.* 2013;**34**(11):1208–1210.
60. Johnson J, King A, Voskertchian A, et al. The impact of chlorhexidine gluconate bathing on skin bacterial burden of neonates admitted to the neonatal intensive care unit. ID Week 2016. New Orleans: IDSA; 2016.
61. Timsit JF, Schwebel C, Bouadma L, et al. Chlorhexidine-impregnated sponges and less frequent dressing changes for prevention of catheter-related infections in critically ill adults: a randomized controlled trial. *JAMA.* 2009;**301**(12):1231–1241.
62. National Health Service. Broviac lines for central venous access—a guide for neonatal staff. 2014. Available at: https://www.networks.nhs.uk/nhs-networks/southern-west-midlands-newborn-network/documents/Attachment%2014%20SWMNN%20Broviac%20lines%202012.pdf. Accessed November 16, 2016.
63. Lai NM, Lai NA, O'Riordan E, Chaiyakunapruk N, Taylor JE, Tan K. Skin antisepsis for reducing central venous catheter-related infections. *Cochrane Database Syst Rev.* 2016;**7**:CD010140.
64. Centers for Disease Control and Prevention. Updated recommendations on the use of chlorhexidine-impregnated dressings for prevention of intravascular catheter-related infections (2017). 2017. Available at: https://www.cdc.gov/infectioncontrol/guidelines/bsi/c-i-dressings/recommendations.html. Accessed April 5, 2018.
65. Balain M, Oddie SJ, McGuire W. Antimicrobial-impregnated central venous catheters for prevention of catheter-related bloodstream infection in newborn infants. *Cochrane Database Syst Rev.* 2015;(9):CD011078.
66. Taylor JE, Tan K, Lai NM, McDonald SJ. Antibiotic lock for the prevention of catheter-related infection in neonates. *Cochrane Database Syst Rev.* 2015;(6):CD010336.
67. Schoot RA, van Ommen CH, Stijnen T, et al. Prevention of central venous catheter–associated bloodstream infections in paediatric oncology patients using 70% ethanol locks: a randomised controlled multi-centre trial. *Eur J Cancer.* 2015;**51**(14):2031–2038.

68. Oliveira C, Nasr A, Brindle M, Wales PW. Ethanol locks to prevent catheter-related bloodstream infections in parenteral nutrition: a meta-analysis. *Pediatrics.* 2012;**129**(2):318–329.
69. Mermel LA, Alang N. Adverse effects associated with ethanol catheter lock solutions: a systematic review. *J Antimicrob Chemother.* 2014;**69**(10):2611–2619.
70. Chhim RF, Crill CM, Collier HK, et al. Ethanol lock therapy: a pilot infusion study in infants. *Ann Pharmacother.* 2015;**49**(4):431–436.
71. Merrill KC, Sumner S, Linford L, Taylor C, Macintosh C. Impact of universal disinfectant cap implementation on central line–associated bloodstream infections. *Am J Infect Control.* 2014;**42**(12):1274–1277.
72. Dudeck MA, Edwards JR, Allen-Bridson K, et al. National Healthcare Safety Network report, data summary for 2013, device-associated module. *Am J Infect Control.* 2015;**43**(3):206–221.
73. Foglia E, Meier MD, Elward A. Ventilator-associated pneumonia in neonatal and pediatric intensive care unit patients. *Clin Microbiol Rev.* 2007;**20**(3):409–425, Table of Contents.
74. Cocoros NM, Kleinman K, Priebe GP, et al. Ventilator-associated events in neonates and children—a new paradigm. *Crit Care Med.* 2016;**44**(1):14–22.
75. Cernada M, Aguar M, Brugada M, et al. Ventilator-associated pneumonia in newborn infants diagnosed with an invasive bronchoalveolar lavage technique: a prospective observational study. *Pediatr Crit Care Med.* 2013;**14**(1):55–61.
76. Klompas M, Branson R, Eichenwald EC, et al. Strategies to prevent ventilator-associated pneumonia in acute care hospitals: 2014 update. *Infect Control Hosp Epidemiol.* 2014;**35**(8):915–936.
77. Azab SF, Sherbiny HS, Saleh SH, et al. Reducing ventilator-associated pneumonia in neonatal intensive care unit using "VAP prevention bundle": a cohort study. *BMC Infect Dis.* 2015;**15**:314.
78. Weber CD. Applying adult ventilator-associated pneumonia bundle evidence to the ventilated neonate. *Adv Neonatal Care.* 2016;**16**(3):178–190.
79. Weems MF, Wei D, Ramanathan R, Barton L, Vachon L, Sardesai S. Urinary tract infections in a neonatal intensive care unit. *Am J Perinatol.* 2015;**32**(7):695–702.
80. Quach C, Moore D, Gonzales M, Perpete C, Lafond M. The Montreal Children's Hospital Infection Control Service annual report (2015–2016). Montreal: McGill University, 2016.
81. Araujo da Silva AR, Zingg W, Dramowski A, Bielicki JA, Sharland M. Most international guidelines on prevention of healthcare-associated infection lack comprehensive recommendations for neonates and children. *J Hosp Infect.* 2016;**94**(2):159–162.
82. Lo E, Nicolle LE, Coffin SE, et al. Strategies to prevent catheter-associated urinary tract infections in acute care hospitals: 2014 update. *Infect Control Hosp Epidemiol.* 2014;**35**(5):464–479.

4 | Surgical Site Infections

AQSA SHAKOOR, WILLIAM MIDDLESWORTH, AND LISA SAIMAN

Background

Burden of surgical site infections

Surgical site infections (SSIs) not only increase morbidity and health-care costs, they also impose emotional and physical burdens on patients and families. There is a scarcity of consensus among physicians and institutions for SSI prevention guidelines for children. This chapter will address existing SSI prevention strategies for the pediatric population following general surgery, spine surgery for scoliosis, neurosurgical ventricular shunts, and cardiovascular surgery, and will examine knowledge gaps and unresolved issues.

The SSI risk for patients undergoing a general surgical procedure is specific to the type of surgery, degree of contamination of the operative field, and underlying patient risk factors (both modifiable and non-modifiable), which will be discussed in more detail in the following sections. In a matched cohort study of pediatric patients with and without an SSI following various surgical procedures, those with an SSI had an increased average length of stay of 10.6 days and an associated $27,288 increase in cost.[1]

The prevalence of SSIs after spine surgery is dependent on the etiology of scoliosis. Patients with non-idiopathic scoliosis have a significantly higher rate of SSIs than those with idiopathic scoliosis (6.3–13.1% vs. 0.5–2.6%, respectively).[2–5] An SSI after spine surgery often requires multiple reoperations, readmissions, and/or longer hospital stays.[2,6] The resultant financial burden is considerable, with estimates ranging from $26,977 to $961,722.[7]

The risk of SSI following initial neurosurgical ventricular shunt placement is significantly lower than that associated with revisions and repeat procedures: 4.1–20.5% vs. 14.6–51.7%, respectively.[8–14] Overall, the risk of infection was shown to be highest in the first eight weeks after a shunt procedure, and the risk decreased substantially after six months.[15] The risk of shunt failure increases by approximately 24% with each subsequent shunt replacement, resulting in a rising cumulative risk of SSI.[10]

SSI rates after pediatric cardiac surgery range from 2.6% to 6.3%.[16–18] SSIs in this population result in prolonged antibiotic use, reoperations, longer hospital and intensive care unit (ICU) stays, longer duration of mechanical ventilation, and increased inotropic support.[19] The financial cost of mediastinal SSIs is not well documented in children, but in adults, costs associated with mediastinitis are estimated to be as high as $299,237 per patient.[20]

Case definitions for surgical site infections

Clear case definitions are essential for effective surveillance and quality improvement initiatives for SSIs. The Centers for Disease Control and Prevention (CDC) National Healthcare Surveillance Network (NHSN) has established case definitions for SSIs (Table 4.1).[21] Mandatory reporting of SSIs, primarily in adults, is based on these definitions. However, mandatory reporting of SSIs in the pediatric population is not currently widespread, and NHSN definitions have not taken pediatric-specific issues into account. As discussed in this chapter, it is likely that the current case definitions do not fully capture the burden of SSIs following scoliosis repair or cardiac surgery. However, the current NHSN case definition for ventriculoperitoneal (VP) shunt infections does include the spectrum of infections such as wound incision infections, osteomyelitis, intra-abdominal infections, as well as meningitis and ventriculitis.[21] Similarly, the Hydrocephalus Clinical Research Network (HCRN) also has a relatively expanded spectrum of potential infectious complications that include: (1) identification of organisms (culture or Gram stain) from cerebrospinal fluid (CSF), wound swab, or pseudocyst fluid; (2) shunt erosion (wound breakdown with visible shunt hardware); (3) abdominal

TABLE 4.1 CDC National Healthcare Surveillance Network Surgical Site Infection Case Definitions

TYPE OF SSI *Timing* **LOCATION**	CRITERIA
Superficial Infection *Within 30 days of procedure* **Involves only skin and subcutaneous incision tissue**	At least one of following: a. Purulent drainage from superficial incision. b. Organisms isolated from aseptically obtained fluid or tissue from superficial incision. c. Superficial incision deliberately opened by surgeon or designee (culture results not part of this criterion); AND At least one of following: a. Pain or tenderness, b. Localized swelling, c. Redness, d. Heat (culture-negative specimen does not meet this criterion); OR Superficial incisional SSI diagnosed by surgeon or designee.
Deep Infection *Within 90 days of procedure* **Involves deep soft tissues (e.g., fascial and muscle layers) of incision**	At least one of following: a. Purulent drainage from deep incision, b. Deep incision spontaneously dehisces or deliberately opened by surgeon or designee (culture-positive or not cultured), AND At least one of following: a. Fever (>38°C), b. Localized pain or tenderness (culture-negative specimen does not meet this criterion), c. Abscess or other evidence of infection involving deep incision noted on direct exam, during invasive procedure, imaging test, or histopathology.
Organ/Space Infection *Within 90 days of procedure* **Involves any part of body opened or manipulated during procedure**	At least one of following: a. Purulent drainage from drain placed in organ/space, b. Organisms isolated from aseptically obtained fluid or tissue in organ/space, c. Abscess or other evidence of infection involving organ/space noted on direct exam, during invasive procedure, imaging test or histopathology; AND Meets at least one criterion for specific organ/space infection site (see http://www.cdc.gov/nhsn/PDFs/pscManual/17pscNosInfDef_current.pdf).

pseudocyst (with or without positive culture); or (4) positive blood cultures in patient with a ventriculoatrial shunt.[22]

Pathogenesis of surgical site infections

SSIs are the result of cumulative insults to the surgical field. The first insult is tissue damage, whether from sharp dissection such as incision, mechanical pressure from retractors, or ischemic injury from disruption of vascular supply. Tissue disruption causes inflammation, thrombosis, and/or tissue hypoxia. Second, microbial contamination of the operative field can establish infection of the vulnerable incision site or the tissues. Endogenous sources of contamination include colonizing flora from the patient's skin, mucous membranes, or viscera. Exogenous sources of contamination include the contaminated environment, staff, air or surgical instruments, as well as distal sources such as hematogenous infections that may subsequently infect the wound.[23] Microbial contamination is usually from bacteria, but it can also be from yeast or mold. Contamination with $>10^5$ microorganisms per gram of tissue in the surgical field is associated with a significant increase in SSIs.[24] Furthermore, the quantity of bacteria necessary to produce an SSI is much lower (e.g., 10^2 staphylococci per gram of tissue) in the presence of foreign material, such as on silk sutures.[25,26] Third, the extent of tissue disruption also correlates with the SSI rate.[23] Following elective, primary closure of an incision, without transection of mucous membranes (so-called clean surgical procedures), the SSI rate is ~2%. Following urgent or emergency surgical procedures of the gastrointestinal tract, respiratory tract, or biliary tract (so-called clean-contaminated procedures), the SSI rate is <10%. The SSI rate increases to 20% or higher for emergency surgical procedures complicated by contamination from perforated organs or penetrating trauma.[27,28]

In addition to the risks associated with tissue disruption, there are also preoperative, intraoperative, and postoperative risk factors for SSIs (Table 4.2). These can be further classified as non-modifiable (e.g., patient age or etiology of the disease process) or modifiable (e.g., surgeon's skill or skin disinfection), as described in Table 4.3. Modifiable risk factors are potentially amenable to SSI-preventive strategies as described herein for different surgical subspecialties. Additional risk factors specific to general surgery, spine surgery for scoliosis, neurosurgical ventricular shunts, and cardiovascular surgery are discussed following each case presentation in this chapter.

TABLE 4.2 Examples of Pre-, Intra-, and Postoperative Risk Factors for Surgical Site Infections

TIMING	HOST FACTORS	OR ENVIRONMENT	MICROBIAL FACTORS
Preoperative	Malnutrition Obesity Fecal or urinary incontinence Prior surgeries	Proper disinfection and sterilization of instruments, implants, and equipment Proper hand hygiene Maintenance of sterile field OR traffic	Colonizing flora; e.g., MRSA Presence of underlying infection (e.g., urinary tract infection, meningitis, infected prostheses)
Intraoperative	Blood loss/ Transfusion Requirements Hypothermia	Surgeon skill Length of procedure Maintenance sterile field Maintenance of temperature and humidity levels in OR OR traffic	Microbial contamination from entry into GI, respiratory, or biliary tracts
Post-operative	Prolonged immobility Hematoma/ seroma around surgical site Fecal or urinary incontinence	N/A	Presence of open cavity (e.g., chest or abdomen) Disruption of sterile dressing

Overview of SSI-reduction efforts

In the late 1980s, the Department of Veterans Affairs (VA) came under scrutiny for high postoperative mortality rates. This led to Public Law 99-166, mandating VA hospitals to report surgical outcomes annually while also promoting the development of databases documenting preoperative risks and postoperative outcomes. As a result of these efforts, the VA hospitals had a 47% decrease in postoperative mortality and 43% decrease in morbidity from 1991 to 2006.[29] The National Surgical Quality Improvement Program (NSQIP), started in 1994, instituted quality improvement initiatives aimed to reduce the rate of SSIs in the adult patient population. Initiatives for children, however, have not been as well coordinated.

SSI reduction has been accomplished through the implementation of bundle strategies, which are a group of evidence-based preventative interventions implemented together to provide maximal benefit. The evidence for bundle strategies has primarily been derived from adult patient populations. Elements of a perioperative bundle include the use of

TABLE 4.3 Examples of Potentially Modifiable and Non-Modifiable Risk Factors for Surgical Site Infections

TYPE OF SURGERY	MODIFIABLE RISK FACTORS	NON-MODIFIABLE RISK FACTORS
General Surgery	Maintenance of sterile field Institutional volume of cases Maintenance of core body temperature Optimal antibiotic prophylaxis	Malnutrition* Obesity* Co-morbidities Colonizing flora; e.g., MRSA*
Spine Surgery	Use of allograft bone Number of spinal levels fused	Non-idiopathic scoliosis Non-ambulatory status Functional status of patient Colonizing flora; e.g., MRSA*
Neuroventriculo-peritoneal Shunt	Postoperative CSF leak Seroma/hematoma around shunt tract Duration of surgery >90 minutes	Age/prematurity Gastrostomy tube Meningitis or intraventricular hemorrhage
Cardiac Surgery	Intraoperative hypothermia Delayed sternal closure Duration postoperative antibiotics Postoperative bleeding	Cardiopulmonary bypass Exposure to blood products

*Could be modified for elective surgery.

clippers rather than razors, skin disinfection with chlorhexidine gluconate (CHG) prior to incision, and appropriate selection, timing, and duration of perioperative antibiotics.

Recently, success with pediatric-specific prevention bundles (derived from data obtained in adult patients) has been reported.[30,31] These efforts focus on Class 1 (clean wound) and Class 2 (clean-contaminated wound) rather than Class 3 (contaminated wound) or Class 4 (dirty-infected wound).[32] For example, Solutions for Patient Safety—a national network composed of over 100 children's hospitals aimed at patient safety initiatives, advocates no razors, preoperative CHG bathing, and delivering preoperative antibiotics within 60 minutes of incision.[33] Nonetheless, implementation challenges and knowledge gaps remain and will be described here, using illustrative cases.

Clinical Scenario 1: General Surgery

A 10-week old female, born at 32 weeks' gestation with birthweight of 1450 grams, developed necrotizing enterocolitis (NEC) requiring laparotomy. Ten centimeters of terminal ileum were resected and a diverting enterostomy with mucous fistula was created. Her postoperative course was uneventful. She is now postoperative day 3 from ileostomy reversal and has become febrile to 38.9°C. Her exam is notable for erythema around the previous ostomy site and there is concern for an SSI.

Questions

What are the common pathogens associated with SSIs following general surgical procedures? What risk factors contributed to the infection? What are the challenges in addressing the risk factors? What evidence-based prevention measures and bundles are available for pediatric patients undergoing general surgery?

Key Challenges

There are a specific challenges associated with the prevention of SSIs following general surgical procedures.

Pathogens Causing Surgical Site Infections following General Surgical Procedures

To optimize perioperative antibiotic prophylaxis, it is essential to assess trends in the microorganisms causing SSIs and their susceptibility patterns. These trends may be different in children with prolonged hospitalizations prior to surgery or who are immunocompromised.

As described before, endogenous flora from a patient's own skin, mucous membranes, or hollow viscera are the most common sources of pathogens for SSIs. Following general surgical procedures, SSIs result from exposure of the wound to the flora of specific body sites. The endogenous flora of skin and mucous membranes are predominantly aerobic Gram-positive cocci (e.g., *Staphylococcus aureus* and coagulase-negative staphylococci). In contrast, the endogenous flora of the gastrointestinal tract consist of Gram-negative bacilli (e.g., *Escherichia coli*), Gram-positive cocci (e.g., enterococcal spp.), and anaerobes (e.g., *Bacillus fragilis*). The flora of the biliary tract, perineum, or groin consist of Gram-negative bacilli and anaerobic bacteria. While yeast and molds are rarely associated with SSIs, these have been identified in immunocompromised patients.[34,35] Additionally, the surgical team or operating room environment can be sources of exogenous flora, most commonly Gram-positive cocci (e.g., staphylococci and streptococci).

Risk factors Contributing to SSIs Following General Surgery

Malnutrition, obesity, or multiple comorbidities such as hepatic or renal insufficiency, and bowel or urinary incontinence, are risk factors for SSI following general surgery as well as subspecialty surgical procedures. Additional risk factors include transfusions of packed red blood cells (pRBC), which can have immunomodulatory effects, such as decreasing helper-to-suppressor T-lymphocyte ratios, defective antigen presentation, decreasing natural killer cell function, and reducing cell-mediated immunity.[36] The rate of SSI has been shown to double in patients requiring a transfusion. While patients requiring transfusions commonly have a higher percentage of contaminated or dirty/infected wounds, higher American Society of Anesthesiology (ASA) scores, and a higher percentage of emergency cases, perioperative transfusion remains an independent risk factor for SSI after controlling for these variables.[37] Furthermore, the volume of transfused pRBC correlated directly with risk of SSI and 30-day mortality.[38]

The risk of SSIs is also related to birthweight, and published incidence rates probably underestimate the true burden of SSIs in the neonatal population. While 36% of infants in the neonatal ICU (NICU) undergoing surgical procedures are very low birthweight (VLBW) infants weighing <1500 grams at birth,[39] studies of SSIs typically exclude VLBW infants or include very few VLBW infants in their analysis.[40,41] Hence, the incidence of SSIs in the NICU population may be systematically underestimated, which may restrict our ability to determine risk factors for SSIs in this unique population.

Accuracy of Risk Stratification for SSIs

Traditional risk stratification according to wound class, developed for adult patients, may not adequately risk-adjust for the pediatric population. In support of that, the Pediatric National Surgical Quality Improvement Project (NSQIP-P) database retrospectively studied 10,424 surgical procedures to stratify the SSI risk following general surgical procedures in children.[42] Cases were categorized as clean (e.g., pyloromyotomy), clean/contaminated (e.g., ostomy reversal or cholecystectomy for biliary dyskinesia), contaminated (e.g., cholecystectomy for cholecystitis or appendectomy for non-perforated appendicitis [NPA]), and dirty (e.g., appendectomy for perforated appendicitis). The SSI rate was higher (6.9%) following ostomy reversal (categorized as clean/contaminated) than the SSI rate (2.1%) following appendectomy for NPA (categorized as contaminated). Additionally, the SSI rate following appendectomy for perforated appendicitis (categorized as contaminated) was only 9.9% compared to the SSI rate of >20% following contaminated surgical procedures in the adult population. These observations highlight the limitations of the current wound classification for risk stratification for SSIs in children. Thus, large, multicenter studies, particularly in the era of bundle strategies to prevent SSIs, should be performed to better estimate the SSI risk following specific types of surgery in children.

Appropriate Perioperative Prophylaxis

The Clinical Guidelines for Antimicrobial Prophylaxis in Surgery are standardized perioperative antimicrobial prophylaxis guidelines for adults and children.[43] However, most recommendations for children represent expert opinion or are extrapolated from data in adult populations. This highlights the need for research aimed to optimize perioperative prophylaxis for children, especially for high-risk populations like neonates.

Suboptimal timing or incorrect dosing of preoperative antibiotics are risk factors for SSIs. In a retrospective study of 5,023 pediatric patients undergoing general, cardiac, or spine surgery, inappropriate timing, defined as administering the antibiotic more than one hour prior to surgical incision or following incision, or administration of an inadequate dose, defined as a dose below the recommended dose per kilogram, were independent risk factors for SSIs.[44] Children for whom antibiotics were administered incorrectly had a 1.7-fold increased risk of SSI compared with children who received antibiotics within the recommended guidelines.

Chlorhexidine Gluconate vs. Povidone Iodine vs. Alcohol as Skin Disinfection

CHG is a water-soluble, cationic biguanide that binds to the negatively charged bacterial cell wall, altering the bacterial cell osmotic equilibrium.[45] It is prepared in concentrations of 0.25%, 0.5%, 1%, 2%, and 4% in aqueous or alcohol media.[46] At low concentrations, CHG affects membrane integrity, and at high concentrations, CHG results in cell death secondary to precipitation of cytoplasmic contents.[47] Povidone iodine (PI) functions as an electron end acceptor, thereby reducing the microorganisms' ability to generate adenosine triphosphate (ATP),[48] impairing protein synthesis and altering cell membrane structure.[46] CHG achieves a greater reduction in the density of skin flora and has longer residual activity than PI.[49,50]

There has been substantial debate regarding the relative efficacy of CHG vs. PI as preoperative skin disinfection for reducing SSIs. A Cochrane review, published in 2015, analyzed randomized controlled trials comparing the efficacy of various preoperative skin disinfectants in adult patients undergoing clean surgical procedures.[51] Among the five studies that compared iodine-containing products with CHG-containing products, only one study demonstrated superiority of 0.5% CHG in reducing risk of SSIs. This was the third Cochrane review on this topic failing to demonstrate superiority of CHG as a preoperative skin disinfection. Recently, the CDC Healthcare Infection Control Practices Advisory Committee (HICPAC) guidelines recommended that skin preparation in the operating room be performed using an alcohol-based agent.[52]

The SSI bundle advocated by Solutions for Patient Safety does include preoperative bathing (the night before and/or day of surgery) with a CHG-containing products (wipes or soap), or plain soap and water. Randomized controlled trials that compared CHG baths with soap or placebo did not find that CHG baths reduced SSIs.[53] It is feasible that certain populations might benefit more from CHG bathing; for example, patients with urinary and/or fecal incontinence, as they are more likely to have higher concentrations of pathogenic flora on their skin.

Suggested Approaches and Approach to the Clinical Scenario

As part of the preoperative discussion regarding surgical options, the benefits and risks (including SSIs) are explained to the parents of the infant described in this case vignette. She is at a higher risk of developing an SSI given her immunological vulnerabilities, the presence of comorbidities such as prematurity and fragile skin, and potential colonization with multidrug-resistant pathogens due to her relatively prolonged hospitalization. Despite parenteral nutrition, she could also be malnourished. While the immunomodulatory implications of pRBC transfusions have not been delineated for SSIs in neonates, it is feasible that this effect would be additive with the physiologically immunosuppressed state of this neonate. Furthermore, abdominal surgery and multiple surgical procedures, as in the case of our patient, are associated with increased rates of SSIs in the NICU population.[54]

As previously described, the NSQIP-P risk classification for a clean-contaminated surgery, such as an ostomy reversal, underestimates the SSI risk in the pediatric population.[42] The pediatric surgical risk calculator described later in this chapter calculated that she had a slightly higher than average risk of developing an SSI (5.6% vs. 4.2%).

Using SSI Prevention Bundles

The Cincinnati Children's Hospital Medical Center (CCHMC) developed an interdisciplinary protocol to prevent SSIs in Class 1 (clean) and Class 2 (clean/contaminated) surgical wounds, as shown in Handout 4.1.[55] This protocol focuses on ensuring adequate perioperative skin preparation, perioperative antibiotic administration (including re-dosing for prolonged cases), as well as intra- and postoperative temperature control. Implementation of this protocol was associated with a decrease in SSIs by 64%: from 1.5 to 0.54 per 100 surgical procedures. Increasing compliance with the protocol and SSI reductions occurred for both same-day and inpatient surgery.

Calculating SSI Risk

The American College of Surgeons National Surgical Quality Improvement Program-Pediatric (ACS-NSQIP-P) developed a pediatric surgical risk calculator to estimate patient-specific probability of postoperative adverse events using data from 181,353 cases performed at 67 hospitals, including 382 Current Procedural Terminology (CPT) codes representing all surgical subspecialties.[56] The user can enter 18 preoperative variables, including demographic characteristics, comorbid conditions, and surgical procedures, into the risk calculator, and a logistical regression model is used to calculate risk of adverse outcomes. These outcomes include mortality, composite morbidity (any defined morbidity), SSI, venous thromboembolism, reintubation, cardiac events, pneumonia, renal insufficiency/failure, and urinary tract infection. Kraemer et al. demonstrated excellent discrimination for morbidity, mortality, and other complication parameters collected by the risk calculator.[56]

Unresolved Issues

Because of limited evidence in children, there is a lack of consenus around some strategies for the prevention of SSIs after following general surgical procedures.

HANDOUT 4.1 Cincinnati Children's Hospital Medical Center Surgical Site Infection Bundle for General Surgery

OR Room #: ______________

Date of Surgery: ______________

Surgeon: ______________

Anesthesiologist: ______________

Patient Sticker

1. Antibiotic Administered <60 mins prior to incision	Yes	No	Comment		
2. Prep — CHG Wash	At Home	In Patient	Not Done	N/A	
OR Prep Used	Chloraprep	Duraprep	Alcohol	Betadine Scrub or Prep	Other
3. Method of Hair Removal	Not needed	Clippers	Disposable Razor		
4. OR Temp on Patient Arrival (goal 75°F)	°F		Comment		
5. Patient Temperature	SDS or IP (°C)	Temp on incision (°C)	Temp on Arrival to PACU/ICU (°C)		
6. Oxygen Administration @ 60% FiO2 per Protocol — OR @ 60% FiO2 intra-op	Yes	No	Comment		
Oxygen post-operative	O2 in PACU (L/min)	O2 4 hrs Post-op (L/min)	O2 in PACU/ICU (L/min)		

Appropriate antimicrobial prophylaxis

Based on our hospital's perioperative antibiotic protocol shown in Table 4.4, this infant received a preoperative dose of ampicillin-sulbactam (50 mg/kg), which was continued for 24 hours after surgery. This prophylaxis will have activity against most Gram-positive organisms, Gram-negative bacilli, and anaerobes. Given her prolonged hospitalization, however, it is possible that her skin and gastrointestinal (GI) tract flora have developed resistance to ampicillin-sulbactam.

TABLE 4.4 New York-Presbyterian Morgan Stanley Children's Hospital High-Risk General Surgery Antimicrobial Prophylaxis

SURGERY TYPE	PRIMARY ANTIBIOTIC PROPHYLAXIS (AGENT AND DOSE)	ALTERNATIVE (E.G., PENICILLIN ALLERGY)	POSTOPERATIVE DURATION
Appendectomy, complicated	Piperacillin + tazobactam (100 mg/kg/dose, max 4.5 g)	Ciprofloxacin (10 mg/kg/dose, max 400 mg) *AND* Metronidazole (7.6 mg/kg/dose, max 500 mg)	Up to 2 weeks
Appendectomy, uncomplicated	Ampicillin + sulbactam (50 mg/kg/dose, max 3.375 g)	Ciprofloxacin (10 mg/kg/dose, max 400 mg) *AND* Metronidazole (7.6 mg/kg/dose, max 500 mg)	24 hours
Esophageal	Ampicillin + sulbactam (50 mg/kg/dose, max 3.375 g)	Clindamycin (10 mg/kg/dose, max 900 mg) *AND* Gentamicin (2.5 mg/kg/dose, no max)	24 hours
Gastric	Cefazolin (30 mg/kg/dose, max 2 g)	Vancomycin (15 mg/kg/dose, max 1000 mg) *OR* Clindamycin (10 mg/kg/dose, max 900 mg)	1 dose 6–8 hours after last intraoperative dose

(continued)

TABLE 4.4 Continued

SURGERY TYPE	PRIMARY ANTIBIOTIC PROPHYLAXIS (AGENT AND DOSE)	ALTERNATIVE (E.G., PENICILLIN ALLERGY)	POSTOPERATIVE DURATION
Gastrointestinal or biliary	Ampicillin + sulbactam (50 mg/kg/dose, max 3.375 g)	Clindamycin (10 mg/kg/dose, max 900 mg) *AND* Gentamicin (2.5 mg/kg/dose)	24 hours
Genitourinary	Cefazolin (30 mg/kg/ dose, max 2 g)	Clindamycin (10 mg/kg/dose, max 900 mg) *AND* Gentamicin (2.5 mg/kg/dose)	1 post-op dose within 24 hours of surgery end time
Gynecological	Cefazolin (30 mg/kg/ dose, max 2 g)	Clindamycin (10 mg/kg/dose, max 900 mg) *AND* Gentamicin (2.5 mg/kg/dose)	1 post-op dose within 24 hours of surgery end time
Skin and Soft Tissue	Cefazolin (30 mg/kg/ dose, max 2 g)	Vancomycin (15 mg/kg/dose, max 1000 mg) *OR* Clindamycin (10 mg/kg/dose, max 900 mg)	None
Thoracic	Cefazolin (30 mg/kg/ dose, max 2 g)	Vancomycin (15 mg/kg/dose, max 1000 mg) *OR* Clindamycin (10 mg/kg/dose, max 900 mg)	24 hours
Vascular	Cefazolin (30 mg/kg/ dose, max 2 g)	Clindamycin (10 mg/kg/dose, max 900 mg)	None

Chlorhexidine Gluconate in Neonates

While skin antisepsis with CHG is used widely in adults and children two months of age and older, there are no specific guidelines for infants less than two months of age.[57] The U.S. Food and Drug Administration (FDA) states that CHG should be used with care in premature infants or infants under two months of age as these products may cause irritation or chemical burns in these patients.

Topical CHG absorption has been described in preterm infants with measurable serum CHG concentrations (1.6–206 ng/ml amounts) observed, with the highest concentrations detected two to three days following exposure.[58] Neurotoxicity is a theoretical concern, as CHG has been shown to inhibit L1 cell adhesion–mediated neurite growth of cerebellar granule neurons in *in vitro* models.[47] The clinical significance of this observation is unknown.

Case 2: Spine Surgery for Scoliosis Repair

A 12-year-old girl with cerebral palsy and spastic quadriplegia underwent an uneventful posterior spinal fusion from T6 to L3 one month ago. She now presents to the Emergency Department with pain, fever, and purulent drainage from incision site.

Questions

What are the common pathogens associated with spinal fusion infections? What factors may have contributed to the infection? What evidence-based prevention measures and bundles are available for pediatric patients undergoing spine surgery?

Key Challenges

There are specific challenges associated with the prevention of SSIs after spinal fusion procedures.

Common Pathogens associated with Spinal Fusion Infections

SSI in patients with *idiopathic* scoliosis are caused by Gram-positive skin flora such as staphylococci and *Propionibacterium acnes*.[3,59] Additional pathogens are recovered in *non-idiopathic* scoliosis patients, including Gram-positive skin flora, Gram-negative bacilli, and enterococci organisms, as well as polymicrobial infections.[3,4,6] This suggests that the skin of these patients has a higher degree of skin colonization with GI flora and genitourinary pathogens, thereby increasing the risk of SSIs from these potentially more virulent flora.

Risk Factors for SSIs following Scoliosis Surgery

As mentioned before, patients with non-idiopathic scoliosis are at a higher risk of SSIs than those with idiopathic scoliosis.[5] Among patients with non-idiopathic scoliosis, ASA score ≥ 2, non-ambulatory status, urinary or bowel incontinence, and higher degree of cognitive impairment are associated with an increased SSI risk.[2,6,60,61] Children with non-idiopathic scoliosis who also have myelomeningocele and cerebral palsy had higher rates of SSIs when compared to children with non-idiopathic scoliosis associated with other etiologies. While malnutrition is not consistently defined in the orthopedic literature, several proxy measures for poor nutritional status such as body mass index, albumin, and lymphocyte counts have been associated with SSIs.[61,62] Hypothermia, intraoperative blood loss, and blood transfusion have also been implicated as risk factors, although definitive studies are lacking in this population.[61]

Impact of Number of Spinal Levels Fused

Fusion of more than 10 levels is a risk factor for a deep SSI following scoliosis surgery.[61,63] This was corroborated in a retrospective study that demonstrates that longer fusions were associated with readmissions and repeat operations.[64] It is likely that confounding variables exist, which include fecal incontinence, malnutrition, or non-ambulatory status in the patients requiring a higher number of spinal fusions, placing them at higher risk of infections.

Suggested Approaches and Approach to the Clinical Scenario

Non-modifiable risk factors in this patient that increase her risk of a SSI include cerebral palsy, non-ambulatory status, and fecal incontinence. The use of institutional perioperative prophylaxis, guided by local resistance patterns, preoperative CHG bathing, and using a preoperative checklist may reduce her risk.

We provide examples of perioperative antimicrobial prophylaxis strategies and checklists used to reduce SSIs among children undergoing scoliosis repair in Tables 4.5 and 4.6 and Handout 4.2. Input from institutional infectious disease and pharmacy specialists is essential in order to construct perioperative protocols that incorporate local epidemiological trends.

Implementing Standardized Perioperative Antibiotic Regimens

Institution #1—Non-idiopathic scoliosis

The Morgan Stanley Children's Hospital of New York–Presbyterian Hospital created a standardized, perioperative, antimicrobial prophylaxis regimen for children undergoing surgery for non-idiopathic scoliosis

TABLE 4.5 New York–Presbyterian Morgan Stanley Children's Hospital Perioperative Antibiotic Prophylaxis Regimen for Spine Surgery

ANTIBIOTIC	IV DOSAGE	PREOPERATIVE TIMING	REDOSING	POSTOPERATIVE PROPHYLAXIS
Cefazolin (if no β-lactam allergy and no MRSA colonization)	30 mg/kg ± 10%, max 2000 mg	Within 60 min of incision	If surgery ≥4 hours Timing: 4 h ± 30 mins from previous dose	Discontinue within 24 h Redosing interval: every 8 h
Vancomycin (if β-lactam allergy and/or MRSA colonization)	15 mg/kg ± 10%, max 1000 mg	Within 120 min of incision	If surgery ≥8 hours Timing: 8 h ± 30 mins from previous dose	Discontinue within 24 h Redosing interval: every 8 h
Tobramycin*	2.5 mg/kg ± 10%	Within 60 min of incision	If surgery ≥8 hours Timing: 8 h ± 30 mins from previous dose	Discontinue within 24 h Redosing interval: every 8 h

* If Tobramycin allergy, give Gram-negative coverage on case-by-case basis.

(Table 4.5).[65] The choice of tobramycin for Gram-negative pathogens was based on susceptibility patterns of the SSI pathogens of this patient population at this institution. During the study period, adherence to bundle strategies (which included perioperative antibiotics as well as

TABLE 4.6 The Children's Hospital of Los Angeles Preoperative Antibiotics Protocol for Adolescent Idiopathic Scoliosis

TIMING	ANTIBIOTICS
Preoperative	1. Vancomycin (15 mg/kg; maximum 1000 mg) administered within 1 hour of incision. 2. Ceftazidime (50 mg/kg; maximum 2000 mg) administered within 20–30 minutes of incision.
Intraoperative	1. Re-dose vancomycin (15 mg/kg IV every 12 hours; maximum 1000 mg) and ceftazidime (50 mg/kg every 8 hours; maximum 2000 mg). 2. Irrigation with or without detergent, at surgeon's discretion, using 5 liters of pulsatile lavage irrigation.
Postoperative	1. Vancomycin (15 mg/kg IV every 12 hours; maximum 1000 mg) and ceftazidime (50 mg/kg every 8 hours; maximum 2000 mg) continued for 24 hours. 2. After 24 hours of vancomycin, cefazolin (20 mg/kg IV every 8 hours; maximum 2000 mg) until postoperative day 3.

HANDOUT 4.2 Texas Children's Hospital Spine Study Group Surgical Site Infection Bundle for Spine Surgery

Preoperative:

- Sign on door restricting traffic
- Ensure preoperative antibiotics
- Clip hair, as needed
- Remove dirt, debris, adhesive material
- Apply Chloraprep to surgical field and do not wash off
  - Wait 3 minutes
- Scrub hands with Avagard
- Double glove
  - # double gloved ________
- Use Ioban draping

Intraoperative:

- # scrubbed in case __________
- Re-dose antibiotics
  - Ancef every 4 hours
  - Alternative: _____

Postoperative:

- Irrigate with Bacitracin at end of procedure
  - Amount ______ liter(s)
- Change outer gloves at end of irrigation and before bone graft placement
- Sprinkle vancomycin powder into surgical bed
  - Amount ______ gram(s)
- Close incision with antibiotic impregnated sutures
- Dressing
  - "Mud flap" as needed-

  Post-op orders with at least one dose of same antibiotic
- Drain placement
  - Location: _________
  - Betadine soak

Patient Sticker

Surgeon: ___________________________

Date of surgery: ____________________

Person completing form: ______________

Surgeon sign-off: ____________________

Diagnosis:

- Idiopathic	- Scoliosis	- Initial surgery
- Congenital	- Spondylosis	- Revision surgery
- Neuromuscular	- Fracture	- Post-infection
- Degenerative	- Spinal cord injury	- Other: ______
- Trauma	- Other: _____	
- Other: _____		

Operative Time	**Spinal Level**	**Graft**
- < 2hours	- Cervical	- Autograft
- 2-4 hours	- Thoracic	- Allograft
- 4-6 hours	- Lumbar	- BMP
- 6-8 hours	- Sacrum	- Other:
- >8 hours	- Pelvis	

Elective blood loss: ________________________

Total # in room: ___________________________

other elements) improved, and SSIs rates declined. An association was identified between under-dosing of pre- and intraoperative antibiotics and SSIs among patients undergoing fusion procedures.

Institution #2—Idiopathic scoliosis

The Children's Hospital of Los Angeles implemented a protocol for adolescent patients with idiopathic scoliosis (AIS).[59] The most commonly isolated pathogen at their institution was coagulase-negative staphylococcus. Based on this local epidemiology, perioperative antibiotics were changed from cefazolin alone to ceftazidime and vancomycin (Table 4.6). Following implementation of these guidelines, the rate of debridement for SSI decreased from 11% to 0.7%.

Institution #3—Importance of appropriate timing

A nested case–control study at Johns Hopkins Hospital found that patients who received preoperative antibiotic prophylaxis either more than 60 minutes *before* incision or *after* incision had an increased risk of deep SSIs.[63] This analysis took into account previous spine surgery, presence of a complex medical condition, and the number of vertebrae fused.

Using Perioperative Checklist

The Texas Children's Hospital Spine Study Group used quality improvement methodologies to create a perioperative checklist to reduce SSIs in children undergoing scoliosis surgery (Handout 4.2).[66] The checklist addressed factors thought to increase the risk of SSIs, such as the etiology of scoliosis, initial versus revision surgery, and type of graft used. The annual SSI rate prior to implementing the checklist ranged from 3.4 to 8.9% (mean 5.8%), and after its implementation, decreased to 2.2%.

Unresolved Issues

As with general surgical procedures, there is limited evidence for some strategies proposed for the prevention of SSIs after following spinal fusion procedures.

Limitation of Case Definitions

Efforts thus far have focused only on tracking SSIs after corrective surgeries, while infectious rates specifically in procedures such as growing rod procedures are under-reported. For example, when performing growing rod procedures for scoliosis repair, the rod is accessed repeatedly to lengthen the rod and allow the thoracic cavity to grow. As these lengthening procedures are not associated with fusion, an SSI following lengthening the growing rod would not "count" in current CDC NHSN case definitions. Though these SSIs do not match the CDC NHSN case definitions, institutional efforts should be made to track these complications as well, and assess for possible SSI prevention strategies.

Choosing Perioperative Prophylaxis for Scoliosis Repair

Perioperative prophylaxis for scoliosis repair has not been standardized for drug selection and dosing, or for intraoperative redosing. As a result, prophylactic antibiotic regimens vary widely. Among 37 U.S. children's hospitals, 52% used broad-spectrum antibiotics for preoperative antibiotic prophylaxis in idiopathic scoliosis (most commonly isolated pathogens being Gram-positive skin flora in these SSIs), while only 37% of hospitals utilized broad-spectrum antibiotics for prophylaxis in non-idiopathic scoliosis (most commonly isolated organisms being Gram-positive and Gram-negative pathogens).[67] The overuse of broad-spectrum antibiotics in idiopathic scoliosis and their underuse in non-idiopathic scoliosis is an area for improvement in establishing proper prophylaxis guidelines.

Utility of Vancomycin in the Surgical Bed

The efficacy of topical vancomycin applied to the surgical bed is unproven. While one randomized controlled trial of adult patients undergoing spine surgery demonstrated that the addition of vancomycin applied to the surgical site did not lower the SSI rate,[68] another, retrospective, cohort study demonstrated a significant reduction in SSI rates, from 2.6% in patients who did not receive a local application of vancomycin powder to 0.2% in those who did.[69] The utility of topical vancomycin in the pediatric population has not been systematically studied.

Case 3: Ventriculoperitoneal Shunt Infection

A 45-day-old, ex-34-week male presents to the Emergency Department for evaluation of fever. He had undergone a ventriculoperitoneal (VP) shunt placement one month ago for congenital hydrocephalus. He had a normal physical exam, and his skin was without any breakdown over the tunneled VP shunt. CSF Gram stain returns with Gram-positive cocci in clusters.

Questions

What are the common pathogens associated with VP shunt infections? What factors may have contributed to the infection? What evidence-based prevention measures and bundles are available for pediatric patients undergoing surgery?

Key Challenges

There are a specific challenges associated with the prevention of SSIs following insertion of neuroventricular shunts.

Common Pathogens associated with VP shunt infections

S. aureus and coagulase-negative staphylococci, including *S. epidermidis,* are the most common causes of SSIs associated with neurosurgical ventricular shunts.[70–72] Additional SSI pathogens include *P. acnes, Streptococcus pneumoniae,* viridans streptococci, *E. coli, Klebsiella* spp., and mixed flora.[72]

Risk Factors for Neurosurgical Ventricular Shunt Infections

Prematurity, younger age, lower birthweight, and younger gestational age are risk factors for SSIs following insertion of neuroventricular shunts.[8,9,70,73–76] The association of SSIs with prematurity probably reflects an increased risk of shunt failure, revisions, and subsequent infections in infants with hydrocephalus due to intraventricular hemorrhage or meningitis.[73,75,76] The Hydrocephalus Clinical Research Network found that a first shunt revision was associated with a threefold to fourfold increased risk of infection, whereas two or more revisions were associated with a sixfold to 13-fold increased risk.[8] Each revision is likely to be a new opportunity to introduce bacteria into a previously instrumented field with subsequent entry of microorganisms into the CSF.

The skin of infants in the NICU is more likely to be colonized with pathogenic skin flora, thereby increasing the risk of infection.[73,74] Prospective quantification of skin flora revealed a greater bacterial burden in neonates who developed VP shunt infections.[77] Furthermore, coagulase-negative staphylococci that demonstrated increased adherence to shunt material were more commonly detected in neonates than in older children.[77]

Comorbidities such as chronic respiratory conditions,[75] cardiac surgery,[9] and gastrostomy tubes are also associated with an increased SSI risk.[8] While gastrostomy may be a surrogate for existing comorbidities, it is also possible that a gastrostomy provides a portal of entry for skin and enteric flora to infect the shunt.

Suggested Approaches and Approach to the Clinical Scenario

The infant in Case 3 has several risk factors for postoperative shunt infection, including prematurity and an extended hospital stay with potential colonization by pathogenic flora. Use of a checklist to enhance compliance with bundle elements, as utilized by the Hydrocephalus Clinical Research Network (HCRN), could reduce the risk of infections. Improved skin disinfection, antibiotic prophylaxis, and management of comorbid conditions could reduce SSIs.

Using a Perioperative Checklist and Protocols

The HCRN implemented a care bundle in four pediatric neurosurgical centers, as shown in Figure 4.1; the overall SSI rate decreased from 8.8% to 5.7% using the case definition described earlier.[22] Elements of their protocol included recommendations for limiting traffic in the operating room (OR), CHG shampoo, perioperative antibiotics (including those injected into the shunt reservoir), double-gloving by the surgical team, and use of antibiotic-impregnated sutures. All surgeons who performed more than 40 procedures (10 of the 15 surgeons in the study) lowered their infection rates when they implemented all of the bundle strategies. Thus, compliance with each bundle component should be monitored, and adherence reinforced.

Unresolved Issues

More data are needed to support several specific strategies that have been suggested for the prevention of SSIs after neuroventricular shunt insertion.

Optimal Perioperative Prophylaxis

The optimal perioperative prophylaxis regimen remains unknown. Due to the concerns regarding resistant Gram-positive skin flora such as cefazolin-resistant coagulase-negative staphylococci, some experts have advocated for vancomycin prophylaxis. The optimal dose remains uncertain, as does the need for penetration into cerebrospinal fluid.

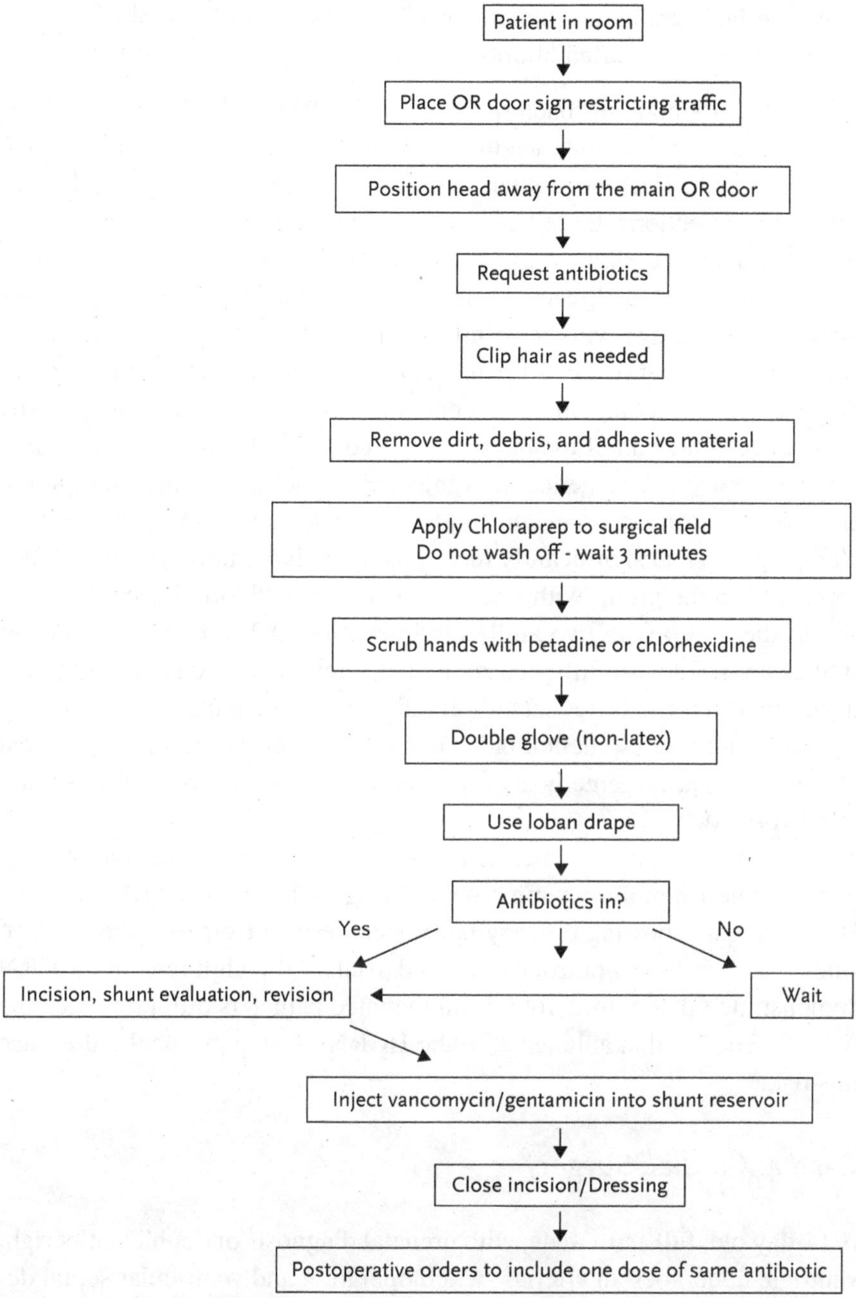

FIGURE 4.1 The Hydrocephalus Clinical Research Network surgical site infection bundle for ventriculoperitoneal shunts.

Antibiotic Injection around and in VP Shunts and Antimicrobial-Impregnated or coated Shunts

Biofilms (containing bacteria) can form on both the luminal and the outer surfaces of the shunt, leading to shunt infections.[78] Such biofilms are very difficult to treat, necessitating removal of the shunt for cure. To prevent shunt infections, there has been great interest in injecting antibiotics in and around the shunt during placement. In a randomized controlled trial evaluating the efficacy of injected antibiotics among infants less than one year of age with congenital hydrocephalus, three regimens were compared: intravenous cefotaxime (conventional therapy), conventional therapy plus vancomycin, and gentamicin injected in and around the shunt once at the end of the insertion procedure, and conventional therapy plus vancomycin, and gentamicin injected in and around the shunt at the end of the insertion procedure and one week later.[71] The conventional therapy group had significantly more postoperative shunt infections (6/20) compared to the group with one intraoperative antibiotic injection (1/20) and to the group with two antibiotic injections (0/20). Large multicenter studies are needed to fully determine the safety and efficacy of antibiotic injection. If it is used, frequent observations for potential adverse effects of injectable antibiotics, including local reactions such as irritation, chemical meningitis, and the emergence of multidrug-resistant organisms, should be performed.

There has been much interest in the use of antimicrobial-coated (e.g., minocycline-rifampin) or impregnated (e.g., silver) VP shunt catheters. However, data showing efficacy have been derived from non-randomized studies rather than controlled clinical trials.[79] In children, the HCRN demonstrated that antimicrobial-impregnated catheters did not reduce the risk of SSIs, but that adherence to the HCRN 11-step protocol did reduce this risk.[80]

Case 4: Cardiac Surgery

A 14-day old, full-term male, with prenatal diagnosis of double outlet right ventricle undergoes an arterial switch operation and ventricular septal defect repair with delayed sternal closure. On postoperative day (POD) 1, he develops bleeding requiring a chest washout. On POD 3, his chest is closed. On POD 5, he develops fever to 38.6^{0}C and rising white blood cell (WBC) count. Blood and urine cultures are obtained, and vancomycin and piperacillin-tazobactam are started. On POD 7, his sternal wound dehisces, and cultures are positive for methicillin-resistant *Staphylococcus aureus* (MRSA).

Questions

What are the common pathogens associated with cardiac surgery infections? What factors may have contributed to the infection? What evidence-based prevention measures and bundles are available for children undergoing cardiac surgery?

Key Challenges

There are specific challenges association with the prevention of SSIs after cardiac surgery.

Common Pathogens associated with SSIs After Cardiac Surgery

SSIs following cardiac surgery are predominantly caused by Gram-positive skin flora such as *S. aureus*, including MRSA and *S. epidermidis*. Gram-negative bacilli and fungi are less commonly seen.[81–84] In adult cardiac surgery patients, SSIs caused by MRSA were associated with a 12-fold increase in 90-day postoperative mortality compared to patients without an SSI.[85]

Risk Factors for SSIs following Cardiac surgery

Risk factors for SSIs following cardiac surgery include younger age (specifically <30 days), a higher ASA score, longer ICU stay, and longer preoperative stay.[83,86] Postoperative bleeding requiring transfusion or chest washout may increase the risk of infection due to manipulation of a previously sterile field.[86]

Unique to cardiac surgery, cardiopulmonary bypass is associated with a reduction in T-lymphocytes and T-helper cells which demonstrate impaired mitogen response.[87,88] Intraoperative hypothermia may impair chemotaxis and phagocytosis, macrophage motility, antibody production, and the oxidative antimicrobial activity of neutrophils.[89] Furthermore, hypothermia may cause vasoconstriction[90] and decrease the partial pressure of oxygen in tissues. These factors can adversely affect collagen deposition and reduce collagen cross-links, both oxygen-dependent steps, ultimately compromising wound healing.[91]

Delayed sternal closure (DSC) is a well-established technique that aims to minimize postoperative respiratory and hemodynamic instability in post-cardiac surgery patients. While this life-saving maneuver confers obvious benefits, the risk of SSIs in DSC has been documented to range from 6.7% to 13.7%.[92–94] Potential risk factors for SSI specifically in patients with DSC include age less than 30 days, greater dependence on parenteral nutrition, receipt of stress dose steroids, use of extracorporeal membrane oxygenation, multiple DSC events, and the diagnosis of hypoplastic left heart syndrome.[82,92–94]

Some experts have advocated obtaining mediastinal cultures in infants with DSC. In a survey conducted at 38 pediatric centers, the centers that obtained routine mediastinal cultures had lower SSI rates than those that did not.[95] While subsequent management of positive cultures was not discussed, the authors postulated that positive mediastinal cultures led to interventions such as antibiotics or mediastinal washouts that then led to improved outcomes. Further studies are needed to investigate the association between surveillance mediastinal cultures and SSIs, and to define optimal management.

Suggested Approaches and Approach to the Clinical Scenario

The neonate just described is at an increased risk of developing a SSI due to his young age, postoperative complications, delayed sternal closure, and blood transfusion.

Pre-, intra- and postoperative Bundle Strategies

Izquierdo-Blasco et al. implemented pre-, intra-, and postoperative measures to prevent SSIs in children undergoing cardiac surgery requiring cardiopulmonary bypass (Box 4.1).[81] Implementation of this protocol was associated with reducing the incidence of SSIs from 10.9–1.92%.[81] These investigators introduced aztreonam as perioperative prophylaxis for infants in the NICU because several SSIs were caused by Gram-negative bacilli in this population. This highlights the importance of using local epidemiology to optimize perioperative antibiotic prophylaxis.

Unresolved Issues

Limited pediatric-specific data have contributed to a variable adoption of some strategies for the prevention of SSIs after following cardiac procedures.

BOX 4.1 EXAMPLE PROTOCOL FOR PREVENTION OF SURGICAL SITE INFECTION AFTER CARDIAC SURGERY

I. Non-pharmacological Measures

A. Preoperative

- Bathe or shower with 4% chlorhexidine soap 2 hours prior to surgery.
- Change clothing and bed sheets after bathing.
- If hair has to be removed, use electric clippers with a single-use head on the day of surgery.

B. Intraoperative

- OR used exclusively for clean surgery.
- Daily review of OR air-conditioning.
- Ensure doors closed throughout surgery.
- Antiseptic skin preparation with 2% alcoholic chlorhexidine solution.
- Change surgical gloves after sternotomy and before skin suturing.
- Checklist for compliance of above measures.

C. Postoperative

- Keep sterile dressing on for 48 hours.
- If transthoracic echocardiogram is required, use aseptic technique with sterile ultrasound probe.

II. Antibiotic Prophylaxis

A. Preoperative/Postoperative

- First dose of prophylactic antibiotic to be administered <60 minutes prior to incision.
  - Surgery with sternal closure in the OR:
    - Cefazolin IV 25 mg/kg every 6 hours for 24 hours.
    - Patient with beta-lactam allergy or colonization with MRSA, vancomycin IV 10 mg/kg every 8 hours.
  - Surgery with delayed sternal closure:
    - Cefazolin IV 25 mg/kg every 6 hours AND aztreonam[a] IV 50 mg/kg every 8 hours until 24 hours after sternal closure.

B. Intraoperative

Surgeries lasting more than 3 hours, a repeat dose of the antibiotic should be administered for every 500 mL of cardiopulmonary bypass perfusion.

---

[a] Aztreonam added for Gram-negative bacilli in DSC group based on previous cultures.

Adapted from Izquierdo-Blasco J, Campins-Marti M, Soler-Palacin P, et al. Impact of the implementation of an interdisciplinary infection control program to prevent surgical wound infection in pediatric heart surgery. *Eur J Pediatr.* 2015;174(7):957–963.[81]

Limitations of Case Definitions

Current NHSN case definitions do not capture all SSIs. For example, if an infant has DSC, and mediastinitis develops after chest closure, this SSI would not count because of manipulation of the wound prior to the development of the SSI. Nonetheless, such infections should be tracked and possible prevention strategies should be considered.

Duration of Antimicrobial Prophylaxis

A consortium of the American Society of Health-System Pharmacists, the Infectious Diseases Society of America, the Surgical Infection Society, and the Society of Healthcare Epidemiology of America published consensus guidelines recommending postoperative antimicrobial prophylaxis for 24 hours in adult patients undergoing cardiac surgery.[43] The Society of Thoracic Surgeons recommends 48 hours of postoperative prophylaxis for adult patients.[96] Both guidelines acknowledged a lack of data for the pediatric population and hence did not provide formal recommendations for children. Furthermore, despite the lack of evidence, the practice of continuing antibiotic prophylaxis until thoracostomy tubes and invasive lines have been removed is common in the pediatric population.[83,97,98]

A children's hospital in Oregon implemented a protocol in which postoperative antibiotics were discontinued at 48 hours (the duration of prophylaxis for infants with DSC was left to the discretion of the provider). The mean duration of antibiotics at their institution was reduced from 4.2 to 1.9 days with no associated increase in the incidence of SSIs.[99] A similar study was performed by Columbia University Medical Center in New York, restricting the duration of perioperative antibiotics to 48 hours after neonatal cardiac surgery and to 24 hours after DSC. No increase in SSI rate was observed.[83]

Routine MRSA Screening

Pediatric patients with complex congenital heart disease have multiple interactions with the healthcare system, including cardiac catheterization procedures, surgeries, and admission to ICUs. Adults hospitalized within the previous 12 months are at risk for MRSA colonization.[100] A meta-analysis of MRSA colonization in the NICU and PICU found that its overall prevalence was 1.9% on admission, and that the acquisition rate of MRSA was 4.1%. Furthermore, this analysis found a 24.2 relative risk of MRSA *infection* among MRSA *colonized* patients.[101]

Lack of a standardized practice for obtaining and processing surveillance cultures poses a challenge in assessing MRSA colonization. Issues include the body site from which surveillance cultures are obtained (e.g., nares, umbilicus, groin, axilla, and/or pharynx), and the method of processing the cultures (i.e., culture versus polymerase chain reaction (PCR). Furthermore, if routine preoperative surveillance cultures are positive for MRSA, centers must determine if decolonization will be performed and which method will be used; for example, CHG bathing and/or mupirocin applied to the anterior nares.

Assessing Process and Outcome Measures

Both outcome and process measures can be used to measure the success of SSI prevention programs.

Establishing an Interdisciplinary Team

An interdisciplinary team is crucial to success in reducing SSIs. Team members should include administrative leadership, surgeons, anesthesiologists, nurse practitioners, and physician assistants from the relevant surgical services. It is critical to engage front-line staff, OR nursing leadership and front-line nurses, infection prevention and control staff, infectious disease specialists, information technology personnel, and quality improvement staff. It is crucial to have institutional support from senior leadership who can authorize funding, such as for bathing products and information technology resources, when needed. OR staff are often influential champions of process improvement measures.

Establishing SSI rates

To establish SSI rates, the team must understand the SSI case definitions, including what constitutes the numerator and the denominator. To most accurately identify SSIs (the numerator), multiple methods of detection should be used: for example, results of wound cultures, readmissions, and infectious disease consults for SSI management. Surgeons, nurse practitioners and physician assistants from the relevant surgical services should be engaged to review SSIs and perform root cause analysis; this enhances teamwork and improves an understanding of the case definitions.

Several potential sources exist to establish the number of eligible surgical procedures for calculation of SSI rates (denominators). Surgeons' billing records, OR schedules, and/or International Classification of Diseases (ICD) codes can be used. However, these sources need to be filtered for ineligible cases; for instance, heart transplants or growing rod procedures without fusions (as discussed previously). Information technology resources can be very helpful with this task, but a secondary source of validation should be employed to ensure accuracy in the determination of eligible cases.

Monitoring adherence to preoperative bathing and perioperative prophylaxis

Ensuring adherence to bundle elements such as preoperative bathing and antimicrobial prophylaxis is complex and involves many stakeholders, including patients and families. While measurement of adherence to the appropriate timing of preoperative antibiotics can be done at many institutions using an electronic data query, measurement of adherence to preoperative bathing is more complex. Preoperative bathing may occur at home, in the emergency department, or in inpatient units. To ensure adherence and documentation of adherence, service line champions need to be engaged, as they are most likely to identify barriers to adherence and solutions to overcome those barriers. Others have shown that engaging families also improved preoperative bathing compliance and overall adherence to the institutional protocol.[31] Aggregating adherence rates over time are needed.

Data presentations to key stakeholders

Key stakeholders must be regularly informed about SSI rates and adherence rates to process measures. It is important to have consistent data and consider what data are shared internally versus shared with the public. "Missed" process measures are presented, along with solutions to avoid similar misses in the future. The data must be shared with front-line providers as well.

Summary

SSIs are a major source of preventable morbidity and mortality in the neonatal and pediatric populations. Recognizing *non-modifiable* risk factors such as prematurity, presence of comorbidities, and inherent infectious risks within the surgery itself (such as cardiopulmonary bypasses) aids in identifying high-risk patients. Ultimately, success in reducing SSIs is achieved by addressing *modifiable* risk factors such as antibiotic selection and timing, skin disinfection, nutritional status, and exposure to blood products.

Significant harm in health care arises from the gap between what we know and what we do. One of our aims in this chapter was to demonstrate that adherence to institutional antibiotic protocols and the creation of prevention bundles will lead to a reduction in SSIs in general surgery, spine surgery, VP shunts, and cardiac surgery. It is with great emphasis that we encourage institutions to create an interdisciplinary team consisting of nurses, pharmacists, infectious disease specialists, intensivists, and surgeons to develop their own protocols and bundles, and to monitor implementation, adherence, and outcomes.

Over the past decade, there have been great advances in the creation of pediatric-specific quality improvement initiatives, including the pediatric National Surgical Quality Improvement Program (NSQIP-P), Hydrocephalus Clinical Research Network (HCRN), and Solutions for Patient Safety. While many challenges and knowledge gaps remain, national collaborations, clinical and basic science research, and multidisciplinary initiatives such as those discussed in this chapter offer promising solutions to pediatric SSIs.

References

1. Sparling KW, Ryckman FC, Schoettker PJ, et al. Financial impact of failing to prevent surgical site infections. *Qual Manag Health Care.* 2007;16(3):219–225.
2. Cahill PJ, Warnick DE, Lee MJ, et al. Infection after spinal fusion for pediatric spinal deformity: thirty years of experience at a single institution. *Spine (Phila Pa. 1976).* 2010;35(12):1211–1217.
3. Mackenzie WG, Matsumoto H, Williams BA, et al. Surgical site infection following spinal instrumentation for scoliosis: a multicenter analysis of rates, risk factors, and pathogens. *J Bone Joint Surg Am.* 2013;95(9):800–806, S1–S2.
4. Sebaaly A, El Rachkidi R, Yaacoub JJ, Saliba E, Ghanem I. Management of spinal infections in children with cerebral palsy. *Orthop Traumatol Surg Res.* 2016;102(6):801–805.
5. Aleissa S, Parsons D, Grant J, Harder J, Howard J. Deep wound infection following pediatric scoliosis surgery: incidence and analysis of risk factors. *Can J Surg.* 2011;54(4):263–269.
6. Sponseller PD, Jain A, Shah SA, et al. Deep wound infections after spinal fusion in children with cerebral palsy: a prospective cohort study. *Spine (Phila Pa 1976).* 2013;38(23):2023–2027.

7. Hedequist D, Haugen A, Hresko T, Emans J. Failure of attempted implant retention in spinal deformity delayed surgical site infections. *Spine (Phila Pa 1976).* 2009;34(1):60–64.
8. Simon TD, Butler J, Whitlock KB, et al. Risk factors for first cerebrospinal fluid shunt infection: findings from a multi-center prospective cohort study. *J Pediatr.* 2014;164(6):1462–1468 e2.
9. Riva-Cambrin J, Kestle JR, Holubkov R, et al. Risk factors for shunt malfunction in pediatric hydrocephalus: a multicenter prospective cohort study. *J Neurosurg Pediatr.* 2016;17(4):382–390.
10. Kulkarni AV, Rabin D, Lamberti-Pasculli M, Drake JM. Repeat cerebrospinal fluid shunt infection in children. *Pediatr Neurosurg.* 2001;35(2):66–71.
11. Hirsch JF, Renier D, Pierre-Kahn A. Influence of the use of a surgical isolator on the rate of infection in the treatment of hydrocephalus. *Childs Brain.* 1978;4(3):137–150.
12. Renier D, Lacombe J, Pierre-Kahn A, Sainte-Rose C, Hirsch JF. Factors causing acute shunt infection. Computer analysis of 1174 operations. *J Neurosurg.* 1984;61(6):1072–1078.
13. Ronan A, Hogg GG, Klug GL. Cerebrospinal fluid shunt infections in children. *Pediatr Infect Dis J.* 1995;14(9):782–786.
14. Meirovitch J, Kitai-Cohen Y, Keren G, Fiendler G, Rubinstein E. Cerebrospinal fluid shunt infections in children. *Pediatr Infect Dis J.* 1987;6(10):921–924.
15. Mancao M, Miller C, Cochrane B, Hoff C, Sauter K, Weber E. Cerebrospinal fluid shunt infections in infants and children in Mobile, Alabama. *Acta Paediatr.* 1998;87(6):667–670.
16. Sohn AH, Schwartz JM, Yang KY, Jarvis WR, Guglielmo BJ, Weintrub PS. Risk factors and risk adjustment for surgical site infections in pediatric cardiothoracic surgery patients. *Am J Infect Control.* 2010;38(9):706–710.
17. Ben-Ami E, Levy I, Katz J, Dagan O, Shalit I. Risk factors for sternal wound infection in children undergoing cardiac surgery: a case-control study. *J Hosp Infect.* 2008;70(4):335–340.
18. Nateghian A, Taylor G, Robinson JL. Risk factors for surgical site infections following open-heart surgery in a Canadian pediatric population. *Am J Infect Control.* 2004;32(7):397–401.
19. Barker GM, O'Brien SM, Welke KF, et al. Major infection after pediatric cardiac surgery: a risk estimation model. *Ann Thorac Surg.* 2010;89(3):843–850.
20. Alexander JW, Solomkin JS, Edwards MJ. Updated recommendations for control of surgical site infections. *Ann Surg.* 2011;253(6):1082–1093.
21. Centers for Disease Control and Prevention National Healthcare Safety Network. Surveillance for Surgical Site Infection (SSI) Events, available at: https://www.cdc.gov/nhsn/pdfs/pscmanual/9pscssicurrent.pdf. Accessed October 31, 2018.
22. Kestle JR, Riva-Cambrin J, Wellons JC, 3rd, et al. A standardized protocol to reduce cerebrospinal fluid shunt infection: the Hydrocephalus Clinical Research Network Quality Improvement Initiative. *J Neurosurg Pediatr.* 2011;8(1):22–29.
23. Mangram AJ, Horan TC, Pearson ML, Silver LC, Jarvis WR. Guideline for Prevention of Surgical Site Infection, 1999. Centers for Disease Control and Prevention (CDC) Hospital Infection Control Practices Advisory Committee. *Am J Infect Control.* 1999;27(2):97–132; quiz 3–4; discussion 96.

24. Krizek TJ, Robson MC. Evolution of quantitative bacteriology in wound management. *Am J Surg.* 1975;130(5):579–584.
25. Elek SD, Conen PE. The virulence of Staphylococcus pyogenes for man; a study of the problems of wound infection. *Br J Exp Pathol.* 1957;38(6):573–586.
26. James RC, Macleod CJ. Induction of staphylococcal infections in mice with small inocula introduced on sutures. *Br J Exp Pathol.* 1961;42:266–277.
27. Culver DH, Horan TC, Gaynes RP, et al. Surgical wound infection rates by wound class, operative procedure, and patient risk index. National Nosocomial Infections Surveillance System. *Am J Med.* 1991;91(3B):152S–157S.
28. Cruse PJ, Foord R. The epidemiology of wound infection. A 10-year prospective study of 62,939 wounds. *Surg Clin North Am.* 1980;60(1):27–40.
29. Daley J, Khuri SF, Henderson W, et al. Risk adjustment of the postoperative morbidity rate for the comparative assessment of the quality of surgical care: results of the National Veterans Affairs Surgical Risk Study. *J Am Coll Surg.* 1997;185(4):328–340.
30. Toltzis P, O'Riordan M, Cunningham DJ, et al. A statewide collaborative to reduce pediatric surgical site infections. *Pediatrics.* 2014;134(4):e1174–1180.
31. Schaffzin JK, Harte L, Marquette S, et al. Surgical site infection reduction by the Solutions for Patient Safety Hospital Engagement Network. *Pediatrics.* 2015;136(5):e1353–e1360.
32. Berard F, Gandon J. Postoperative wound infections: the influence of ultraviolet irradiation of the operating room and of various other factors. *Ann Surg.* 1964;160(Suppl 2):1–192.
33. Solutions for Patient Safety. Available at: http://www.solutionsforpatientsafety.org. Accessed October 31, 2018.
34. Bowler PG, Duerden BI, Armstrong DG. Wound microbiology and associated approaches to wound management. *Clin Microbiol Rev.* 2001;14(2):244–269.
35. Kaya D, Aldirmaz Agartan C, Yucel M. Fungal agents as a cause of surgical wound infections: an overview of host factors. *Wounds.* 2007;19(8):218–222.
36. Blajchman MA. Immunomodulatory effects of allogeneic blood transfusions: clinical manifestations and mechanisms. *Vox Sang.* 1998;74(Suppl 2):315–319.
37. Fawley J, Chelius TH, Anderson Y, Cassidy LD, Arca MJ. Relationship between perioperative blood transfusion and surgical site infections in the newborn population: An ACS-NSQIP-Pediatrics analysis. *J Pediatr Surg.* 2016;51(9):1397–1404.
38. Goobie SM, DiNardo JA, Faraoni D. Relationship between transfusion volume and outcomes in children undergoing noncardiac surgery. *Transfusion.* 2016;56(10):2487–2494.
39. Segal I, Kang C, Albersheim SG, Skarsgard ED, Lavoie PM. Surgical site infections in infants admitted to the neonatal intensive care unit. *J Pediatr Surg.* 2014;49(3):381–384.
40. Davenport M, Doig CM. Wound infection in pediatric surgery: a study in 1,094 neonates. *J Pediatr Surg.* 1993;28(1):26–30.
41. Ichikawa S, Ishihara M, Okazaki T, et al. Prospective study of antibiotic protocols for managing surgical site infections in children. *J Pediatr Surg.* 2007;42(6):1002–1007; discussion 7.

42. Oyetunji TA, Gonzalez DO, Gonzalez KW, Nwomeh BC, St. Peter SD. Wound classification in pediatric surgical procedures: Measured and found wanting. *J Pediatr Surg.* 2016;51(6):1014–1016.
43. Bratzler DW, Dellinger EP, Olsen KM, et al. Clinical practice guidelines for antimicrobial prophylaxis in surgery. *Am J Health Syst Pharm.* 2013;70(3):195–283.
44. Shah GS, Christensen RE, Wagner DS, Pearce BK, Sweeney J, Tait AR. Retrospective evaluation of antimicrobial prophylaxis in prevention of surgical site infection in the pediatric population. *Paediatr Anaesth.* 2014;24(9):994–998.
45. Milstone AM, Passaretti CL, Perl TM. Chlorhexidine: expanding the armamentarium for infection control and prevention. *Clin Infect Dis.* 2008;46(2):274–281.
46. Sathiyamurthy S, Banerjee J, Godambe SV. Antiseptic use in the neonatal intensive care unit—a dilemma in clinical practice: an evidence based review. *World J Clin Pediatr.* 2016;5(2):159–171.
47. Milstone AM, Bamford P, Aucott SW, Tang N, White KR, Bearer CF. Chlorhexidine inhibits L1 cell adhesion molecule-mediated neurite outgrowth in vitro. *Pediatr Res.* 2014;75(1–1):8–13.
48. Rackur H. New aspects of mechanism of action of povidone-iodine. *J Hosp Infect.* 1985;6(Suppl A):13–23.
49. Peterson AF, Rosenberg A, Alatary SD. Comparative evaluation of surgical scrub preparations. *Surg Gynecol Obstet.* 1978;146(1):63–65.
50. Aly R, Maibach HI. Comparative antibacterial efficacy of a 2-minute surgical scrub with chlorhexidine gluconate, povidone-iodine, and chloroxylenol sponge-brushes. *Am J Infect Control.* 1988;16(4):173–177.
51. Dumville JC, McFarlane E, Edwards P, Lipp A, Holmes A. Preoperative skin antiseptics for preventing surgical wound infections after clean surgery. *Cochrane Database Syst Rev.* 2013(3):CD003949.
52. Berrios-Torres SI, Umscheid CA, Bratzler DW, et al. Centers for Disease Control and Prevention Guideline for the Prevention of Surgical Site Infection, 2017. *JAMA Surg.* 2017;152(8):784–791.
53. Webster J, Osborne S. Preoperative bathing or showering with skin antiseptics to prevent surgical site infection. *Cochrane Database Syst Rev.* 2006(2):CD004985.
54. Clements KE, Fisher M, Quaye K, O'Donnell R, Whyte C, Horgan MJ. Surgical site infections in the NICU. *J Pediatr Surg.* 2016;51(9):1405–1408.
55. Ryckman FC, Schoettker PJ, Hays KR, et al. Reducing surgical site infections at a pediatric academic medical center. *Jt Comm J Qual Patient Saf.* 2009;35(4):192–198.
56. Kraemer K, Cohen ME, Liu Y, et al. Development and evaluation of the American College of Surgeons NSQIP Pediatric Surgical Risk Calculator. *J Am Coll Surg.* 2016;223(5):685–693.
57. O'Grady NP, Alexander M, Burns LA, et al. Guidelines for the prevention of intravascular catheter-related infections. *Clin Infect Dis.* 2011;52(9):e162–e193.
58. Chapman AK, Aucott SW, Gilmore MM, Advani S, Clarke W, Milstone AM. Absorption and tolerability of aqueous chlorhexidine gluconate used for skin antisepsis prior to catheter insertion in preterm neonates. *J Perinatol.* 2013;33(10):768–771.
59. Myung KS, Glassman DM, Tolo VT, Skaggs DL. Simple steps to minimize spine infections in adolescent idiopathic scoliosis. *J Pediatr Orthop.* 2014;34(1):29–33.

60. Sponseller PD, LaPorte DM, Hungerford MW, Eck K, Bridwell KH, Lenke LG. Deep wound infections after neuromuscular scoliosis surgery: a multicenter study of risk factors and treatment outcomes. *Spine (Phila Pa. 1976).* 2000;25(19):2461–2466.
61. Glotzbecker MP, Riedel MD, Vitale MG, et al. What's the evidence? Systematic literature review of risk factors and preventive strategies for surgical site infection following pediatric spine surgery. *J Pediatr Orthop.* 2013;33(5):479–487.
62. Hatlen T, Song K, Shurtleff D, Duguay S. Contributory factors to postoperative spinal fusion complications for children with myelomeningocele. *Spine (Phila Pa. 1976).* 2010;35(13):1294–1299.
63. Milstone AM, Maragakis LL, Townsend T, et al. Timing of preoperative antibiotic prophylaxis: a modifiable risk factor for deep surgical site infections after pediatric spinal fusion. *Pediatr Infect Dis J.* 2008;27(8):704–708.
64. Jain A, Puvanesarajah V, Menga EN, Sponseller PD. Unplanned hospital readmissions and reoperations after pediatric spinal fusion surgery. *Spine (Phila Pa. 1976).* 2015;40(11):856–862.
65. Salsgiver E, Crotty J, LaRussa SJ, et al. Surgical site infections following spine surgery for non-idiopathic scoliosis. *J Pediatr Orthop.* 2017;37(8):e476–e83.
66. Ryan SL, Sen A, Staggers K, Luerssen TG, Jea A, Texas Children's Hospital Spine Study Group. A standardized protocol to reduce pediatric spine surgery infection: a quality improvement initiative. *J Neurosurg Pediatr.* 2014;14(3):259–265.
67. McLeod LM, Keren R, Gerber J, et al. Perioperative antibiotic use for spinal surgery procedures in US children's hospitals. *Spine (Phila Pa 1976).* 2013;38(7):609–616.
68. Tubaki VR, Rajasekaran S, Shetty AP. Effects of using intravenous antibiotic only versus local intrawound vancomycin antibiotic powder application in addition to intravenous antibiotics on postoperative infection in spine surgery in 907 patients. *Spine (Phila Pa 1976).* 2013;38(25):2149–2155.
69. Sweet FA, Roh M, Sliva C. Intrawound application of vancomycin for prophylaxis in instrumented thoracolumbar fusions: efficacy, drug levels, and patient outcomes. *Spine (Phila Pa 1976).* 2011;36(24):2084–2088.
70. Davis SE, Levy ML, McComb JG, Masri-Lavine L. Does age or other factors influence the incidence of ventriculoperitoneal shunt infections? *Pediatr Neurosurg.* 1999;30(5):253–257.
71. Moussa WM, Mohamed MA. Efficacy of postoperative antibiotic injection in and around ventriculoperitoneal shunt in reduction of shunt infection: A randomized controlled trial. *Clin Neurol Neurosurg.* 2016;143:144–149.
72. Kestle JR, Garton HJ, Whitehead WE, et al. Management of shunt infections: a multicenter pilot study. *J Neurosurg.* 2006;105(3 Suppl):177–181.
73. Spader HS, Hertzler DA, Kestle JR, Riva-Cambrin J. Risk factors for infection and the effect of an institutional shunt protocol on the incidence of ventricular access device infections in preterm infants. *J Neurosurg Pediatr.* 2015;15(2):156–160.
74. Bruinsma N, Stobberingh EE, Herpers MJ, Vles JS, Weber BJ, Gavilanes DA. Subcutaneous ventricular catheter reservoir and ventriculoperitoneal drain-related infections in preterm infants and young children. *Clin Microbiol Infect.* 2000;6(4):202–206.

75. Simon TD, Hall M, Riva-Cambrin J, et al. Infection rates following initial cerebrospinal fluid shunt placement across pediatric hospitals in the United States. Clinical article. *J Neurosurg Pediatr.* 2009;4(2):156–165.
76. Tuli S, Drake J, Lawless J, Wigg M, Lamberti-Pasculli M. Risk factors for repeated cerebrospinal shunt failures in pediatric patients with hydrocephalus. *J Neurosurg.* 2000;92(1):31–38.
77. Pople IK, Bayston R, Hayward RD. Infection of cerebrospinal fluid shunts in infants: a study of etiological factors. *J Neurosurg.* 1992;77(1):29–36.
78. Dawod J, Tager A, Darouiche RO, Al Mohajer M. Prevention and management of internal cerebrospinal fluid shunt infections. *J Hosp Infect.* 2016;93(4):323–328.
79. Konstantelias AA, Vardakas KZ, Polyzos KA, Tansarli GS, Falagas ME. Antimicrobial-impregnated and -coated shunt catheters for prevention of infections in patients with hydrocephalus: a systematic review and meta-analysis. *J Neurosurg.* 2015;122(5):1096–1112.
80. Kestle JR, Holubkov R, Douglas Cochrane D, et al. A new Hydrocephalus Clinical Research Network protocol to reduce cerebrospinal fluid shunt infection. *J Neurosurg Pediatr.* 2016;17(4):391–396.
81. Izquierdo-Blasco J, Campins-Marti M, Soler-Palacin P, et al. Impact of the implementation of an interdisciplinary infection control program to prevent surgical wound infection in pediatric heart surgery. *Eur J Pediatr.* 2015;174(7):957–963.
82. Adler AL, Smith J, Permut LC, McMullan DM, Zerr DM. Significance of positive mediastinal cultures in pediatric cardiovascular surgical procedure patients undergoing delayed sternal closure. *Ann Thorac Surg.* 2014;98(2):685–690.
83. Murray MT, Corda R, Turcotte R, Bacha E, Saiman L, Krishnamurthy G. Implementing a standardized perioperative antibiotic prophylaxis protocol for neonates undergoing cardiac surgery. *Ann Thorac Surg.* 2014;98(3):927–933.
84. Katayanagi T. Nasal methicillin-resistant *S. aureus* is a major risk for mediastinitis in pediatric cardiac surgery. *Ann Thorac Cardiovasc Surg.* 2015;21(1):37–44.
85. Engemann JJ, Carmeli Y, Cosgrove SE, et al. Adverse clinical and economic outcomes attributable to methicillin resistance among patients with *Staphylococcus aureus* surgical site infection. *Clin Infect Dis.* 2003;36(5):592–598.
86. Turcotte RF, Brozovich A, Corda R, et al. Health care-associated infections in children after cardiac surgery. *Pediatr Cardiol.* 2014;35(8):1448–1455.
87. Markewitz A, Faist E, Weinhold C, et al. Alterations of cell-mediated immune response following cardiac surgery. *Eur J Cardiothorac Surg.* 1993;7(4):193–199.
88. Markewitz A, Faist E, Niesel T, Lang S, Weinhold C, Reichart B. Changes in lymphocyte subsets and mitogen responsiveness following open-heart surgery and possible therapeutic approaches. *Thorac Cardiovasc Surg.* 1992;40(1):14–18.
89. van Oss CJ, Absolom DR, Moore LL, Park BH, Humbert JR. Effect of temperature on the chemotaxis, phagocytic engulfment, digestion and O2 consumption of human polymorphonuclear leukocytes. *J Reticuloendothel Soc.* 1980;27(6):561–565.
90. Sessler DI. Temperature monitoring and perioperative thermoregulation. *Anesthesiology.* 2008;109(2):318–338.
91. Jonsson K, Jensen JA, Goodson WH, 3rd, et al. Tissue oxygenation, anemia, and perfusion in relation to wound healing in surgical patients. *Ann Surg.* 1991;214(5):605–613.

92. Harder EE, Gaies MG, Yu S, et al. Risk factors for surgical site infection in pediatric cardiac surgery patients undergoing delayed sternal closure. *J Thorac Cardiovasc Surg.* 2013;146(2):326–333.
93. Tabbutt S, Duncan BW, McLaughlin D, Wessel DL, Jonas RA, Laussen PC. Delayed sternal closure after cardiac operations in a pediatric population. *J Thorac Cardiovasc Surg.* 1997;113(5):886–893.
94. Bowman ME, Rebeyka IM, Ross DB, Quinonez LG, Forgie SE. Risk factors for surgical site infection after delayed sternal closure. *Am J Infect Control.* 2013;41(5):464–465.
95. Woodward CS, Son M, Calhoon J, Michalek J, Husain SA. Sternal wound infections in pediatric congenital cardiac surgery: a survey of incidence and preventative practice. *Ann Thorac Surg.* 2011;91(3):799–804.
96. Edwards FH, Engelman RM, Houck P, Shahian DM, Bridges CR, Society of Thoracic Surgeons. The Society of Thoracic Surgeons Practice Guideline series: antibiotic prophylaxis in cardiac surgery, part I: duration. *Ann Thorac Surg.* 2006;81(1):397–404.
97. Knoderer CA, Anderson EM, Cox EG. Survey of congenital heart surgeons' preferences for antimicrobial prophylaxis for pediatric cardiac surgery patients. *Am J Health Syst Pharm.* 2008;65(21):2008–2010.
98. Alvarez P, Fuentes C, Garcia N, Modesto V. Evaluation of the duration of the antibiotic prophylaxis in paediatric postoperative heart surgery patients. *Pediatr Cardiol.* 2012;33(5):735–738.
99. Bath S, Lines J, Loeffler AM, Malhotra A, Turner RB. Impact of standardization of antimicrobial prophylaxis duration in pediatric cardiac surgery. *J Thorac Cardiovasc Surg.* 2016;152(4):1115–1120.
100. Hidron AI, Kourbatova EV, Halvosa JS, et al. Risk factors for colonization with methicillin-resistant *Staphylococcus aureus* (MRSA) in patients admitted to an urban hospital: emergence of community-associated MRSA nasal carriage. *Clin Infect Dis.* 2005;41(2):159–166.
101. Zervou FN, Zacharioudakis IM, Ziakas PD, Mylonakis E. MRSA colonization and risk of infection in the neonatal and pediatric ICU: a meta-analysis. *Pediatrics.* 2014;133(4):e1015–1023.

5 | *Clostridioides difficile* and Norovirus

THOMAS J. SANDORA

Background

Clostridioides difficile

The incidence of *Clostridioides difficile* infection (CDI) in hospitalized children has increased in recent decades.[1–3] In 2013, the Centers for Disease Control and Prevention (CDC) declared CDI to be an immediate public health threat requiring urgent action.[4] Fulminant disease and complications of CDI such as prolonged hospitalization and mortality are less common among affected children than adults, but these complications do occur in pediatric patients.[5,6] *C. difficile* is an important cause of diarrhea among pediatric inpatients[7,8] and can also cause outbreaks in this setting.[9,10]

Risk factors for CDI in children are similar to those for adults and include antibiotic exposure (the most important modifiable risk factor), hospitalization, immunodeficiency (including malignancy and transplantation), inflammatory bowel disease, enteral feeding tubes, and the use of acid-suppressing medications (such as proton pump inhibitors and histamine receptor antagonists).[2,11–17]

C. difficile is a spore-forming bacterium. The spores are resistant to routine environmental cleaning with detergents and can survive in the environment for months.[18,19] After the spores are ingested, they convert to the vegetative form in the colon; the organism can then produce clinical disease that is mediated by toxin production and manifests primarily as diarrhea. In healthcare settings, *C. difficile* can easily be transmitted on the hands of healthcare workers, either from direct patient care activities or through contact with a contaminated environment.[20,21]

Norovirus

Noroviruses are a group of non-enveloped single-stranded RNA viruses that are the most common cause of epidemic gastroenteritis worldwide. In the United States, approximately 20 million illnesses attributable to norovirus occur each year.[22] The strains that infect humans belong to genogroups GI, GII, and GIV; over the last 15 years, GII.4 strains have emerged as the cause of the majority of outbreaks worldwide.[23,24]

Norovirus is highly contagious, with an estimated infectious dose as low as 18 viral particles.[25] It has been estimated that during peak viral shedding, each gram of stool may contain as many as 5 billion infectious doses.[22] Humans are the only reservoir, and transmission occurs either person-to-person or through ingestion of contaminated food and water. Healthcare facilities are the most commonly reported settings of norovirus outbreaks in industrialized countries,[22] and outbreaks in these settings can be recurrent and prolonged.[26]

Clinical Scenario

Infection preventionists at a tertiary care medical center have noted an increase in positive *C. difficile* tests in pediatric patients. The most recent case is a six-month-old infant in the neonatal intensive care unit (NICU) with intestinal failure and new increased colostomy output. A *C. difficile* test was sent and is positive, but the infant also tested positive for norovirus.

Questions

Does this infant have true CDI, or is he colonized with the organism? Are there recommendations for healthcare personnel or laboratories that could improve the appropriateness of *C. difficile* testing in children? Should isolation precautions be implemented, and if so, how long should they be continued? What are the pediatric-specific nuances to evidence-based recommendations for the prevention of CDI? What are the key strategies to prevent norovirus transmission in a pediatric healthcare setting?

Key Challenges

Clostridioides difficile

C. difficile poses several challenges in healthcare settings in which infants and children may receive care. Perhaps the most important of these challenges is reliably distinguishing colonization from infection in children under two years of age. Many studies have shown that asymptomatic colonization with *C. difficile* is common among young children, especially those less than 12 months of age.[27–34] These colonizing strains can be either toxigenic or non-toxigenic, although colonization with non-toxigenic strains is more common.[34–38] Colonization rates are highest among neonates, in whom studies have documented the presence of the organism in 30–70% of infants in the first year of life.[39–41] Colonization rates in this age group are higher among formula-fed infants compared with breastfed infants.[29,42–44] Over the first two years of life, colonization rates slowly fall; the presumption is that the gradual development of the eventual adult colonic microflora results in the eviction of *C. difficile* as a commensal organism.[40] By the time children are two years of age, colonization rates are approximately 0–3%, similar to the rate seen among adults.[40] Of note, the risk of colonization among inpatients increases with the duration of hospitalization.[20]

The primary challenge that results from high colonization rates among young children is that positive tests for *C. difficile* in children under two years old may represent colonization even when diarrhea is present. Multiple studies have found that, in young children with diarrhea who test positive for *C. difficile*, another pathogen (most commonly viral) that can explain the symptoms can be identified frequently if careful investigation is undertaken.[28,45,46] Some children's hospitals restrict *C. difficile* testing in patients less than 12 months of age for this reason.[47] Experts have argued that true CDI in children under two years of age is very rare, and that it is especially unlikely in infants under one year old unless there is Hirschsprung disease or another severe motility disorder.[48]

A related challenge is deciding which pediatric patients with diarrhea should be tested for CDI. Only patients with clinically significant diarrhea should be tested, because testing patients without diarrhea only identifies colonization and decreases the test's positive predictive value.[49] In adults, clinically significant diarrhea has often been defined as the passage of three or more loose or watery bowel movements in a 24-hour period[50,51]; however, strict criteria cannot be applied to all cases, and the hallmark is a sustained change in bowel movement consistency and/or frequency without other identified causes.[49] There is no validated definition of clinically significant diarrhea in children. The Society for Healthcare Epidemiology of America (SHEA) compendium of strategies to prevent CDI in acute care hospitals recommends that, because of the high prevalence of asymptomatic carriage of toxigenic *C. difficile*, testing is not advised for children less than one year old, and that testing in young children should be accompanied by testing for alternative causes of diarrhea, especially norovirus and rotavirus.[49]

A final set of challenges associated with CDI is defining the optimal prevention strategies, although these challenges are similar for healthcare settings that provide care to adults. Areas of ongoing debate include strategies for hand hygiene and environmental disinfection as well as the approach to isolation precautions. The SHEA compendium recommends hand hygiene be performed using either soap and water or an alcohol-based hand hygiene product when caring for patients with CDI in routine or endemic settings.[49] However, in outbreak or hyperendemic settings, soap and water should be used preferentially.[49] Alcohol is not sporicidal, but it is superior for hand hygiene against organisms that do not form spores. Gloves are effective at preventing *C. difficile* contamination of the hands,[20] and studies have not demonstrated increases in CDI rates associated with the introduction of alcohol-based hand rubs.[52–54] Facilities must make their own risk assessment in balancing the potential benefits of soap and water handwashing in removing spores from the hands against the potential decrease in hand hygiene adherence when soap and water is the preferred method.[55] Similarly, data are conflicting as to whether inactivation of environmental spores is necessary to prevent transmission of *C. difficile* in endemic settings, although a prior room occupant with CDI has been found to be an independent risk factor for *C. difficile* acquisition in the hospital.[56] Contamination is found frequently on surfaces such as bedrails, overbed tables, and floors, in addition to patient care equipment (e.g., thermometers and stethoscopes) and frequently touched items (e.g., call buttons, doorknobs, and infusion pumps).[19,49] The SHEA compendium recommends that facilities consider using a 1:10 dilution of sodium hypochlorite or other product with an Environmental Protection Agency (EPA)-approved claim for *C. difficile* sporicidal activity in outbreak and hyperendemic settings.[49]

Finally, while contact precautions are recommended for patients with CDI to prevent transmission of the organism,[49] the optimal duration of isolation precautions remains unknown. The SHEA compendium and CDC currently recommend continuing contact precautions for the duration of illness (i.e., until diarrhea ceases).[49,57] However, patients with *C. difficile* are known to shed the organism after resolution of symptoms, and this shedding can last for several weeks or longer.[58] Therefore, some experts have suggested continuing contact precautions for at least 48 hours after diarrhea resolves, and potentially until hospital discharge if CDI incidence remains higher than institutional goals despite adoption of standard prevention measures.[49]

Norovirus

Norovirus presents a number of challenges in the healthcare environment. The inability to cultivate norovirus *in vitro* has hampered efforts to study topics such as susceptibility to antiseptic and disinfectant agents, but surrogate viruses (such as feline calicivirus) have often been used for this purpose. Hand hygiene is the most important method to prevent norovirus transmission. However, evidence suggests that alcohol-based hand sanitizers at typical ethanol concentrations do not effectively remove norovirus or surrogate viruses from the hands.[59–61] In contrast, soap and water handwashing has been shown to be more effective than alcohol for this purpose.[62] For these reasons, CDC has suggested soap and water as the most effective hand hygiene method when caring for patients with norovirus infection.[22]

Contaminated environmental surfaces can serve as a reservoir for continued transmission of norovirus in healthcare facilities, and studies in pediatric wards have demonstrated the presence of norovirus on a variety of high-touch surfaces, including light switches, door handles, and telephones.[63] However, traditional hospital disinfectants (such as quaternary ammonium compounds) do not effectively inactivate non-enveloped viruses such as norovirus.[64] Sodium hypochlorite (bleach) has improved efficacy at inactivating these viruses[65,66]; for this reason, the CDC norovirus outbreak management guideline recommends that either chlorine bleach solution (at a concentration of 1,000–5,000 parts per million) or another disinfectant registered with the EPA as effective against norovirus be used to disinfect environmental surfaces (after cleaning to remove any organic material such as feces).[22]

Individuals with norovirus gastroenteritis are known to shed virus for a period of time after symptoms resolve. In healthy individuals this shedding may last several weeks, but the peak shedding occurs one to three days after onset of illness.[67] Infants (particularly those less than six months of age) may also shed virus longer than older children.[68] In immunocompromised hosts, this shedding can be prolonged over months to years.[67,69,70] One challenge for infection prevention is determining whether shedding after resolution of symptoms contributes meaningfully to transmission. While chronic shedders could serve as reservoirs for transmission,[71] there is some evidence to suggest that symptomatic patients make the highest contribution to healthcare-associated transmission of norovirus.[72] The assumption is that the presence of symptoms such as vomiting and diarrhea facilitates greater environmental contamination with the virus, facilitating further spread.[73] It remains unknown whether prolonging the duration of isolation precautions in patients at high risk of prolonged shedding (e.g., infants and immunocompromised hosts) can reduce transmission of norovirus in healthcare settings. However, the CDC outbreak management guideline does recommend that hospitalized patients with norovirus be isolated until 24–48 hours after symptom resolution, and that healthcare personnel with norovirus gastroenteritis be excluded from work during their illness and for 48–72 hours following the resolution of their symptoms.[22]

A final challenge in pediatric healthcare settings is preventing transmission of norovirus during gatherings in which food is served. While norovirus can cause infections throughout the year, there is a seasonal pattern of increased activity during the winter months.[22] Since several holidays occur during this timeframe, it is common for hospitals caring for children to stage activities such as holiday gatherings that could pose a risk for transmission of norovirus related to shared food sources and close contact between individuals. Best practice for these events includes exclusion of individuals with active vomiting or diarrhea, as well as strategies such as employing food servers and wrapping ready-to-eat items to minimize bare-handed contact with these foods.[74]

Suggested Approaches

Clostridioides difficile

The SHEA compendium offers a set of recommended strategies for the prevention of CDI.[49] Table 5.1 summarizes these core strategies. In addition to the basic prevention measures, healthcare professionals who work in settings where children are cared for should consider the following approaches:

- Perform CDI surveillance using the same definitions as for adults:
  - Hospital-onset CDI (HO-CDI): for laboratory-identified events (as defined by CDC), case occurs more than three days after admission to the facility; express rate as number of cases per 10,000 patient days (at a minimum, all hospitals should perform surveillance for HO-CDI).
  - Community onset, healthcare facility-associated (CO-HCFA) CDI: cases occurring within 30 days after discharge from a healthcare facility.

TABLE 5.1 Core Strategies for the Prevention of CDI

PREVENTION STRATEGY	RATIONALE
Encourage appropriate use of antimicrobials.	Antibiotic exposure is the most important modifiable risk factor for CDI.
Use contact precautions for patients with CDI (single room preferred).	Gloves and gowns prevent contamination of hands and clothing of healthcare workers.
Ensure cleaning and disinfection of equipment and the environment.	Surfaces and equipment contaminated with *C. difficile* spores are potential reservoirs for transmission.
Implement a lab-based alert system to notify infection prevention and clinical staff about newly diagnosed CDI cases.	Initiating contact precautions in a timely manner can reduce transmission risk.
Conduct surveillance for CDI and report the data to key stakeholders.	Sharing data increases awareness and can help empower needed changes in prevention strategies.
Provide education about CDI to healthcare personnel, environmental service personnel, and patients and families.	Teaching about modes of transmission, risk factors, and prevention strategies may help reduce CDI rates and risk of transmission.
Measure compliance with hand hygiene and contact precautions.	Auditing process measures facilitates targeted education and interventions, and sharing these data can drive performance improvement.

  - Community-associated (CA) CDI: cases occurring either more than 30 days after discharge or present on admission (i.e., the event occurs prior to day 4 of hospitalization).
- Exclude cases under two years of age from surveillance data (because these positive tests probably represent colonization rather than true CDI).
- Create a laboratory policy to reject requests to test formed stool specimens for *C. difficile* (i.e., only test diarrheal stool).
- Restrict routine *C. difficile* tests in patients <12 months of age unless in an outbreak situation, or if the child has an underlying severe chronic gastrointestinal motility disorder (or, if permitted, provide specific language with the result indicating that positive tests in this age group probably represent colonization rather than infection).
- In children with diarrhea who are one to two years of age, only test for *C. difficile* after other infectious and non-infectious causes of diarrhea have been excluded (e.g., norovirus, rotavirus).

- In patients receiving laxatives or stool softeners, consider discontinuing these medications for at least 24 hours and monitoring stool output and consistency prior to sending a *C. difficile* test (to avoid detecting colonization in patients whose diarrhea may be related to the use of these medications).
- Ensure that an antimicrobial stewardship program (ASP) is in place, and include CDI rates as a key outcome measure for the ASP to track.
- During outbreaks or in hyperendemic settings, perform hand hygiene with soap and water as the preferred method when exiting the room of a patient with CDI.
- During CDI outbreaks or in hyperendemic settings, use a sporicidal disinfectant or diluted sodium hypochlorite for environmental disinfection.
- Create an algorithm for discontinuation of contact precautions to assist infection preventionists and clinical staff (Figure 5.1 displays one example of such an algorithm).

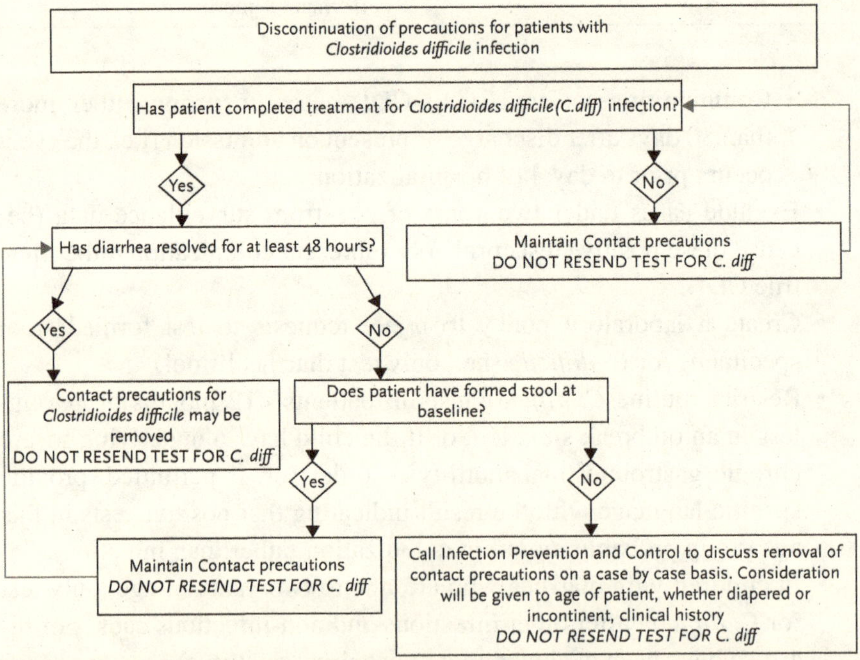

FIGURE 5.1 Example algorithm for discontinuation of isolation precautions.

Norovirus

The key strategies for preventing norovirus transmission and outbreaks in healthcare settings are based on general principles of sound infection prevention practices. Table 5.2 summarizes the most important steps to curb the spread of norovirus in healthcare facilities. In addition to these prevention measures, healthcare professionals who work in settings where children receive care should consider the following steps:

TABLE 5.2 Suggested Steps to Prevent Spread of Norovirus

PREVENTION STRATEGY	RATIONALE
Wash hands with soap and water for a minimum of 20 seconds before and after contact with infected patients.	Alcohol-based hand rubs are less effective at removing norovirus from the hands.
Use contact precautions for patients with norovirus gastroenteritis and continue isolation until 24–48 hours after resolution of symptoms.	Peak shedding occurs in the first 1–3 days after onset of symptoms but can continue after symptoms resolve.
Do not cohort symptomatic patients with patients who do not have gastroenteritis; during outbreaks, consider cohorting staff so that those caring for patients with symptomatic gastroenteritis do not care for patients without gastroenteritis.	Minimize transmission from those with symptomatic gastroenteritis to unaffected individuals.
Disinfect potentially contaminated environmental surfaces using chlorine bleach or another EPA-registered disinfectant with a label claim against norovirus.	Quaternary ammonium compounds are less effective at inactivating norovirus.
Exclude healthcare workers with suspected norovirus gastroenteritis from work during illness and for 48–72 hours after resolution of symptoms.	Minimize risk of transmission to patients by excluding affected staff during peak shedding timeframe.
Ensure food safety procedures are followed during outbreaks or periods of increased norovirus circulation.	Minimizing bare-hands contact with ready-to-eat foods can reduce the risk of transmission.
Report all outbreaks promptly to public health officials.	Early identification and notification facilitates understanding of local epidemiology and implementation of control measures.

- Remind clinical staff to promptly notify Infection Prevention and Control when multiple cases of gastroenteritis are seen among patients or healthcare workers in a given area.
- Develop a visual reminder for staff to wash their hands with soap and water upon exiting the room of a patient with suspected norovirus infection (e.g., post a handwashing sign on the door).
- Audit hand hygiene practices and adherence to contact precautions and regularly provide these data to clinical staff.
- Ensure that the facility has an adequate supply of disinfectant with an EPA label claim against norovirus, and deploy this disinfectant promptly to units with cases of norovirus, with a focus on increasing frequency of cleaning (especially for bathrooms and high-touch surfaces).
- Work with Occupational Health Services personnel to reinforce return-to-work policy (exclusion for 48–72 hours after resolution of symptoms) for employees and clinical staff after an episode of gastroenteritis.
- At the onset of norovirus season (typically late fall or early winter), send a reminder notification to all staff about basic food safety measures (e.g., using individually wrapped food items at group gatherings). Handout 5.1 is provided as an example of such a communication.

Approach to the Clinical Scenario

In the scenario outlined at the beginning of this chapter, the six-month-old infant in the NICU is likely to be colonized asymptomatically with *C. difficile*, and norovirus is the more likely etiology of the increased colostomy output. Staff caring for the patient should be reminded to perform hand hygiene using soap and water. Contact precautions should be instituted because of the presence of diarrhea (and the positive test for norovirus), but they would not be directed specifically at prevention of *C. difficile* transmission in this context. The isolation precautions could be removed 24–48 hours after the diarrhea has resolved.

HANDOUT 5.1 Example Staff Communication Messaging to Decrease Norovirus

Alert: Norovirus

S	Infection Prevention & Control would like to remind staff that **norovirus** season has arrived. **Norovirus** is circulating in the community and has caused at least one large outbreak, according to public health officials.
B	Norovirus, the most common cause of gastroenteritis in the U.S., typically circulates every winter and spring and can cause outbreaks of Gl illness (nausea, vomiting, diarrhea) among patients and staff. Norovirus is extremely contagious—as few as 18 viral particles may be sufficient to cause infection. Infection is characterized by nausea, vomiting, and diarrhea. Symptoms usually begin 1–2 days after exposure (often very acutely) and last about 24–72 hours. Transmission is person-to-person; virus is passed in the stool and vomitus of infected people from onset of illness until at least several days after symptoms resolve.
A	• Hand hygiene is key to preventing transmission of norovirus. Handwashing with soap and water for at least 20 seconds is preferred over alcohol-based hand sanitizers, when available. • Patients with Gl illness consistent with or confirmed as norovirus should be maintained on contact precautions until 24–48 hours after complete resolution of symptoms. Family members of patients should not visit common areas (e.g., kitchen, playrooms). • Ill persons should be advised to stay home and increase fluid intake to prevent dehydration until their symptoms have resolved, regardless of whether a specific etiological agent has been identified. • Bathrooms and frequently touched surfaces in the environment of a patient or staff member with norovirus should be disinfected regularly with bleach wipes.
R	**Recommendations for safe food handling to reduce the risk of norovirus transmission**: • Have easy access to soap and water or alcohol-based hand rubs where food is served. • Perform hand hygiene before going through a buffet line, before eating, and before reaching into bowls of individually wrapped or unwrapped items (e.g., cookies, candy). • Pre-packaged, individually wrapped food items for meetings, conferences, and parties are strongly encouraged. • Consider using food servers for holiday events. • Leftover shared food should be discarded and not saved for a later time. • Page Infection Prevention and Control if you become aware of any clusters of Gl illness among patients, staff, or visitors in your work area. **Healthcare workers with presumed norovirus**: • Healthcare providers with presumed norovirus infection may not return to work until 3 days after symptoms resolve.

Unresolved Issues

Clostridiodes difficile

There are several issues related to CDI prevention that remain unresolved. The utility of personal protective equipment (gowns and/or gloves) for family members or visitors to the rooms of patients with CDI is unknown.[49] SHEA has provided expert guidance about isolation precautions for visitors; for visitors of patients with enteric pathogens such as *C. difficile*, the use of contact precautions was suggested as a measure to protect them from acquiring pathogens that can be potentially harmful.[75] However, the guidance document also acknowledged that for parents, guardians, or visitors with extended stays (including overnight visitation, as is common in a pediatric setting), the use of personal protective equipment in this context may not be practical. If family members and visitors perform hand hygiene on exiting the room and do not visit the rooms of other patients, the additional benefit of gowns and gloves for preventing transmission remains unclear. Hand hygiene should be emphasized for these individuals as the primary prevention strategy. A second issue that requires more research is the role of no-touch disinfection technologies such as ultraviolet light or hydrogen peroxide vapor, which are capable of killing spores. Although several studies have shown them to be effective at reducing environmental contamination,[76] the same result can be achieved with manual cleaning with a sporicidal disinfectant. While they may play a role as an adjunct to standard environmental cleaning and disinfection, it remains unclear at this time whether these newer technologies should be incorporated routinely for the prevention of transmission of *C. difficile*.

Norovirus

One important and unresolved issue is whether to extend the duration of contact precautions for norovirus in patients at high risk of prolonged shedding, such as immunocompromised hosts. The rationale for doing so would be to protect other patients who may be at high risk for severe disease (particularly if the index case is on a unit with other immunocompromised patients), given the expectation of prolonged shedding of an extremely contagious virus. If this option is being considered, one strategy adopted by some children's hospitals is to require a negative stool polymerase chain reaction (PCR) test prior to removing isolation precautions. The downside of this approach is that it can result in a child remaining on contact precautions for many months; individualized strategies could be considered (within the context of an institution's existing infection prevention policies) to allow a pediatric patient to have occasional time out of the room under a certain set of guidelines (e.g., trips outside to the garden at times when fewer other patients are expected to be present). In addition, the challenges regarding the use of personal protective equipment for family and visitors in the room of patients with norovirus are similar to those described earlier for *C. difficile*. Hand hygiene with soap and water should be emphasized for family and visitors as the most important strategy to prevent acquisition and spread of norovirus.

References

1. Kim J, Smathers SA, Prasad P, Leckerman KH, Coffin S, Zaoutis T. Epidemiological features of *Clostridium difficile*-associated disease among inpatients at children's hospitals in the United States, 2001–2006. *Pediatrics*. 2008;122(6):1266–1270.
2. Nylund CM, Goudie A, Garza JM, Fairbrother G, Cohen MB. *Clostridium difficile* infection in hospitalized children in the United States. *Arch Pediatr Adolesc Med*. 2011;165(5):451–457.
3. Zilberberg MD, Shorr AF, Kollef MH. Increase in *Clostridium difficile*-related hospitalizations among infants in the United States, 2000–2005. *Pediatr Infect Dis J*. 2008;27(12):1111–1113.
4. Centers for Disease Control and Prevention. Antibiotic resistance threats in the United States, 2013. Available from: https://stacks.cdc.gov/view/cdc/20705. Accessed October 21, 2018.
5. Pokorn M, Radsel A, Cizman M, et al. Severe *Clostridium difficile*-associated disease in children. *Pediatr Infect Dis J*. 2008;27(10):944–946.
6. Sammons JS, Localio R, Xiao R, Coffin SE, Zaoutis T. *Clostridium difficile* infection is associated with increased risk of death and prolonged hospitalization in children. *Clin Infect Dis*. 2013;57(1):1–8.
7. Langley JM, LeBlanc JC, Hanakowski M, Goloubeva O. The role of *Clostridium difficile* and viruses as causes of nosocomial diarrhea in children. *Infect Control Hosp Epidemiol*. 2002;23(11):660–664.
8. Oguz F, Uysal G, Dasdemir S, Oskovi H, Vidinlisan S. The role of *Clostridium difficile* in childhood nosocomial diarrhea. *Scand J Infect Dis*. 2001;33(10):731–733.
9. Han VK, Sayed H, Chance GW, Brabyn DG, Shaheed WA. An outbreak of *Clostridium difficile* necrotizing enterocolitis: a case for oral vancomycin therapy? *Pediatrics*. 1983;71(6):935–941.
10. Brunetto AL, Pearson AD, Craft AW, Pedler SJ. *Clostridium difficile* in an oncology unit. *Arch Dis Child*. 1988;63(8):979–981.
11. Sandora TJ, Fung M, Flaherty K, et al. Epidemiology and risk factors for *Clostridium difficile* infection in children. *Pediatr Infect Dis J*. 2011;30(7):580–584.
12. Tai E, Richardson LC, Townsend J, Howard E, McDonald LC. *Clostridium difficile* infection among children with cancer. *Pediatr Infect Dis J*. 2011;30(7):610–612.

13. Pant C, Anderson MP, Deshpande A, et al. Health care burden of *Clostridium difficile* infection in hospitalized children with inflammatory bowel disease. *Inflamm Bowel Dis*. 2013;19(5):1080–1085.
14. Vesikari T, Isolauri E, Maki M, Gronroos P. *Clostridium difficile* in young children. Association with antibiotic usage. *Acta Paediatr Scand*. 1984;73(1):86–91.
15. Thompson CM, Jr., Gilligan PH, Fisher MC, Long SS. *Clostridium difficile* cytotoxin in a pediatric population. *Am J Dis Child*. 1983;137(3):271–274.
16. Freedberg DE, Lamouse-Smith ES, Lightdale JR, Jin Z, Yang YX, Abrams JA. Use of acid suppression medication is associated with risk for *C. difficile* infection in infants and children: a population-based study. *Clin Infect Dis*. 2015;61(6):912–917.
17. Nylund CM, Eide M, Gorman GH. Association of *Clostridium difficile* infections with acid suppression medications in children. *J Pediatr*. 2014;165(5):979–84 e1.
18. Fekety R, Kim KH, Brown D, Batts DH, Cudmore M, Silva J, Jr. Epidemiology of antibiotic-associated colitis; isolation of *Clostridium difficile* from the hospital environment. *Am J Med*. 1981;70(4):906–908.
19. Gerding DN, Muto CA, Owens RC, Jr. Measures to control and prevent *Clostridium difficile* infection. *Clin Infect Dis*. 2008;46(Suppl 1):S43–S49.
20. McFarland LV, Mulligan ME, Kwok RY, Stamm WE. Nosocomial acquisition of *Clostridium difficile* infection. *N Engl J Med*. 1989;320(4):204–210.
21. Johnson S, Gerding DN, Olson MM, et al. Prospective, controlled study of vinyl glove use to interrupt *Clostridium difficile* nosocomial transmission. *Am J Med*. 1990;88(2):137–140.
22. Division of Viral Diseases, National Center for Immunization and Respiratory Diseases, Centers for Disease Control and Prevention. Updated norovirus outbreak management and disease prevention guidelines. *MMWR Recomm Rep*. 2011;60(RR-3):1–18.
23. Siebenga JJ, Vennema H, Zheng DP, et al. Norovirus illness is a global problem: emergence and spread of norovirus GII.4 variants, 2001–2007. *J Infect Dis*. 2009;200(5):802–812.
24. Iturriza-Gomara M, Lopman B. Norovirus in healthcare settings. *Curr Opin Infect Dis*. 2014;27(5):437–443.
25. Teunis PF, Moe CL, Liu P, et al. Norwalk virus: how infectious is it? *J Med Virol*. 2008;80(8):1468–1476.
26. Centers for Disease Control and Prevention. Recurring norovirus outbreaks in a long-term residential treatment facility—Oregon, 2007. *MMWR*. 2009;58(25):694–698.
27. Bolton RP, Tait SK, Dear PR, Losowsky MS. Asymptomatic neonatal colonisation by *Clostridium difficile*. *Arch Dis Child*. 1984;59(5):466–472.
28. Tang P, Roscoe M, Richardson SE. Limited clinical utility of *Clostridium difficile* toxin testing in infants in a pediatric hospital. *Diagn Microbiol Infect Dis*. 2005;52(2):91–94.
29. Tullus K, Aronsson B, Marcus S, Mollby R. Intestinal colonization with *Clostridium difficile* in infants up to 18 months of age. *Eur J Clin Microbiol Infect Dis*. 1989;8(5):390–393.
30. Tvede M, Schiotz PO, Krasilnikoff PA. Incidence of *Clostridium difficile* in hospitalized children. A prospective study. *Acta Paediatr Scand*. 1990;79(3):292–299.

31. Phua TJ, Rogers TR, Pallett AP. Prospective study of *Clostridium difficile* colonization and paracresol detection in the stools of babies on a special care unit. *J Hyg (Lond).* 1984;93(1):17–25.
32. Donta ST, Myers MG. *Clostridium difficile* toxin in asymptomatic neonates. *J Pediatr.* 1982;100(3):431–434.
33. Elstner CL, Lindsay AN, Book LS, Matsen JM. Lack of relationship of *Clostridium difficile* to antibiotic-associated diarrhea in children. *Pediatr Infect Dis.* 1983;2(5):364–366.
34. Delmee M, Verellen G, Avesani V, Francois G. *Clostridium difficile* in neonates: serogrouping and epidemiology. *Eur J Pediatr.* 1988;147(1):36–40.
35. Rousseau C, Lemee L, Le Monnier A, Poilane I, Pons JL, Collignon A. Prevalence and diversity of *Clostridium difficile* strains in infants. *J Med Microbiol.* 2011;60(Pt 8):1112–1118.
36. Toma S, Lesiak G, Magus M, Lo HL, Delmee M. Serotyping of *Clostridium difficile. J Clin Microbiol.* 1988;26(3):426–428.
37. Larson HE, Barclay FE, Honour P, Hill ID. Epidemiology of *Clostridium difficile* in infants. *J Infect Dis.* 1982;146(6):727–733.
38. Ellis ME, Mandal BK, Dunbar EM, Bundell KR. *Clostridium difficile* and its cytotoxin in infants admitted to hospital with infectious gastroenteritis. *Br Med J (Clin Res Ed).* 1984;288(6416):524–526.
39. Al-Jumaili IJ, Shibley M, Lishman AH, Record CO. Incidence and origin of *Clostridium difficile* in neonates. *J Clin Microbiol.* 1984;19(1):77–78.
40. Jangi S, Lamont JT. Asymptomatic colonization by *Clostridium difficile* in infants: implications for disease in later life. *J Pediatr Gastroenterol Nutr.* 2010;51(1):2–7.
41. Tamma PD, Sandora TJ. *Clostridium difficile* infection in children: current state and unanswered questions. *J Pediatric Infect Dis Soc.* 2012;1(3):230–243.
42. Borriello SP. 12th C. L. Oakley lecture. Pathogenesis of *Clostridium difficile* infection of the gut. *J Med Microbiol.* 1990;33(4):207–215.
43. Penders J, Stobberingh EE, van den Brandt PA, van Ree R, Thijs C. Toxigenic and non-toxigenic *Clostridium difficile*: determinants of intestinal colonisation and role in childhood atopic manifestations. *Gut.* 2008;57(7):1025–1026.
44. Stark PL, Lee A, Parsonage BD. Colonization of the large bowel by *Clostridium difficile* in healthy infants: quantitative study. *Infect Immun.* 1982;35(3):895–899.
45. El Feghaly RE, Stauber JL, Tarr PI, Haslam DB. Viral co-infections are common and are associated with higher bacterial burden in children with *Clostridium difficile* infection. *J Pediatr Gastroenterol Nutr.* 2013;57(6):813–816.
46. Lukkarinen H, Eerola E, Ruohola A, et al. *Clostridium difficile* ribotype 027-associated disease in children with norovirus infection. *Pediatr Infect Dis J.* 2009;28(9):847–848.
47. Kociolek LK, Sandora TJ. National variability in surveillance, testing, and infection prevention for *Clostridium difficile* infection in pediatric populations. *Am J Infect Control.* 2013;41(10):933–935.
48. Faust SN, Wilcox MH, Banaszkiewicz A, Bouza E, Raymond J, Gerding DN. Lack of evidence for an unmet need to treat *Clostridium difficile* infection in infants aged

<2 years: expert recommendations on how to address this issue. *Clin Infect Dis.* 2015;60(6):912–918.

49. Dubberke ER, Carling P, Carrico R, et al. Strategies to prevent *Clostridium difficile* infections in acute care hospitals: 2014 update. *Infect Control Hosp Epidemiol.* 2014;35(6):628–645.
50. Johnson S, Louie TJ, Gerding DN, et al. Vancomycin, metronidazole, or tolevamer for *Clostridium difficile* infection: results from two multinational, randomized, controlled trials. *Clin Infect Dis.* 2014;59(3):345–354.
51. Dubberke ER, Han Z, Bobo L, et al. Impact of clinical symptoms on interpretation of diagnostic assays for *Clostridium difficile* infections. *J Clin Microbiol.* 2011;49(8):2887–2893.
52. Boyce JM, Ligi C, Kohan C, Dumigan D, Havill NL. Lack of association between the increased incidence of *Clostridium difficile*-associated disease and the increasing use of alcohol-based hand rubs. *Infect Control Hosp Epidemiol.* 2006;27(5):479–483.
53. Kaier K, Hagist C, Frank U, Conrad A, Meyer E. Two time-series analyses of the impact of antibiotic consumption and alcohol-based hand disinfection on the incidences of nosocomial methicillin-resistant *Staphylococcus aureus* infection and *Clostridium difficile* infection. *Infect Control Hosp Epidemiol.* 2009;30(4):346–353.
54. Knight N, Strait T, Anthony N, et al. *Clostridium difficile* colitis: a retrospective study of incidence and severity before and after institution of an alcohol-based hand rub policy. *Am J Infect Control.* 2010;38(7):523–528.
55. Boyce JM, Pittet D, Healthcare Infection Control Practices Advisory Committee, HICPAC/APIC/SHEA/IDSA Task Force. Guideline for hand hygiene in health-care settings. Recommendations of the Healthcare Infection Control Practices Advisory Committee and the HICPAC/SHEA/APIC/IDSA Hand Hygiene Task Force. Society for Healthcare Epidemiology of America/Association for Professionals in Infection Control/Infectious Diseases Society of America. *MMWR Recomm Rep.* 2002;51(RR-16):1–45, quiz CE1–4.
56. Shaughnessy MK, Micielli RL, DePestel DD, et al. Evaluation of hospital room assignment and acquisition of *Clostridium difficile* infection. *Infect Control Hosp Epidemiol.* 2011;32(3):201–206.
57. Siegel JD, Rhinehart E, Jackson M, Chiarello L, Health Care Infection Control Practices Advisory Committee. 2007 Guideline for isolation precautions: preventing transmission of infectious agents in healthcare settings. Available from: https://www.cdc.gov/hicpac/2007IP/2007isolationPrecautions.html. Accessed October 21, 2018.
58. Sethi AK, Al-Nassir WN, Nerandzic MM, Bobulsky GS, Donskey CJ. Persistence of skin contamination and environmental shedding of *Clostridium difficile* during and after treatment of *C. difficile* infection. *Infect Control Hosp Epidemiol.* 2010;31(1):21–27.
59. Sickbert-Bennett EE, Weber DJ, Gergen-Teague MF, Sobsey MD, Samsa GP, Rutala WA. Comparative efficacy of hand hygiene agents in the reduction of bacteria and viruses. *Am J Infect Control.* 2005;33(2):67–77.
60. Kampf G, Grotheer D, Steinmann J. Efficacy of three ethanol-based hand rubs against feline calicivirus, a surrogate virus for norovirus. *J Hosp Infect.* 2005;60(2):144–149.
61. Lages SL, Ramakrishnan MA, Goyal SM. In-vivo efficacy of hand sanitisers against feline calicivirus: a surrogate for norovirus. *J Hosp Infect.* 2008;68(2):159–163.

62. Liu P, Yuen Y, Hsiao HM, Jaykus LA, Moe C. Effectiveness of liquid soap and hand sanitizer against Norwalk virus on contaminated hands. *Appl Environ Microbiol.* 2010;76(2):394–399.
63. Gallimore CI, Taylor C, Gennery AR, et al. Contamination of the hospital environment with gastroenteric viruses: comparison of two pediatric wards over a winter season. *J Clin Microbiol.* 2008;46(9):3112–3115.
64. Doultree JC, Druce JD, Birch CJ, Bowden DS, Marshall JA. Inactivation of feline calicivirus, a Norwalk virus surrogate. *J Hosp Infect.* 1999;41(1):51–57.
65. Duizer E, Bijkerk P, Rockx B, De Groot A, Twisk F, Koopmans M. Inactivation of caliciviruses. *Appl Environ Microbiol.* 2004;70(8):4538–4543.
66. Girard M, Ngazoa S, Mattison K, Jean J. Attachment of noroviruses to stainless steel and their inactivation, using household disinfectants. *J Food Prot.* 2010;73(2):400–404.
67. Glass RI, Parashar UD, Estes MK. Norovirus gastroenteritis. *N Engl J Med.* 2009;361(18):1776–1785.
68. Murata T, Katsushima N, Mizuta K, Muraki Y, Hongo S, Matsuzaki Y. Prolonged norovirus shedding in infants < or = 6 months of age with gastroenteritis. *Pediatr Infect Dis J.* 2007;26(1):46–49.
69. Bok K, Green KY. Norovirus gastroenteritis in immunocompromised patients. *N Engl J Med.* 2012;367(22):2126–2132.
70. Henke-Gendo C, Harste G, Juergens-Saathoff B, Mattner F, Deppe H, Heim A. New real-time PCR detects prolonged norovirus excretion in highly immunosuppressed patients and children. *J Clin Microbiol.* 2009;47(9):2855–2862.
71. Sukhrie FH, Siebenga JJ, Beersma MF, Koopmans M. Chronic shedders as reservoir for nosocomial transmission of norovirus. *J Clin Microbiol.* 2010;48(11):4303–4305.
72. Sukhrie FH, Teunis P, Vennema H, et al. Nosocomial transmission of norovirus is mainly caused by symptomatic cases. *Clin Infect Dis.* 2012;54(7):931–937.
73. Teunis PF, Sukhrie FH, Vennema H, Bogerman J, Beersma MF, Koopmans MP. Shedding of norovirus in symptomatic and asymptomatic infections. *Epidemiol Infect.* 2015;143(8):1710–1717.
74. Barclay L, Park GW, Vega E, et al. Infection control for norovirus. *Clin Microbiol Infect.* 2014;20(8):731–740.
75. Munoz-Price LS, Banach DB, Bearman G, et al. Isolation precautions for visitors. *Infect Control Hosp Epidemiol.* 2015;36(7):747–758.
76. Otter JA, Yezli S, Perl TM, Barbut F, French GL. The role of "no-touch" automated room disinfection systems in infection prevention and control. *J Hosp Infect.* 2013;83(1):1–13.

6 | Prevention of Infections with Multidrug-Resistant (MDR) Organisms

LORRY G. RUBIN AND GHOLAMABBAS AMIN OSTOVAR

Background

Multidrug-resistant organisms (MDROs) are a major concern in pediatric inpatients because infections with these pathogens may cause infections that are severe and difficult to treat because of a limited armamentarium of antimicrobial agents. For most infections, antimicrobial therapy is initiated empirically prior to the results of cultures and susceptibility testing, and commonly prescribed empiric choices lack activity against MDR pathogens. This may result in a delay of initiation of antimicrobial therapy active against the pathogen and an increase in morbidity and mortality. Therefore, prevention of transmission and infection with MDROs is of paramount importance. Although a number of microorganisms can be categorized as MDR, this chapter will focus upon methicillin-resistant *Staphylococcus aureus* (MRSA), MDR Gram-negative bacilli (GNB), and vancomycin-resistant enterococci (VRE).

Certain principles for prevention of MDR infections are applicable for all pathogens. The first line of prevention of MDR infections is prevention of exposure. Preventing exposure requires adherence to standard infection prevention practices, including hand hygiene before and after contact with the patient or the patient care environment. Direct or indirect contact between MDR-colonized or -infected patients and other patients should be minimized. This may involve identification of colonized and/or infected patients and implementation of contact isolation precautions. As patients move between units in a single healthcare facility and between facilities, MDR status should be communicated.

Prevention of colonization is central to prevention of infection because colonization is generally a prerequisite to infection. An important and potentially modifiable risk factor for colonization is antimicrobial therapy, because antimicrobial therapy disrupts the microbiome of the skin and mucosal sites, resulting in an enhanced susceptibility to colonization with microorganisms to which the patient is exposed. Creation of an ecological void with antimicrobial therapy potentiates colonization by endogenous and exogenous bacteria, including MDROs. A reduction in use of antimicrobials, particularly those with broad spectrum effectiveness, via antimicrobial stewardship efforts is of paramount importance to maintain colonization resistance to MDROs and prevent MDRO transmission. Routine and directed environmental cleaning may also play an important role in prevention of transmission.

Control measures to prevent infection with MDROs may be divided into two categories: (1) vertical—pathogen-specific interventions; and (2) horizontal—general interventions to broadly decrease pathogen transmission (Table 6.1).[1] A "horizontal" approach is a broad-based approach to reducing infections due to all pathogens, but it may be effective in decreasing infection and carriage with the MDRO(s) of interest. A pathogen-specific "vertical" approach tends to be comparatively resource-intensive and may be most appropriate in an outbreak situation and for implementation for a limited period of time. Whether pathogen-specific vertical interventions or general horizontal interventions are more effective is a debated issue, and effectiveness and cost-effectiveness may vary with the pathogen and hospital or hospital unit.

Clinical Scenario

Over the last month, two patients in a pediatric intensive care unit developed healthcare-associated methicillin-resistant *Staphylococcus aureus* (MRSA) bacteremia, and another developed a sternal wound infection with MRSA. A fourth patient has been identified as "MRSA-colonized," based on the results of an endotracheal tube culture obtained on hospital day 7. The pediatric intensivist is concerned because MRSA has rarely been identified in clinical cultures in this unit. She asks if surveillance cultures should be performed to determine the burden of MRSA in the unit. The mother of the patient with a surgical site infection wants to know how long her toddler must remain in isolation.

TABLE 6.1 Horizontal vs. Vertical Approach in MDRO Prevention

	HORIZONTAL APPROACH GENERAL INTERVENTION FOR MANY PATHOGENS	VERTICAL APPROACH INTERVENTIONS SPECIFIC FOR A PARTICULAR PATHOGEN
Potential Effect	Reduce overall nosocomial infections due to a range of pathogens	Reduce nosocomial infections with a particular pathogen(s)
Resource Utilization	Modest or marked	Marked
Indication	General increase in healthcare-associated infections due to multiple pathogens	Outbreak due to particular pathogen
Examples of Potential Components of Intervention	• Increased adherence to components of standard precautions; e.g., hand hygiene • Enhanced standard precautions; e.g., routine gown and gloves • Enhanced environmental cleaning; e.g., increase frequency of cleaning high-touch surfaces • Antimicrobial stewardship enhancements • Implementation of "bundles" of interventions to decrease categories of nosocomial infection	• Isolation precautions for patients colonized or infected with the specific pathogen • Screening patients and/or staff for the MDRO of interest • Decolonization (if feasible) • Inclusion of components of horizontal approach (see adjacent column) related to hand hygiene, isolation precautions, and environmental cleaning

Questions

Is this a MRSA outbreak? When should surveillance cultures for MRSA be performed? What anatomical sites should be screened? What is the role of decolonization for patients infected or colonized with MRSA? When can isolation precautions for MRSA be discontinued?

Key Challenges

1. For patients on contact isolation precautions due an MDRO, it is unclear if parents/caregivers should use gowns and gloves, given the probability that they were previously exposed to the pathogen and the impracticality of continuously wearing gloves and a gown for a caregiver essentially living in the room of the patient.

2. The use of contact isolation precautions poses unique challenges in a family-centered care model and for delivery of developmentally appropriate care. The risk/benefit of the use of these precautions in the absence of an ongoing outbreak or a draining lesion is unclear.
3. The duration of contact isolation precautions and criteria to discontinue precautions are not well defined, given that colonization can be prolonged and that there are cost and potential risks with the continued use of contact isolation precautions.
4. The relative roles of horizontal infection prevention strategies to decrease nosocomial infections (including those caused by MDROs) overall and vertical infection control strategies that target a specific MDRO are unclear.

Suggested Approaches

Methicillin-Resistant *Staphylococcus aureus* (MRSA)

Definition and Mechanism of Resistance

Methicillin resistance in *S. aureus* is caused by acquisition of the *mecA* gene that encodes a penicillin-binding protein, PBP2a, to which these drugs have decreased affinity. Despite this common feature, MRSA strains are heterogeneous, varying in resistance to non-β lactam antimicrobials, as well as in their propensity to colonize, cause invasive infection, and cause outbreaks of infection. Many MRSA strains belong to clonal groups defined by pulse field gel electrophoresis patterns of chromosomal DNA, e.g., USA100.

Epidemiology of MRSA Infection

S. aureus, including MRSA, is a major cause of healthcare-associated infection (HAI) in pediatric patients, particularly those in pediatric and neonatal intensive care units (ICUs) and surgical patients, and is frequently responsible for healthcare-associated outbreaks. However, in most reports, methicillin-susceptible *S. aureus* (MSSA) strains comprise the majority of *S. aureus* strains causing HAI in hospitalized children. For example, in reports of *S. aureus* infections in two different neonatal intensive care units (NICUs) during eight-year periods during the 2000s, 28% of *S. aureus* infections were caused by MRSA.[2,3] In 149 NICUs participating in the National Nosocomial Infections Surveillance System between 1995 and 2004, 23% of *S. aureus* infections were caused by MRSA.[4] Interventions designed specifically to reduce MRSA infections—that is, surveillance and contact isolation precautions with or without decolonization—may have played some role in reducing the proportion of MRSA among *S. aureus* infections in some NICUs. However, at a NICU with no MRSA-specific interventions other than contact isolation for babies with MRSA isolated from a clinical culture, the proportion of MRSA was low. During 2015 and 2016 at a level 4 NICU at a children's hospital in New York, the percentages of MRSA among all *S. aureus* infections and blood culture isolates were 16% and 19%, respectively (L. Rubin, unpublished observation). Although it represents an outlier experience, Huang et al. reported that, since 1998, over 90% of *S. aureus* isolates in a NICU in Taiwan were MRSA.[5]

Historically, MRSA was first recognized in inpatients with HAIs, and these strains are termed HA-MRSA. During the mid-1990s, distinct clones of MRSA arose in community settings and are termed community-associated MRSA (CA-MRSA).[6] CA-MRSA strains usually exhibit resistance to fewer antimicrobial agents than HA-MRSA strains. In recent years, CA-MRSA strains have become common causes of hospital-onset MRSA infections, including in NICUs. For example, from 2000 to 2008 in a NICU in New York, there was a gradual change in the predominant clones from HA-MRSA to CA-MRSA strains, with "USA300" emerging as the predominant CA-MRSA clone.[7] In another NICU, carriage of CA-MRSA was higher than with HA-MRSA.[8] MRSA strains vary in their propensity to cause clinical infections. In a study in a single NICU, babies colonized with HA-MRSA were significantly more likely to develop MRSA infections than those colonized with CA-MRSA.[8]

Risk Factors for MRSA Infection

Colonization with MRSA is considered to be a prerequisite for infection. Huang et al. compared MRSA carriage strains to clinical infection strains in individual babies in a NICU using pulsed-field gel electrophoresis and found a high correlation between colonizing strains and infecting strains, suggesting that colonizing strains are the reservoir for MRSA infections in infants.[5] Although there are multiple risk factors for MRSA infection in hospitalized children, colonization appears to be the most important one. In a meta-analysis of studies conducted primarily during the decade that started in 2000, patients in a NICU or PICU who were colonized with MRSA on admission had a relative risk of 24.2 for developing an MRSA infection during hospitalization.[9] Other NICU studies report that detection of MRSA carriage at any time during hospitalization is a risk factor for subsequent MRSA infection. In one NICU study, the risk of MRSA infection in colonized babies was 10.2%, compared to a risk of infection of 2.3% in non-colonized babies.[10] Another study found a strong association between colonization and subsequent infection with MRSA.[11] In a study of both MRSA and MSSA in a Hawaiian NICU, *S. aureus* colonization was strongly predictive of subsequent invasive infection, with infection developing in 14% of colonized infants and 0.2% of non-colonized infants.[12]

Other risk factors for MRSA infection in NICUs include overcrowding and poor adherence to hand hygiene by healthcare personnel.[13]

Colonization with MRSA

Pediatric patients in an ICU can be colonized with MRSA upon admission. In a meta-analysis of studies of colonization of MRSA in PICUs and NICUs on admission, the prevalence of MRSA colonization was 1.5% on admission to the NICU, and 3.0% on admission to a PICU.[9] Among babies in NICUs, outborn babies had a higher MRSA carriage rate upon admission than inborn babies, but outborn babies were older than inborn babies at the time of testing. Although most MRSA carriage in babies in a NICU is related to acquisition in the NICU, a small proportion of MRSA carriage in newborns is related to vertical transmission from mother to baby.[11] In a study of women pregnant at 34–36 weeks' gestation, anogenital colonization with MRSA was detected in 3.8% of women (and an additional 12.8% carried MRSA in their nares).[14] At-birth MRSA colonization was found in 2.5% of their infants, implying that there is a high transmission rate from anogenitally colonized women to their newborn infants.[14] Early MRSA colonization of newborns has also been reported following primary cesarean section.[12] Thus, acquisition of MRSA can occur early and may be vertically transmitted.

Acquisition of MRSA during ICU hospitalization accounts for a substantial proportion of the burden of MRSA colonization of PICU and NICU patients. In a meta-analysis of MRSA colonization studies, the acquisition rate of MRSA colonization was 4.1% during a NICU or PICU stay. In the NICU population alone, 6.1% of patients acquired MRSA during their stay, rates that were higher than the rates on admission.[9] In one NICU, 25% of babies acquired MRSA over the course of their NICU hospitalization.[10] In a longitudinal study of MRSA colonization and infection in a single NICU "weekly colonization pressure," defined as the ratio between the number of MRSA-positive patient-days/week and the total number of patient-days/week, correlated with MRSA transmission in the unit[15]; similar observations have also been made in an adult medical ICU.[16] In another NICU, an inverse correlation between hand hygiene adherence and MRSA colonization rate was identified.[17] Additionally, the average patient census correlated with MRSA prevalence; each additional patient in an average census was associated with a 31% greater MRSA colonization rate, an observation that was limited to the subset of patients located in single-patient rooms. Differences in MRSA carriage rates based on whether babies were housed in single rooms or in large open rooms with 9 or 14 beds were not observed. Risk factors significantly associated with MRSA carriage in NICU patients specifically include birthweight less than 1500 g, and prematurity with gestational age less than 32 weeks.[10,12] Isolated reports have documented MRSA transmission to babies during a NICU hospitalization via contaminated expressed breast milk or from contact with a family member.[18]

The duration of MRSA carriage in colonized pediatric inpatients is unclear but is probably prolonged. Among babies in a NICU, the median duration of MRSA colonization was 15.5 and 35 weeks in babies not colonized and colonized with MRSA at time of hospital discharge, respectively.[19]

Laboratory Screening for Colonization with MRSA

Monitoring the rate of clinical cultures yielding MRSA is an insensitive method for assessing the burden of MRSA in a pediatric unit. Supplementing clinical cultures with screening for carriage of MRSA significantly increases detection of MRSA-colonized pediatric patients. For example, in a PICU, the addition of weekly nasal swab screening cultures resulted in a greater than twofold higher detection of MRSA-colonized children than detection using clinical cultures alone.[20] In a NICU in which weekly nasal swab screening cultures were performed, only 12% of MRSA-colonized babies were initially detected by clinical cultures.[21]

Screening ICU patients for MRSA carriage is not a universal practice. Screening and instituting contact isolation precautions of colonized patients has reduced MRSA infection in an outbreak situation[22] but has not been shown to consistently reduce the endemic MRSA infection rate.[19] If these measures are combined with decolonization treatment, reduction in MRSA rates have been observed, but the data are limited.[2] If performed, screening can be serially performed on all patients in a unit, performed periodically, or performed only at the time when a cluster of MRSA infections occurs. Some degree of screening is performed in most NICUs, but a weekly universal screening program is less commonly employed. In a 2009 survey of U.S. NICUs with fellowship training programs, of 91 respondents, 55% of NICUs screened all patients upon admission, and 72% conducted periodic point prevalence screening.[23] In a 2006 consensus statement on the issue of MRSA in NICUs, a group of public health and hospital personnel in Chicago recommended that "infants in the NICU should be screened periodically to detect MRSA colonization. The frequency of screening should increase (e.g., to once per week) when clusters of colonization are detected; after evidence suggests a halt in transmission, it may decrease to a lower frequency (e.g., to once per month) until the investigation is over."[24] Notably, hospitals in Chicago were subject to Illinois state regulation mandating surveillance for MRSA in ICUs. In a follow-up survey of NICUs in Chicago, approximately one-half of NICUs performed weekly surveillance for MRSA and one-half performed no additional surveillance following testing upon admission.[25] None of the six PICUs in Chicago performed additional routine surveillance cultures after admission. An ongoing screening program in a NICU at Johns Hopkins Hospital in Baltimore performs weekly screening cultures on all neonates plus cultures on admission for neonates admitted from home or transferred from another hospital.[26]

In studies of detection of MRSA carriage in children, there have been variations in both the body sites sampled and the laboratory detection method employed. There is a consensus that in neonates the nares should be swabbed. In some studies, a variety of other sites were swabbed, with the umbilicus the most commonly sampled extra-nasal site in neonates. Huang et al. studied cultures of nares, umbilicus, postauricular area, axillae, and perineum and concluded that sampling of both nares and umbilicus is optimal.[5] In another study, cultures of both nares and umbilicus increased the sensitivity of MRSA detection compared to nares culture alone, although the negative predictive value of a nares culture alone was 99.4%.[25] Nasal and umbilical swabs can be cultured together to reduce the cost compared to culturing the swabs separately. In a meta-analysis of studies of MRSA carriage in pediatric patients, sampling solely the nares of NICU patients yielded a prevalence of MRSA colonization of 1.7%, which was not statistically different from the colonization rates of screening policies that included one or more additional sites.[9]

In most studies of patients in a PICU, the nares have been the site used for screening for MRSA carriage. In PICU patients, culturing nares and groin increased the sensitivity of MRSA detection, but the negative predictive value of a nares culture alone was 99%.[25] In one study of MRSA colonization upon admission to a PICU, recovery of MRSA from a pharyngeal swab, 92.6%, was significantly more sensitive than a nasal swab, 63.1%.[27]

MRSA detection can be performed by culture or a nucleic acid amplification test (NAAT). Swabs can be cultured by plating on selective media that allow rapid identification of MRSA colonies with or without prior incubation in enrichment broth.[14,25,28] Cultures on chromogenic media can be read at 18–24 hours, although sensitivity is generally higher after 48 hours of incubation.[28] An alternative to culture is detection using a NAAT, such as a polymerase chain reaction (PCR)-based assay, specific for MRSA. Such assays have the advantage of a rapid turnaround time. A meta-analysis of surveillance programs performed in NICUs and PICUs found that use of PCRs yielded an MRSA prevalence similar to the MRSA colonization detected by culture methods.[9] Culture has the advantage of isolate availability for molecular typing and antimicrobial susceptibility testing, although specimens positive using a NAAT can be reflexed to culture. Thus, either culture or NAAT testing is an acceptable method for MRSA carriage surveillance.

Prevention and Control of MRSA Infection

Principles of prevention and control of an MRSA outbreak are summarized in Box 6.1. When considering an infection prevention initiative focused specifically on reduction of MRSA infections, it is important to compare the cost and potential impact of an initiative designed to decrease both MRSA and MSSA infections. For example, a NICU that expanded a long-established screening and decolonization program for MRSA to include MSSA screening and decolonization observed a significant reduction in clinical isolates of MSSA as well as MSSA infections.[29]

Use of contact isolation precautions and hand hygiene

Contact isolation precautions with use of gowns and non-sterile gloves are generally appropriate for patients colonized or infected with MRSA, particularly in a NICU. In addition, cohorting of colonized/infected patients is advisable, along with cohorting of caregivers, if feasible. In units in which new admissions are tested for MRSA carriage, contact isolation precautions are sometimes instituted until the test for MRSA carriage proves negative. In most centers, patients with MRSA colonization or infection remain in contact isolation for the duration of hospitalization

BOX 6.1 MRSA OUTBREAK MANAGEMENT

1. Monitor rate of MRSA infection and clinical isolation of MRSA in pediatric units of interest. For units in which screening for MRSA carriage is routine, review MRSA carriage prevalence and new acquisitions for a significant increase over baseline.
2. If the infection rate is high, if there is a significant increase in infection rate or carriage rate from baseline, or if fatal infections occur, create line listings of cases. Factors to be entered include room location, clinical service caring for patient, patient major diagnoses, equipment used to care for patient (breast pump, ventilator), and personnel caring for infected patients.

   Examine line listings for commonalities. Assess environment of infected patients for possible sources.
3. Enlist/ensure administrative support for multidisciplinary management of outbreak.
4. Ensure overcrowding does not exist, or remedy overcrowding.
5. Reinforce horizontal precautions already in place, including adherence to hand hygiene and contact isolation precautions for MRSA-colonized or -infected patients, and enhance environmental cleaning and perform testing to ensure adequacy of cleaning. Document results of surveys of adherence to hand hygiene and contact isolation precautions, and environmental testing effectiveness.
6. Communicate with local health department, who may provide assistance with management of outbreak.
7. Request that the microbiology laboratory save isolates. Arrange molecular typing for epidemiological comparison of isolates to determine relatedness of isolates and the possibility of a common source.
8. Contact isolation precautions of colonized and infected patients. If feasible, cohort by location and caregivers.
9. Consider screening of patients in the unit for carriage of MRSA, if not already performed.
10. Consider decolonization of colonized and infected patients with nasal (and umbilical for babies younger than 30 days of age or residing in NICU) application of mupirocin ointment twice a day for five days.
11. Consider chlorhexidine-based washes from neck down for MRSA decolonization in children, except for premature infants younger than four weeks of age. Experience with and safety of chlorhexidine body washes in premature infants and neonates are limited.
12. Consider culturing of environment if particular areas or particular equipment are implicated in MRSA transmission.
13. Consider culture of selected hospital personnel if epidemiological data implicate one or a group of hospital personnel in transmission. Suggest mupirocin nasal and chlorhexidine washes of colonized hospital personnel. Consider furlough of colonized personnel from patient care assignments if feasible.

and upon readmission. If decolonization is attempted, it is reasonable to remove precautions if three consecutive surveillance cultures separated by at least one week (and obtained when the patient is not receiving antimicrobial therapy with activity against MRSA) are negative.[30] In a study in adults, a single negative PCR test had a high negative predictive value for the absence of MRSA carriage.[31] However, cases of recolonization of babies with MRSA during the same hospitalization have been documented. Following an outbreak in one NICU, active surveillance for MRSA carriage, along with extensive healthcare personnel involvement and education, continuous hand-hygiene training, and with contact isolation precautions for MRSA-colonized or infected babies was associated with a significant fivefold reduction of MRSA infections and number of episodes of MRSA bacteremia (as well a significant ~50% reduction in bloodstream infections with all bacteria).[22]

Decolonization with topical mupirocin

Nasal application of mupirocin ointment is the most common regimen prescribed for decolonization of MRSA-colonized inpatients. Some regimens included mupirocin application to other sites, including the umbilical stump and abraded skin.[12] In a 2009 survey related to practices in NICUs, 37% of respondents reported the use of mupirocin to decolonize all or a subgroup of MRSA-colonized or -infected neonates.[20]

Nasal mupirocin applied twice daily for five days is effective in eradicating nasal carriage of MRSA in approximately two-thirds of neonates.[10,21] In a meta-analysis of studies, this intervention was associated with a lower acquisition rate compared with those that did not use this intervention, but the difference was not significant.[9] This intervention has been associated with a decrease in overall MRSA carriage in a NICU, and there have been trends toward a reduction in rates of MRSA infection (or at least a reduction in rates of clinical cultures growing MRSA).[21] Among colonized babies who were treated with mupirocin, 3.2% developed an MRSA infection compared to infection in 16.2% of an MRSA-colonized control group not treated within mupirocin. Among mupirocin-treated MRSA-colonized babies who subsequently developed MRSA infection, all cases occurred in those in whom the decolonization regimen failed to eradicate MRSA carriage. In an experience with universal use of mupirocin prophylaxis, one NICU applied mupirocin to the nares, umbilicus, and abraded skin of all babies during their entire stay and found a significantly decreased rate of *S. aureus* (both MSSA and MRSA) infection of 0.40 infections per 1,000 hospital days compared to a rate of 1.82 prior to implementation of mupirocin use.[12] However, the program was implemented when there was an increased rate of MRSA infection that prompted the implementation of the decolonization program. In contrast, investigators at another institution concluded that nasal mupirocin treatment of babies and staff was not effective in eradicating MRSA in their NICU, but the effectiveness of this treatment in preventing clinical infection was uncertain because of the study design, and the number of patients with clinical infection was low.[32] A cost-effectiveness analysis of screening for MRSA with or without decolonization in NICUs concluded that a practice of screening, isolation, and decolonization was more cost-effective than screening and isolation alone, assuming the decolonization intervention reduces the MRSA infection rate.[33]

Use of mupirocin ointment to decolonize patients has generally been studied as one component of a bundle of interventions that may include contact isolation, emphasis on adherence to hand hygiene, enhanced environmental cleaning, and in some cases, surveillance cultures of personnel. Furthermore, use of mupirocin in a NICU or PICU setting has not been subjected to a randomized control trial. Thus, the use of mupirocin decolonization for reducing the rate of MRSA infection in NICUs is promising, but the direct role of the mupirocin intervention is uncertain.

In NICUs using mupirocin for decolonization programs, mupirocin-resistance has not generally emerged as a significant problem. In a NICU that used nasal mupirocin for several years, only 3 of 84 (3.6%) tested MRSA isolates acquired during NICU hospitalization exhibited low-level mupirocin resistance, and none had high-level resistance.[26] In a NICU with a program of universal mupirocin application, no mupirocin-resistant MRSA (or MSSA) isolates were detected.[12] However, a cluster of MRSA infections caused by a mupirocin-resistant strain has occurred in a NICU despite low mupirocin use (L. Rubin, unpublished observation). In a multicenter study in NICUs, MRSA-colonized babies treated with nasal mupirocin were not found to be at an increased risk of development of a subsequent Gram-negative infection.[34]

Chlorhexidine washes to reduce MRSA colonization and infection

Washing with chlorhexidine-impregnated cloths, with or without nasal mupirocin, has decreased the incidence of MRSA infections in adult ICUs.[35,36] Some pediatric centers have implemented chlorhexidine washes in patients in PICUs, commonly as an element of a bundle to decrease vascular catheter-related bloodstream infections. Most decolonization regimens in NICUs have not included body washes with chlorhexidine-impregnated cloths, or their use was limited.[20,21] Use in newborns and in premature neonates has been limited[37] because of contact dermatitis, concerns of potential toxicity caused by absorption of chlorhexidine through immature skin, and a previous U.S. Food and Drug Administration (FDA) product label that stated it should not be used in premature or low birthweight infants or children less than two months of age. However, in 2012, the FDA modified the labeled indications for chlorhexidine gluconate cloths or solutions to read "Use with care in premature infants or infants under 2 months of age. These products may cause irritation or chemical burns" (FDA website, http://www.fda.gov/Safety/MedWatch/SafetyInformation/Safety-RelatedDrugLabelingChanges/ucm307387.htm). Furthermore, there is a theoretical concern about the potential negative effects of chlorhexidine on the developing microbiome. In a 2014 survey of NICU Fellowship Program Directors, the majority of NICUs use chlorhexidine for skin preparation for vascular catheter placement or maintenance, but only 8–16% used chlorhexidine body washes routinely, for presurgical use, or MRSA decolonization.[38] In one NICU, topical chlorhexidine baths using chlorhexidine cloths were used in conjunction with nasal mupirocin for MRSA-colonized babies, but use was limited to infants >36 weeks gestational age or >4 weeks chronological age.[2] In another NICU, use of chlorhexidine washes in babies with birthweights more than 1000 grams and with a central venous catheter or with birthweights less than 1000 grams who were 28 days of age or older was associated with a reduction in the rate of catheter-related bloodstream infection, and no adverse effects were reported.[37] Therefore, chlorhexidine washes can be used in conjunction with nasal mupirocin for prevention of MRSA infection in MRSA colonized patients in an ICU but should be used with caution in premature neonates.

Screening of hospital staff for MRSA carriage

Transmission of MRSA within an ICU is most often attributed to transient contamination of the hands of healthcare personnel. Using whole-genome sequencing of *S. aureus* isolates, Price et al. found only a small proportion of transmission events in an adult ICU were related to nasally colonized healthcare personnel.[39] Culture of hospital personnel is generally not performed but can be considered in an outbreak situation if epidemiological data suggest that one or a group of hospital personnel may be implicated in transmission of MRSA. In one NICU with a high prevalence of MRSA colonization among NICU patients, an MRSA carriage prevalence of ~8% was found among the healthcare personnel.[15] Following an outbreak of MRSA infection in a PICU, a colonization prevalence among 61 nurses and physicians was 26.2%, with pulsed-field gel electrophoresis showing two major clusters of MRSA in staff and in patients.[40] In contrast, in a NICU with a cluster of infections caused by mupirocin-resistant MRSA, surveillance cultures of 471 personnel revealed nasal carriage of MRSA and nasal carriage of mupirocin-resistant MRSA in only 0.85% and 0.21%, respectively (L. Rubin, unpublished observations). However, in none of the outbreaks could investigators determine if there was transmission of MRSA from staff to patients. In some outbreaks, all personnel, or personnel in whom carriage is documented, have been treated with nasal application of mupirocin ointment,[32] with or without chlorhexidine-based washes, in an attempt at decolonization. If feasible, colonized personnel who are implicated in transmission should be furloughed from patient care assignments until decolonization is documented.

Multidrug-Resistant Gram-Negative Bacilli (MDR GNB)

Definition and Mechanism of Resistance

β-lactam antibiotics have been the mainstay for treatment of infections caused by GNB. Bacterial production of β-lactamase enzymes is the most important mechanism of resistance of GNB to β-lactam antibiotics.[41] Hundreds of β-lactamases with varying specificities for particular β-lactam antibiotics have been identified, and new enzymes continue to emerge. GNB that produce a β-lactamase enzyme that encodes resistance to multiple β-lactam antimicrobials, including third generation cephalosporin antimicrobials, are termed extended spectrum β-lactamase (ESBL) producers. GNB that produce an ESBL and/or exhibit resistance to multiple classes of antimicrobials are termed MDR GNB. Carbapenem-resistant GNB, particularly carbapenem-resistant enterobacteriaceae (CRE) that elaborate a carbapenemase have recently emerged and are of particular clinical concern. These CRE isolates are resistant to all β-lactam antibiotics, including carbapenems, as well as most other classes of antimicrobials, often through the acquisition of plasmids encoding multiple drug class resistance. Therefore, there are few options for effective antimicrobial therapy of patients infected with CRE.

Various classification schemes have been developed for β-lactamases,[42,43] but a classification scheme for extended spectrum β-lactamases proposed by Giske may be the most clinically useful (Table 6.2).[44] The majority of MDR GNB are members of the following genera or species: *Escherichia coli, Klebsiella pneumoniae, Acinetobacter baumannii, Pseudomonas aeruginosa, Enterobacter* species, and *Citrobacter* species. MDR GNB have become increasingly prevalent, and monitoring and controlling infections caused by these organisms has become an important part of infection control programs.

Understanding mechanisms of patient GNB acquisition is essential for designing effective infection control practices. There are two main modes of becoming colonized with MDR GNB. Transmission of a fully resistant organism to a patient can occur from healthcare personnel who have transient or persistent carriage, visitors, the patient's environment, or shared equipment. Another mechanism of acquisition is the emergence of MDR in GNB already colonizing the patient. In this case, emergence of resistance occurs by de-repression of chromosomal β-lactamase genes, such as

TABLE 6.2 Classification Scheme for Extended Spectrum β-lactamases

ESBL CLASS	EXTENDED SPECTRUM β-LACTAMASE ENZYME EXAMPLES	TYPICAL ANTIBIOTIC RESISTANCE	LABORATORY DETECTION
Class A ESBLs ($EBSLS_A$)	TEM- ESBLs SHV-ESBLs	Resistant to extended-spectrum cephalosporins and clavulanic acid inhibition	Detectable by phenotypic methods
Miscellaneous ESBLs ($ESBL_M$ including plasmid mediated β-lactamases)	$ESBL_{M\text{-}C}$ (plasmid-mediated AmpC) like CMY and FOX $ESBL_{M\text{-}D}$ (OXA-ESBL) OXA-10 group	Resistant to extended-spectrum cephalosporins	Genetic methods are usually needed for detection
$ESBL_{CARBA}$ (ESBL enzymes with hydrolytic activity against carbapenems)	$ESBL_{CARBA\text{-}A}$: examples include KPC and IMI 1 and 2 $ESBL_{CARBA\text{-}B}$: examples include IMP $ESBL_{CARBA\text{-}D}$ (OXA-carbapenemases)	Resistant against at least one carbapenem and all extended-spectrum cephalosporins	Detectable with genetic or phenotypic analysis

AmpC, that are expressed upon exposure to certain stressors. Alternatively, GNB can acquire resistance through acquisition of a mobile genetic element such as a plasmid encoding an ESBL.[45,46]

Epidemiology of MDR GNB Infection

Although ESBL-producing bacteria were reported initially from patients in acute care hospitals, by the turn of the 21st century, they were prevalent in chronic care facilities and outpatient settings, and in all age groups. CRE were initially reported in acute care facilities and were associated with prolonged hospital stays, prior hospital stays, recent exposure to extended-spectrum antibiotics, and invasive devices. However, they are no longer limited to acute care facilities and are reported from other facilities and from the community.[45,47,48]

Risk Factors for Infection with MDR GNB

Other than colonization with MDR GNB, there are limited data on other risk factors for MDR GNB infection in pediatrics patients. In NICUs, independent risk factors for MDR GNB infection are VLBW, extreme prematurity, underlying renal disease, and prolonged antibiotic exposure, particularly to third-generation cephalosporins and carbapenems.[49] Outside the NICU, case–control studies found underlying neurological comorbidity, chronic medical conditions, prior treatments with immunosuppressive agents, prolonged length of hospital stay, and previous antimicrobial treatment (with extended-spectrum cephalosporins) to be risk factors for infection with ESBL-producing organisms.[50] In another study, chronic medical conditions, frequent hospital admissions, and a history of recurrent infections were risk factors for infection or colonization with ESBL-producing bacteria.[51] In a multi-center matched case–control study, risk factors for colonization or infection with CRE were exposure to antibacterials with antipseudomonal activity during the previous three months, prior surgery, and mechanical ventilation.[52]

Colonization with MDR GNB

Acquisition of MDR GNB can occur from other patients, healthcare personnel, or the environment. International travel has been identified as a risk factor for acquisition of ESBL-enterobacteriaceae in children.[47] Maternal colonization with ESBL enterobacteriaceae is a major risk factor for colonization of newborn infants.[53,54] In a study on vertical transmission of ESBL *E. coli*, 36% of infants born to women colonized at 36 weeks gestation were found to be colonized at the age of two weeks.[55] In another study of VLBW infants and their mothers, 8.6% of colonized infants were found to be related to a colonized mother.[54]

Laboratory Screening for Colonization with MDR GNB

Enterobacteriaceae colonize the lower gastrointestinal tract; rectal, perirectal, or stool cultures are used to identify colonized individuals.[45,56] Surveillance cultures for MDR GNB may be obtained as an integral part of an infection control program. Culturing the specimen on selective media or chromogenic media is more efficient and more rapid than culturing surveillance specimens on non-selective media followed by susceptibility testing of selected colonies.[57]

Prevention and Control of MDR GNB Infections

Many of the strategies for the prevention of MDR GNB infections are similar to those used for prevention of MRSA.

Contact isolation precautions for colonization/Infection with MDR GNR

Identifying patients colonized with MDR GNB and instituting contact isolation precautions may reduce the risk of transmission to other patients, particularly in the NICU.[55,58] The Centers for Disease Control and Prevention (CDC) recommends contact isolation precautions for inpatients with infection or colonization with any MDR GNB, including ESBL-producing GNB.[57] During a four-year study in a NICU, Benenson et al. performed weekly fecal cultures for ESBL-producing *K. pneumoniae* on neonates staying for more than seven days.[58] Neonates with a positive culture were placed in contact isolation precautions and were cohorted to receive care by designated nurses separately from other neonates. These interventions were associated with a decrease in the acquisition of ESBL-producing *K. pneumoniae*. In a separate retrospective descriptive review, once-weekly screening compared to on-demand cultures was associated with a decrease in secondary cases and infections.[59]

Effectiveness of screening methods has been studied mostly in high-risk patients (e.g., NICU patients) and/or in the setting of an outbreak.[45]

Although contact isolation precautions are generally appropriate for babies in a NICU with ESBL-producing GNB, for inpatient units with a high endemic rate of ESBL-producing bacteria, preemptive screening may be impractical. Screening patients for ESBL-producing GNB places a burden on the microbiology laboratory and infection preventionists.[45]

Furthermore, there is no conclusive evidence of effectiveness of contact isolation precautions in reducing transmission and infection rates. Therefore, the role of contact isolation for carriers of ESBL-producing GNB is unsettled, particularly in units where endemic colonization rates with these microorganisms are high.[45,60]

Colonization with MDR GNB typically persists for a prolonged period of time. Repeating cultures to evaluate clearance of colonization may be considered after an interval of several months without hospitalization, antimicrobial therapy, or presence of invasive devices.[61] In a study on duration of colonization in newborns colonized with ESBL-producing enterobacteriaceae after discharge from a NICU, some infants remain colonized throughout the first year of life.[55]

Patients who are colonized or infected with CRE should be placed on contact isolation.[56] Following a healthcare-associated case of CRE, active surveillance is recommended by the CDC.[56] The risk of infection among CRE carriers is variable, based on factors such as patient population and type of organism.[45] In an adult study by Schechner et al., 8.8% of newly colonized patients developed a subsequent CRE infection.[62] In another study, 9% of adult patients colonized with carbapenem-resistant *Klebsiella pneumoniae* developed clinical infection.[63] Prevention of colonization is therefore a key prevention strategy.

Environmental decontamination for MDR GNB

The immediate environment of a patient colonized with MDR GNB becomes contaminated.[45,64] Rooms occupied by these patients should be cleaned and disinfected with Environmental Protection Agency–approved disinfectants on a daily basis and upon discharge and transfer of the patient.[65] Newer technologies such as ultraviolet C irradiation and hydrogen peroxide vaporizers have been used to decontaminate areas.

Adjunctive measures to reduce infections with MDR GNB

Adherence to standard precautions that includes an emphasis on hand hygiene before and after contact with a patient or his environment, with reeducation and monitoring of adherence, should be helpful in reducing transmission of MDR GNB. Establishment of an antimicrobial stewardship program to decrease usage of broad-spectrum antimicrobials and reduce overall antimicrobial use, along with monitoring adherence to this program, is important and can result in a reduction in the number of patients colonized and infected with MDR GNB.[66] Providing practitioners with timely feedback on antimicrobial use has a positive effect on adherence to stewardship guidelines.[67]

Data on using antimicrobials for decolonization of pediatric carriers are very limited. In a study of adult carriers of carbapenem-resistant *K. pneumoniae*, use of a regimen of oral solutions of gentamicin and polymyxin E for seven days was associated with a significant decrease in positive rectal cultures after two and six weeks.[68] However, in a study on six preterm newborns, selective digestive decolonization with a five-day course of amikacin and polymyxin was not effective.[69] Concerns about emerging resistance has led most to abandonment of oral antimicrobial therapy to effect decolonization.[45]

Vancomycin-Resistant Enterococci

Definition and Mechanism of Resistance

Enterococci are normal flora in the colon. *Enterococcus faecalis* and *Enterococcus faecium* are the enterococcal species most commonly isolated from clinical specimens. Enterococci acquire genetic elements, including plasmids, insertion sequences, and transposons that result in antimicrobial resistance to multiple agents. Vancomycin binds to the D-Ala-D-Ala terminal end of the pentapeptide portion of the *N*-acetylglucosamine–*N*-acetylmuramic acid precursor of cell wall peptidoglycan with high affinity, leading to inhibition of synthesis of the cell wall. Vancomycin resistance results from the acquisition of genes that encode synthesis of D-Ala-D-Lac or D-Ala-D-Ser pentapeptide precursors of peptidoglycan with low affinity for vancomycin.[70] The vancomycin resistance (Van) operon may be carried on a plasmid or chromosome.[71] Among the nine variable ligase genes in the operon, *VanA* and *VanB* are the most common genes associated with human cases of VRE infection. *VanA* is plasmid-borne, results in high-level vancomycin resistance, and is found in *E. faecium* strains,[72,73] while *VanB* acquisition results in a variable level of vancomyin resistance. Vancomycin resistance is defined by the Clinical and Laboratory Standards Institute as a minimum inhibitory concentration to vancomycin of greater than or equal to 32 μg/mL. Most of the vancomycin-resistant strains causing infections are *E. faecium*, with *E. faecalis* composing a smaller proportion.[74,75]

Epidemiology of VRE Infection

Although HA-VRE infection is relatively common among adults in an ICU, the incidence of VRE infection in pediatric patients appears to be lower. However, data in pediatric populations are limited. In a university hospital in Turkey over a five-year period, VRE infections occurred in ~1% of children in a PICU, ~3% of pediatric oncology inpatients, and 0.36% of babies in a NICU.[76–78] Bloodstream infection was the most common clinical manifestation of VRE infection in each unit, followed by urinary tract infection (UTI) and central nervous system (CNS) infection.[76–78] Crude in-hospital mortality was higher in neonates who developed a systemic VRE infection.[78] In a study from the U.S. National Healthcare Safety Network that included primarily adults, VRE ranked as the second most common pathogen of nosocomial infection after staphylococci.[74]

Risk Factors for VRE Infection

In a NICU with an outbreak of VRE infection, a logistic regression analysis revealed the receipt of glycopeptides after detection of VRE colonization as an independent risk factor for the development of systemic VRE infection in colonized neonates.[79] Similarly, in a PICU, glycopeptide use after detection of VRE colonization was a risk factor for developing VRE infection.[76]

Colonization with VRE

In both adults and children, VRE colonization is an important risk factor for VRE infection. Asymptomatic colonization with VRE is approximately ten times more common than infection. Colonization with VRE is more likely to result in clinical infection than colonization with antimicrobial-susceptible enterococci. In a NICU in Turkey, weekly screening for VRE by culture of rectal swabs showed a prevalence of carriage that varied widely from 1.9% to 30.3% annually over the course of five years.[78] In a NICU in Greece with a case of VRE bacteremia, colonization was common, with a peak prevalence of 40%.[79] Upon multivariate analysis, administration of at least one second-line antimicrobial agent, typically vancomycin or teichoplanin, and hospitalization during the first month of the study period during which a high VRE prevalence was documented were identified as independent risk factors for VRE colonization. In adults, risk factors for VRE colonization and infection include prior antimicrobial use, exposure to surfaces contaminated with VRE, exposure to other patients with VRE (especially roommates), presence of invasive devices, severity of illness, admission to an ICU, prolonged hospital stay, and residence in a long-term care facility.[80] VRE infection developed in approximately 10% of VRE-colonized children in an ICU or an oncology service, but only 3% of colonized babies in a NICU.[76–78] Colonization pressure—the proportion of VRE-positive patient days on a particular unit—is significantly associated with VRE acquisition.[81]

The duration of carriage in adults is prolonged and may persist for years.[82] In a meta-analysis that used a mathematical model estimate, the median time to clearance of VRE colonization was 26 weeks.[83] Therefore, there is little utility in repeating cultures soon after detection to evaluate clearance of colonization. Repeat cultures may be considered about six months after an interval without hospitalization, antimicrobial therapy, or presence of invasive devices.

Laboratory Screening for VRE Colonization

Active screening for VRE colonization can be performed on stool or rectal swabs by culture or NAAT. The burden of VRE can also be estimated by testing specimens submitted for *C. difficile* testing.[71] In adults, rectal swab culture (77%) had a much higher yield than pharyngeal swabs (11%).[84] However, a single rectal VRE screening culture can have a sensitivity of less than 50% despite the use of chromogenic selective agar.[85] Stool has a higher yield than rectal swab. A variety of chromogenic selective agars have been developed for the detection of colonization with vancomycin-resistant *E. faecium* and *E. faecalis*, including chromID VRE agar.[71] Chromogenic agar media have a higher sensitivity and specificity than bile esculin azide agar containing vancomycin.[71] Commercial NAATs have been developed to detect *vanA* +/– *vanB* from stool and rectal swab specimens (e.g., Roche LightCycler VRE detects *vanA/vanB;* Cepheid Xpert detects *vanA* or *vanA/vanB*). Although the turnaround time is faster than with the chromogenic agar media, the performance of NAATs is lower than with chromogenic agar. These tests have a high negative predictive value, but vary in positive predictive value. The positive predictive value may be proportional to the prevalence of VRE in the population tested and the presence of *vanA* and/or *vanB* in other bacterial species.[71]

Prevention and Control of VRE Infection

In hospitals, VRE can be transmitted via contact with healthcare personnel and the environment. VRE may persist in the hospital environment for a prolonged period of time.[82] Hands of healthcare personnel are important vectors of patient-to-patient VRE transmission, and adequate hand hygiene has been shown to reduce acquisition of VRE by 47%.[85,86] VRE can survive on and be found on many objects and surfaces in the hospital environment. Components of a program to prevent infection with VRE may include the following:

1. An enhanced emphasis on hand hygiene, with enhanced education and adherence monitoring;
2. Monitoring clinical specimens for VRE and instituting contact isolation precautions when detected;
3. Rectal/stool surveillance cultures with contact isolation precautions for colonized patients;
4. Enhanced environmental cleaning; and
5. Antimicrobial stewardship.[86]

The CDC recommends contact isolation for inpatients with infection or colonization with VRE.[87] Contact isolation includes a single-patient room, dedicated equipment, and gown and gloves for contact with the patient or his/her environment, and may also include cohorting of patients and personnel. Contact isolation is indicated for patients with VRE infection, particularly if the patient has a draining wound or secretions with VRE. However, the use of contact isolation for VRE carriers has been debated due to the lack of unequivocal data on effectiveness of contact isolation in limiting transmission and infection rates, as well as the cost of implementing contact isolation precautions and the potentially negative effect on patient care.[80] A limited effect of contact isolation for VRE-colonized patients is evident in adult units with a high rate endemic rate of carriage. In two adult hospitals in California, there was no significant difference in the rate of VRE detection after use of contact isolation for patients with VRE was discontinued, although the use of chlorhexidine washes was expanded to all patients during the period of discontinuation of contact isolation.[88]

Active surveillance with screening for VRE colonization is most clearly indicated as part of an overall response to a VRE outbreak that includes contact isolation, enhanced environmental cleaning, and enhanced education of hospital personnel. Routine screening for VRE can be considered in high-risk units such as oncology, transplant, intensive care, or burn units with ongoing cases of VRE infection, but it is generally not indicated for an entire hospital.[89]

Environmental cleaning to prevent VRE infections

VRE can survive exposure to certain disinfectants and to heat. Automated mobile ultraviolet (UV) units are a newer technology that is effective against many bacteria, including VRE, in hospital rooms and is active against bacteria on high-touch surfaces. However, the surface to be disinfected must be directly in line with the emitted UV rays.[80]

VRE decolonization

Decolonization is generally not recommended, but it can be considered in patient populations in whom VRE infection is associated with high morbidity and mortality. Examples of such populations may include liver transplant recipients and patients with hematologic malignancies. Regimens that have been used in adults include oral bacitracin, vancomycin, and novobiocin. Another protocol used bowel preparation with polyethylene glycol, oral linezolid, oral daptomycin, and oral *Lactobacillus rhamnosus*.[90]

Antimicrobial stewardship

To minimize the risk of VRE infection, Healthcare Infection Control Practices Advisory Committee (HICPAC) guidelines recommend minimizing the use of vancomycin, third-generation cephalosporin antimicrobials, and antimicrobials with anaerobic activity such as metronidazole, because these agents are associated with an increased risk of VRE colonization and infection.[57]

Fecal transplant

The gastrointestinal (GI) tract is often a reservoir of MDR bacteria, particularly VRE and MDR GNB. The feces of patients with dysbiosis, such as those with *C. difficile* infection, have a reduced bacterial diversity, a larger proportion of Proteobacteria such as *E. coli* and *Klebsiella*, and a larger number of antibiotic-resistance genes than that of normal persons.[91] Successful fecal microbial transplant for treatment of recurrent *C. difficile* infection has resulted in a reduction of antibiotic-resistance genes in the feces.[91] This is presumably the result of reestablishing a healthy gut microbiome that provides colonization resistance against MDR pathogens. In contrast, Sohn et al. performed fecal transplants on three patients with *C. difficile* and VRE colonization and did not observe eradication of VRE carriage.[92] These findings and case reports suggest that fecal transplants or potentially other interventions to restore the gut microbiome can eradicate some but not all MDR bacteria.[93,94]

Approach to the Clinical Scenario

The situation described in the clinical scenario suggests an increase in clinical cases of MRSA infection and may constitute an outbreak. To determine if there has truly been an outbreak, the current rate of clinical MRSA infection, measured as infections per 1,000 hospital days or percentage of PICU patients with an infection, should be compared to the baseline rate of infection. Assuming there has been an increase in infection rate, the first strategy should be an analysis of the adherence to basic infection control measures, including hand hygiene, isolation precautions, and environmental cleaning. Reeducation of relevant personnel and documentation of adherence to these measures is important. Subsequently, obtaining surveillance cultures of all patients in the unit is reasonable as a component of outbreak investigation, as patients with unrecognized colonization may serve as reservoirs for transmission. Expert guidance from the Society for Healthcare Epidemiology of America (SHEA) describes surveillance cultures as a "special approach" to be employed if MRSA transmission continues despite reliable implementation of basic measures.[30] Culture or NAATs for MRSA from a swab from the anterior nares is typically utilized for surveillance, although one study has suggested that in PICU patients, pharyngeal swabs have a higher sensitivity for detection of MRSA.[27] Topical decolonization, also identified by SHEA as a special approach, has been shown to reduce the subsequent risk of infection in colonized patients, and some studies have demonstrated reductions in transmission. A typical decolonization strategy includes intranasal mupirocin application twice daily for five days, with or without daily bathing with chlorhexidine gluconate. The duration of contact isolation precautions for MRSA continues to be an area of debate. In the absence of a decolonization strategy, colonization is typically prolonged for many months. There are no established criteria for discontinuation of contact isolation precautions, but one strategy is to discontinue precautions after three negative weekly swabs, obtained in the absence of topical or systemic antimicrobial therapy with activity against MRSA or possibly a single negative NAAT for MRSA.

Unresolved Issues

1. The effectiveness of contact isolation precautions for patients with MDROs in general, including MRSA and MDR GNB, is an unresolved issue. A related unresolved question is the optimum duration of contact isolation after successful treatment, particularly in settings where there is no ongoing outbreak and in which there is a relatively high prevalence of colonization with the MDRO (e.g., MRSA) in the community.
2. The indications for, and effectiveness of, routine screening for an MDRO in preventing transmission and infection has been an ongoing area of controversy.
3. The use of universal decolonization for MRSA with routine nasal mupirocin application and/or routine chlorhexidine bathing is an unsettled issue, as is the risk for development of resistance to mupirocin and chlorhexidine.
4. The balance of safety and effectiveness of chlorhexidine skin washes in prevention of infections in newborn and premature infants are unsettled issues.
5. The potential role of universal glove and gown use for prevention of MRDO infections is an unsettled issue.
6. The indications for culturing asymptomatic healthcare personnel to identify those who are MRSA-colonized, and the optimal management (e.g., decolonization therapy, follow-up monitoring, furloughing colonized personnel) of MRSA-colonized healthcare personnel have not been established.
7. Studies of the potential role of family members and other close contacts of patients colonized or infected with MRSA in healthcare-associated transmission of MRSA are needed.

References

1. Septimus E, Weinstein RA, Perl TM, Goldmann DA, Yokoe DS. Commentary: Approaches for preventing healthcare-associated infections: go long or go wide? *Infect Control Hosp Epidemiol.* 2014;35(7):797–801.
2. Milstone AM, Budd A, Shepard JW, et al. Role of decolonization in a comprehensive strategy to reduce methicillin-resistant *Staphylococcus aureus* infections in the neonatal intensive care unit: an observational cohort. *Infect Control Hosp Epidemiol.* 2010;31(5):558–560.

3. Carey AJ, Duchon J, Della-Latta P, Saiman L. The epidemiology of methicillin-susceptible and methicillin-resistant *Staphylococcus aureus* in a neonatal intensive care unit, 2000–2007. *J Perinatol.* 2010;30:135–139.
4. Lessa F, Edwards JR, Fridkin SK, Tenover F, Horan T, Gorwitz RJ. Trends in incidence of late-onset methicillin-resistant *Staphylococcus aureus* infection in neonatal intensive care units: data from the National Nosocomial Infections Surveillance System. *Pediatr Infect Dis J.* 2009;28(7):577–581.
5. Huang YC, Chou YH, Su LH, et al. Methicillin-resistant *Staphylococcus aureus* colonization and its association with infection among infants hospitalized in neonatal intensive care units. *Pediatrics.* 2006;118:469–474.
6. David MZ, Daum RS. Community-associated methicillin-resistant *Staphylococcus aureus*: epidemiology and clinical consequences of an emerging epidemic. *Clin Microbiol Rev.* 2010;23:616–687.
7. Carey AJ, Della-Latta P, Huard R, et al. Changes in the molecular epidemiological characteristics of methicillin-resistant *Staphylococcus aureus* in a neonatal intensive care unit. *Infect Control Hosp Epidemiol.* 2010;31(6):613–619.
8. Reich PJ, Boyle MG, Hogan PG, et al. Emergence of community-associated methicillin-resistant *Staphylococcus aureus* strains in the neonatal intensive care unit: an infection prevention and patient safety challenge. *Clin Microbiol Infect.* 2016;22(7):645, e1–e8.
9. Zervou FN, Zacharioudakis IM, Ziakas PD, Mylonakis E. MRSA colonization and risk of infection in the neonatal and pediatric ICU: a meta-analysis. *Pediatrics.* 2014;133(4):e1015.
10. Huang Y-C, Lien R-I, Lin T-Y. Effect of mupirocin decolonization on subsequent methicillin-resistant *Staphylococcus aureus* infection in infants in neonatal intensive care units. *Pediatr Infect Dis J.* 2015;34(3):241–245.
11. Seybold U, Halvosa JS, White N, Voris V, Ray SM, Blumberg HM. Emergence of and risk factors for methicillin-resistant *Staphylococcus aureus* of community origin in intensive care nurseries. *Pediatrics.* 2008;122(5):1039–1046.
12. Delaney HM, Wang E, Melish M. Comprehensive strategy including prophylactic mupirocin to reduce *Staphylococcus aureus* colonization and infection in high-risk neonates. *J Perinatol.* 2013;33:313–318.
13. Andersen BM, Lindemann R, Bergh K, et al. Spread of methicillin-resistant *Staphylococcus aureus* in a neonatal intensive unit associated with understaffing, overcrowding and mixing of patients. *J Hosp Infect.* 2002;50:18–24.
14. Jimenez-Truque N, Tedeschi S, Saye EJ, et al. Relationship between maternal and neonatal *Staphylococcus aureus* colonization. *Pediatrics.* 2012;129:e1252–e1259.
15. Geraci DM, Giuffré M, Bonura C, et al. Methicillin-resistant *Staphylococcus aureus* colonization: a three-year prospective study in a neonatal intensive care unit in Italy. *PLoS ONE.* 2014;9(2):e87760.
16. Merrer J, Santoli F, Appéré-De Vecchi, Tran B, Jonghe BD, Outin H. "Colonization pressure" and risk of acquisition of methicillin-resistant *Staphylococcus aureus* in a medical intensive care unit. *Infect Control Hosp Epidemiol.* 2000;21:718–723.
17. Julian S, Burnham CA, Sellenriek P, Shannon WD, Hamvas A, Tarr Pl, Warner BB. Impact of neonatal intensive care bed configuration on rates of late-onset bacterial

sepsis and methicillin-resistant *Staphylococcus aureus* colonization. *Infect Control Hosp Epidemiol.* 2015;36(10):1173–1182.
18. Behari P, Englund J, Alcasid G, Garcia-Houchins S, Weber S. Transmission of methicillin-resistant *Staphylococcus aureus* to preterm infants through breast milk. *Infect Control Hosp Epidemiol.* 2004;25(9):778–780.
19. Gregory ML, Eichenwald EC, Puopolo KM. Seven-year experience with a surveillance program to reduce methicillin-resistant *Staphylococcus aureus* colonization in a neonatal intensive care unit. *Pediatrics.* 2009;123(5):e790–e796.
20. Milstone AM, Song X, Beers C, Berkowitz I, Carroll KC, Perl TM. Unrecognized burden of methicillin-resistant *Staphylococcus aureus* and vancomycin-resistant *Enterococcus* carriage in the pediatric intensive care unit. *Infect Control Hosp Epidemiol.* 2008;29:1174–1176.
21. Popoola VO, Budd A, Wittig SM, et al. Methicillin-resistant *Staphylococcus aureus* transmission and infections in a neonatal intensive care unit despite active surveillance cultures and decolonization: challenges for infection prevention. *Infect Control Hosp Epidemiol.* 2014;35:412–418.
22. Iacobelli S, Colomb B, Bonsante F. Successful control of a methicillin-resistant *Staphylococcus aureus* outbreak in a neonatal intensive care unit: a retrospective, before-after study. *BMC Infect Dis.* 2013;13:440.
23. Milstone AM, Song X, Coffin S, Elward A; Society for Healthcare Epidemiology of America's Pediatric Special Interest Group. Identification and eradication of methicillin-resistant *Staphylococcus aureus* colonization in the neonatal intensive care unit: results of a national survey. *Infect Control Hosp Epidemiol.* 2010;31(7):766–768.
24. Gerber SI, Jones RC, Scott MV, et al. Management of outbreaks of methicillin-resistant *Staphylococcus aureus* infection in the neonatal intensive care unit: a consensus statement. *Infect Control Hosp Epidemiol.* 2006;27(2):139–145.
25. Lyles RD, Trick WE, Hayden MK, et al. Regional epidemiology of methicillin-resistant *Staphylococcus aureus* among critically ill children in a state with mandated active surveillance. *J Pediatr Infect Dis Soc.* 2016;5(4):409–416.
26. Suwantarat N, Carroll KC, Tekle T, Ross T, Popoola VO, Milstone AM. Low prevalence of mupirocin resistance among hospital-acquired methicillin-resistant *Staphylococcus aureus* isolates in a neonatal intensive care unit with an active surveillance cultures and decolonization program. *Infect Control Hosp Epidemiol.* 2015;36(2):232–234.
27. Nakamura MM, McAdam AJ, Sandora TJ, Moreira KR, Lee GM. Higher prevalence of pharyngeal than nasal *Staphylococcus aureus* carriage in pediatric intensive care units. *J Clin Microbiol.* 2010;48(8):2957–2959.
28. Xu Z, Hou Y, Peters BM, et al. Chromogenic media for MRSA diagnostics. *Mol Biol Rep.* 2016;43(11):1205–1212.
29. Popoola VO, Colantuoni E, Suwantarat N, et al. Active surveillance cultures and decolonization to reduce *Staphylococcus aureus* infections in the neonatal intensive care unit. *Infect Control Hosp Epidemiol.* 2016;37(4):381–387.
30. Calfee DP, Salgado CD, Milstone AM, et al. Strategies to prevent methicillin-resistant *Staphylococcus aureus* transmission and infection in acute care hospitals: 2014 update. *Infect Control Hosp Epidemiol.* 2014:35(7):772–796.

31. Guerrero DM, Wagner M, Carson G, et al. Utility of a single nasal polymerase chain reaction assay in predicting absence of skin and environmental contamination in hospitalized patients with past methicillin-resistant *Staphylococcus aureus*. *Am J Infect Control.* 2016;44:711–713.
32. Lepelletier D, Corvec S, Caillon J, Reynaud A, Rozé J-C, Gras-Leguen C. Eradication of methicillin-resistant *Staphylococcus aureus* in a neonatal intensive care unit: which measures for which success? *Am J Infect Control.* 2009;37:195–200.
33. You JHS, Chan CY, Wong MY, Ip M. Active surveillance and decolonization of methicillin-resistant *Staphylococcus aureus* on admission to neonatal intensive care units in Hong Kong: a cost-effectiveness analysis. *Infect Control Hosp Epidemiol.* 2012;33(10):1024–1030.
34. Pierce R, Bryant K, Elward A, Lessler J, Milstone AM. Bacterial infections in neonates following mupirocin-based MRSA decolonization: a multicenter cohort study. *Infect Control Hosp Epidemiol.* 2017; Jun 5:1–7. doi:10.1017/ice.2017.108.
35. Ridenour G, Lampen R, Federspiel J, Kritchevsky S, Wong E, Climo M. Selective use of intranasal mupirocin and chlorhexidine bathing and the incidence of methicillin-resistant *Staphylococcus aureus* colonization and infection among intensive care unit patients. *Infect Control Hosp Epidemiol.* 2007;28(10):1155–1161.
36. Frost SA, Alogso MC, Metcalfe L, et al. Chlorhexidine bathing and health care-associated infections among adult intensive care patients: a systematic review and meta-analysis. *Crit Care.* 2016;20(1):379.
37. Quach C, Milstone AM, Perpête C, Bonenfant M, Moore DL, Perreault T. Chlorhexidine bathing in a tertiary care neonatal intensive care unit: impact on central line-associated bloodstream infections. *Infect Control Hosp Epidemiol.* 2014;35(2):158–163.
38. Johnson J, Bracken R, Tamma PD, Aucott SW, Bearer C, and Milstone AM. Trends in chlorhexidine use in US neonatal intensive care units: results from a follow-up national survey. *Infect Control Hosp Epidemiol.* 2016;37(9):1116–1118.
39. Price JR, Cole K, Bexley A, et al. Transmission of *Staphylococcus aureus* between health-care workers, the environment, and patients in an intensive care unit: a longitudinal cohort study based on whole-genome sequencing. *Lancet Infect Dis.* 2017;17(2):207–214.
40. Lin YC, Lauderdale TL, Lin HM, Chen PC, Cheng MF, Hsieh KS, Liu YC. An outbreak of methicillin-resistant *Staphylococcus aureus* infection in patients of a pediatric intensive care unit and high carriage rate among health care workers. *J Microbiol Immunol Infect.* 2007;40(4):325–334.
41. Medeiros AA. Evolution and dissemination of β-lactamases accelerated by generations of β-lactam antibiotics. *Clin Infect Dis.* 1997;24 (Suppl 1):S19–S45.
42. Bush K, Jacoby GA, Medeiros AA. A functional classification scheme for β-lactamases and its correlation with molecular structure. *Antimicrob Agents Chemother.* 1995;39:1211–1233.
43. Ambler RP. The structure of β-lactamases. *Philos Trans R Soc Lond B Biol Sci.* 1980;289:321–331.
44. Giske CG, Sundsfjord AS, Kahlmeter G. Redefining extended-spectrum β-lactamases: balancing science and clinical need. *J Antimicrob Chemother.* 2009;63(1):1–4.

45. Adler A, Friedman D, Marchaim D. Multidrug-resistant gram-negative bacilli-infection control implications. *Infect Dis Clin N Am.* 2016;30:967–997.
46. Tal JR, Coyle JR, Katz DE. The complex epidemiology of extended-spectrum beta-lactamase-producing Enterobacteriaceae. *Future Microbiol.* 2015;10:819–839.
47. Strysko JP, Mony V, Cleveland J. International travel is a risk factor for extended-spectrum β-lactamase-producing Enterobacteriaceae acquisition in children: a case–case–control study in an urban U.S. hospital. *Travel Med Infect Dis.* 2016;14(6):568–571.
48. Schwaber MJ, Carmeli Y. Carbapenemase-resistant Enterobacteriaceae: a potential threat. *JAMA.* 2008;300(24):2911–2913.
49. Tsai MH, Chu SM, Hsu JF, et al. Risk factors and outcomes for multidrug-resistant Gram-negative bacteremia in the NICU. *Pediatrics.* 2014;133(2):e322–e329.
50. Logan LK, Meltzer LA, McAuley JB, et al. Extended-spectrum β-lactamase-producing *Enterobacteriaceae* infections in children: a two-center case–case–control study of risk factors and outcomes in Chicago, Illinois. *J Pediatric Infect Dis Soc.* 2014;3(4):312–319. Epub 2014 Mar 19.
51. Blaschke AJ, Korgenski EK, Daly JA, et el. Extended-spectrum beta-lactamase-producing pathogens in a children's hospital: a 5-year experience. *Am J Infect Control.* 2009;37(6):435–441.
52. Chiotos K, Tamma P, Flett KB, et al. Multicenter study of the risk factors for colonization or infection with carbapenemase-resistant *Enterobacteriaceae* in children. *Antimicrob Agents Chemother.* 2017;61(12):e1440–e1417.
53. Retterdal S, Löhr IH, Bernhoff E. Extended-spectrum β-lactamase-producing Enterobacteriaceae among pregnant women in Norway: prevalence and maternal-neonatal transmission. *J Perinatol.* 2015;35:907–912.
54. Denkel LA, Schwab F, Kola A. The mother as most important risk factor for colonization of very low birth weight (VLBW) infants with extended-spectrum β-lactamase-producing Enterobacteriaceae (ESBL-E). *J Antimicrob Chemother.* 2014;69:2230–2237.
55. Strenger V, Feierl G, Resch B. Fecal carriage and intrafamilial spread of extended-spectrum β-lactamase-producing enterobacteriaceae following colonization at the neonatal ICU. *Pediatr Crit Care Med.* 2013;14(2):157–163.
56. Centers for Disease Control and Prevention. Guidance for control of infections with carbapenem-resistant or carbapenemase-producing Enterobacteriaceae in acute care facilities. *MMWR.* 2009;58(10):256–260.
57. Siegel JD, Rhinhart E, Jackson M. Management of multidrug-resistant organisms in health care settings, 2006. Available at: https://www.cdc.gov/hicpac/pdf/guidelines/MDROGuideline2006.pdf. Accessed December 19, 2016.
58. Benenson S, Levi PD, Block C. Continuous surveillance to reduce extended-spectrum β-lactamase *Klebsiella pneumoniae* colonization in the neonatal intensive care unit. *Neonatology.* 2013;103(2):155–160.
59. Rybczynska H, Melander E, Johansson H. Efficacy of a once-a-week screening programme to control extended-spectrum beta-lactamase-producing bacteria in a neonatal intensive care unit. *Scand J Infect Dis.* 2014;46(6):426–432.

60. Harris AD, Kotetishvili M, Shurland S. How important is patient-to-patient transmission in extended-spectrum-beta-lactamse *Escherichia coli* acquisition? *Am J Infect Control.* 2007;35(2):97–101.
61. Siegel JD, Rhinehart E, Jackson M, Chiarello L, and the Healthcare Infection Control Practices Advisory Committee, 2007. Guideline for isolation precautions: preventing transmission of infectious agents in healthcare settings. Available at: http://www.cdc.gov/ncidod/dhqp/pdf/isolation2007.pdf. Accessed November 26, 2016.
62. Schechner V, Kotlovşky T, Kazma M. Asymptomatic rectal carriage of *blaKPC* producing carbapenem-resistant Enterobacteriaceae: who is prone to become clinically infected? *Clin Microbiol Infect.* 2013;19:451–456.
63. Borer A, Saidel-Odes L, Eskira S. Risk factors for developing clinical infection with carbapenem-resistant *Klebsiella pneumoniae* in hospital patients initially only colonized with carbapenem-resistant K *pneumoniae. Am J Infect Control.* 2012;40(5):421–425.
64. Nseir S, Blazejewski C, Lubret R. Risk of acquiring multidrug-resistant Gram negative bacilli from prior room occupants in the intensive care unit. *Clin Microbiol Infect.* 2011;17(8):1201–1208.
65. Guidelines for environmental infection control in health-care facilities recommendations of CDC and the healthcare infection control practices advisory committee (HICPAC). 2003. Available at: http://www.cdc.gov/hai/pdfs/eic_in_hcf_03.pdf. Accessed November 27, 2016.
66. Knudsen JD, Andersen SE. A multidisciplinary intervention to reduce infections of ESBL- and Amp-C producing, gram-negative bacteria at a university hospital. *PLoS ONE.* 2014;9(1):e86457.
67. Ivers NM, Jamtvedt G, Flottrop SA. Audit and feedback: effects on professional practice and healthcare outcomes in hospitals. *Cochrane Database Syst Rev.* 2012;(6):CD000259.
68. Saidel-Odes L, Polachek H, Peled, N. A randomized, double-blind, placebo-controlled trial of selective digestive decontamination using oral gentamicin and oral polymyxin E for eradication of carbapenem-resistant *Klebsiella pneumoniae* carriage. *Infect Control Hosp Epidemiol.* 2012;33(1):14–19.
69. Gutiérrez-Urbón JM, Feal-Cortizas B, Suárez-Lorenzo JM. Failure of a 5 day course of selective digestive decontamination solution in rectal decolonization of ESBL-producing *Klebsiella pneumoniae* in neonates. *J Antimicrob Chemother.* 2016;71(10):2729–2739.
70. Walsh C. Molecular mechanisms that confer antibacterial drug resistance. *Nature.* 2000;406(6797):775–781.
71. Faron ML, Ledeboer NA, Buchan BW. Resistance mechanisms, epidemiology, and approaches to screening for vancomycin-resistant *Enterococcus* in the health care setting. *J Clin Microbiol.* 2016;54(10):2436–2446.
72. Fisher K, Phillips C. The ecology, epidemiology and virulence of *Enterococcus. Microbiology.* 2009;155(pt 6):1749–1757.
73. Werner G, Coque TM, Hammerum AM, et al. Emergence and spread of vancomycin resistance among enterococci in Europe. *Euro Surveill.* 2008;13(47):19046.
74. Sievert DM, Ricks P, Edwards JR, et al.; National Healthcare Safety Network (NHSN) Team and Participating NHSN Facilities. Antimicrobial-resistant pathogens

associated with healthcare-associated infections: summary of data reported to the National Healthcare Safety Network at the Centers for Disease Control and Prevention, 2009–2010. *Infect Control Hosp Epidemiol.* 2013;34(1):1–14.
75. French GL. Enterococci and vancomycin resistance. *Clin Infect Dis.* 1998;27(Suppl 1):S75–S83.
76. Sutcu M, Akturk H, Acar M, et al. Impact of vancomycin-resistant enterococci colonization in critically ill pediatric patients. *Am J Infect Control.* 2016;44(5):515–519.
77. Aktürk H, Sütçü M, Somer A, et al. Results of four-year rectal vancomycin-resistant enterococci surveillance in a pediatric hematology-oncology ward: from colonization to infection. *Turk J Haematol.* 2016;33(3):244–247.
78. Aktürk H, Sütçü M, Somer A, et al. Vancomycin-resistant enterococci colonization in a neonatal intensive care unit: who will be infected? *J Matern Fetal Neonatal Med.* 2016;29(21):3478–3482.
79. Iosifidis E, Evdoridou I, Agakidou E, et al. Vancomycin-resistant *Enterococcus* outbreak in a neonatal intensive care unit: epidemiology, molecular analysis and risk factors. *Am J Infect Control.* 2013;41(10):857–861.
80. Reyes K, Bardossy AC, Zervos M. Vancomycin-resistant Enterococci. Epidemiology, prevention, and control. *Infect Dis Clin N Am.* 2016;30:953–965.
81. Ajao AO, Harris AD, Roghmann MC, et al. Systematic review of measurement and adjustment for colonization pressure in studies of methicillin-resistant *Staphylococcus aureus*, vancomycin-resistant enterococci, and *Clostridium difficile* acquisition. *Infect Control Hosp Epidemiol.* 2011;32(5):481–489.
82. Zirakzadeh A, Patel R. Vancomycin-resistant enterococci: colonization, infection, detection and treatment. *Mayo Clin Proc.* 2006;8(4):529–536.
83. Shenoy ES, Paras ML, Noubary F, Walensky RP, Hooper DC. Natural history of colonization with methicillin-resistant *Staphylococcus aureus* (MRSA) and vancomycin-resistant *Enterococcus* (VRE): a systematic review. *BMC Infect Dis.* 2014;14:177.
84. Lai KK, Kelley AL, Melvin ZS, Belliveau PP, Fontecchio SA. Failure to eradicate vancomycin-resistant enterococci in a university hospital and the cost of barrier precautions. *Infect Control Hosp Epidemiol.* 1998;19(9):647–652.
85. Kaki R., Yu Y., O'Neill C., et al: Vancomycin-resistant *Enterococcus* (VRE) transmission and risk factors in contacts of VRE carriers. *Infect Control Hosp Epidemiol.* 2014;35:876–879.
86. De Angelis G, Cataldo MA, De Waure C, et al. Infection control and prevention measures to reduce the spread of vancomycin-resistant enterococci in hospitalized patients: a systematic review and meta-analysis. *J Antimicrob Chemother.* 2014;69:1185–1192.
87. Centers for Disease Control and Prevention. Recommendations for preventing the spread of vancomycin resistance. Recommendations of the Hospital Infection Control Practices Advisory Committee (HICPAC). *MMWR Recomm Rep.* 1995;44(RR12):1–13.
88. Martin EM, Russell D, Rubin Z, et al. Elimination of routine contact precautions for endemic methicillin-resistant *Staphylococcus aureus* and vancomycin-resistant *Enterococcus*: a retrospective quasi-experimental study. *Infect Control Hosp Epidemiol.* 2016;37(11):1323–1330.

89. Bryce E, Grant J, Scharf S, et al. Horizontal infection prevention measures and a risk-managed approach to vancomycin-resistant enterococci: an evaluation. *Am J Infect Control.* 2015;43(11):1238–1243.
90. Cheng VC, Chen JH, Tai JW, et al. Decolonization of gastrointestinal carriage of vancomycin-resistant *Enterococcus faecium*: case series and review of literature. *BMC Infect Dis.* 2014;14:514.
91. Millan B, Park H, Hotte N, et al. Fecal microbial transplants reduce antibiotic-resistant genes in patients with recurrent *Clostridium difficile* infection. *Clin Infect Dis.* 2016;62(12):1479–1486.
92. Sohn KM, Cheon S, Kim YS. Can fecal microbiota transplantation (FMT) eradicate fecal colonization with vancomycin-resistant enterococci (VRE)? *Infect Control Hosp Epidemiol.* 2016;37(12):1519–1521.
93. Crum-Cianflone NF, Sullivan E, Ballon-Landa G. Fecal microbiota transplantation and successful resolution of multidrug-resistant-organism colonization. *J Clin Microbiol.* 2015;53(6):1986–1989.
94. Singh R, van Nood E, Nieuwdorp M, et al. Donor feces infusion for eradication of extended spectrum beta-lactamase producing *Escherichia coli* in a patient with end stage renal disease. *Clin Microbiol Infect.* 2014;20(11):O977–O978.

7 | Breast Milk Handling and Misadministration

DONNA FISHER

Background

Human milk is the preferred nutritional source for all newborns, including ill infants and premature neonates. The ability of a mother to provide milk for her infant may be hindered by maternal illness or poor milk production, and may be influenced by cultural expectations and personal preferences. The American Academy of Pediatrics recommends exclusive breastfeeding for the first six months of life.[1]

Some infants must be fed expressed breast milk, including those who are too small to feed at the breast, those too ill to be able to nurse, or those who have craniofacial anomalies that prevent suckling.

Clinical Scenario

You are notified by a neonatologist at your institution that a 3-week-old former 24-week preterm infant receiving gavage feeds was fed with the wrong mother's breast milk. The baby had been fed approximately 2 mL of a 5 mL feeding when it was noticed that the label was for a different baby. Feeds have been otherwise tolerated. There have been no recent feeding difficulties or reflux symptoms, and no abdominal distension.

Questions

How do you advise the NICU team? What are potential risks to the infant? What reporting should be done? How do you inform each baby's parents, and what counseling should be provided? What processes and procedures can prevent this error and exposure in the future?

Key Challenges

Administration of breast milk to the incorrect infant is generally treated like a blood and body fluid exposures.[2-5] Human milk must be collected safely and stored properly if it will not be fed immediately to an infant. It may be provided by a newborn's biological mother or from human donors. Hospitals with nurseries and those that provide care to infants and children must have processes in place for safe collection, handling, storage, and administration of breast milk to infants. While childcare centers that provide care and feeding to infants should also have processes in place for receipt, storage, and handling of breast milk,[2] the scope of this discussion will be limited to healthcare institutions.

Infections transmissible in human breast milk

Infectious risks to the newborn from a single feeding of breast milk are not generally measurable; however, studies of viruses and bacteria potentially transmissible in human milk can be used to inform a rational approach when misadministration occurs. When evaluating risk, the age of the newborn at the time of exposure, gestational age at delivery, and the potential effects of such transmission, as well as the health and infectious status of the donor mother (the mother whose breast milk was given to the incorrect infant) also need to be explored. Likewise, the health status of the recipient mother, defined as the mother whose baby received the incorrect breast milk feeding, should be known or obtained.

Infectious agents of concern after an incorrect breast milk feed include human immunodeficiency virus (HIV), hepatitis B virus (HBV), hepatitis C virus (HCV), and cytomegalovirus (CMV). (Please see Table 7.1.)

Human Immunodeficiency Virus (HIV)

HIV can be transmitted in breast milk to a nursing infant of an infected mother, and virus can be detected in both cell-free and cell-associated portions of human breast milk. Many studies have shown that the rate of transmissibility is associated with maternal viral load, and it is drastically decreased in women who are virologically suppressed on highly active antiretroviral therapy. Maternal receipt of antiretroviral therapy is likely to decrease free virus in breast milk, but the presence of cell-associated virus (intracellular HIV DNA) may remain, and may continue to pose a transmission risk.[6]

TABLE 7.1 Pathogens of Concern After Breast Milk Misadministration

PATHOGENS OF IMPORTANCE	TRANSMISSIBLE IN BREAST MILK	KNOWN CASES OF TRANSMISSION FROM SINGLE FEED	FOLLOW-UP TESTING NEEDED	
			MOTHERS—BOTH DONOR AND RECIPIENT	BABY— RECIPIENT
Human immunodeficiency virus	Yes	No	Baseline testing	No; can be offered on case-by-case basis
Hepatitis B virus	No. Hepatitis B surface antigen (HepBsAg) has been detected in milk from HepBsAg-positive mothers, but transmission has not been documented.	No	Baseline testing	Yes, if donor mother positive, baby should be offered HBIG and vaccine. Follow-up serological testing can be done on baby
Hepatitis C virus	No, but risk when blood is present (e.g., when nipples are cracked and bleeding)	No	Baseline testing	No
Cytomegalovirus	Yes—no long-term effects in term infants	No	Not routine—case by case	No—unless other medical indications

In the United States, safe infant feeding alternatives to breast milk are available at low or no cost to all women; therefore, HIV-infected women are advised not to breastfeed their infants.[7] It is therefore unlikely that a breast milk misadministration would involve milk from an HIV-positive women. There have been no documented cases of HIV transmission from a single breast milk exposure.

Hepatitis B

HBV surface antigen can be found in breast milk from a chronically infected mother, but the risk of transmission is low, and the American Academy of Pediatrics does not consider maternal infection to be considered a contraindication to breastfeeding.[8] In this situation, the benefits of breast milk are accepted as outweighing the risks of transmission. Infants born to mothers positive for hepatitis B surface antigen (HBsAg) should have received HBV immunoglobulin (HBIG) and HBV vaccine as soon as possible after delivery, per routine guidelines.[8,9] If breast milk from a HBsAg-positive mother has been inadvertently fed to another infant, there is an actionable response: confirm that the exposed newborn received routine HBV vaccine at birth, and promptly administer HBIG.

Hepatitis C

HCV RNA is detectable in breast milk, but studies have shown that the risk is extremely low to infants of HCV-positive women. In the United States, women with high hepatitis C viral loads, and who may have cracked or bleeding nipples, are advised to temporarily refrain from breastfeeding. Otherwise, women with HCV infection are encouraged to breastfeed. There is no post-exposure prophylaxis or intervention recommended in the event of a possible HCV exposure.[10]

Cytomegalovirus (CMV)

CMV is excreted in milk, and it can be transmitted to a neonate from an infected mother who is shedding virus.[11] Pregnant women are not routinely screened for CMV infection, but seroprevalence rates of 50–65% have been estimated in the United States.[12] Primary infection during pregnancy is associated with increased intrauterine transmission to a fetus, as well as with shedding higher viral load in breast milk.

Postpartum CMV infection can also occur, including via breast milk. In term infants, CMV transmission by breast milk is not usually associated with clinical illness. In preterm infants, postpartum infection transmitted by breast milk has been associated with systemic symptoms, including hepatitis, thrombocytopenia, pneumonitis, and viral sepsis syndromes. Now that preterm infants are only transfused with CMV-negative or leuko-reduced blood products in the neonatal intensive care unit (NICU) setting, human breast milk is the most common mode of postnatal transmission of CMV from a mother to a preterm infant.[13,14]

Freeze–thaw cycling of breast milk decreases or may eliminate viral particles.[15,16] While steps such as freezing or pasteurizing milk have been proposed to decrease transmission from a CMV-positive mother to her own preterm hospitalized infant, neither is employed routinely. There are no accepted, universal guidelines for either prenatal or postnatal screening for CMV, and maternal serostatus is unlikely to be known.

There have been no reported cases of transmission of CMV infection to a preterm infant from a single misadministered aliquot of human breast milk. Most NICUs routinely store expressed maternal breast milk frozen, decreasing the risk. When a breast milk misadministration event occurs, offering testing for the donor mother for CMV can be made on an individual basis, but it should be discussed in the context of a very low-risk event. If a donor mother is to be tested, the recipient baby's mother should also be tested.

Other viral pathogens

Other viruses can also potentially be transmitted via breast milk. Herpes simplex virus and varicella zoster virus can be transmitted via contact with active skin lesions, including on the breast. Similar to HIV, maternal human T-lymphotropic virus (HTLV) I or II infection is considered a contraindication to breastfeeding, but this infection is rare in women born in the United States. Incidence of maternal HTLV virus positivity is highest in some Caribbean and Asian populations.[17] Viruses detected in low levels in maternal breast milk, but which do not pose a contraindication to breastfeeding, include West Nile virus and Zika virus. In these instances, transmission to an infant is extremely uncommon, and benefits of breastfeeding are felt to outweigh the risks.[18,19]

Bacteria

Bacteria are present in human milk, and pumping or other methods of expressing milk are not sterile procedures. Mothers with certain bacterial and viral infections (eg. acute systemic infection, infections of the breast with either bacterial drainage at a skin site or mastitis with drainage) may be advised to temporarily suspend breastfeeding or provide expressed breast milk to decrease exposure of their own infants. There are no data to support routinely culturing milk for bacteria (or viruses or other pathogens) in a single misadministered feeding.[20,21]

Many neonatal units have additional policies to address infection-related precautions and contraindications to breast feeding, and infection control practitioners and pediatric hospital epidemiologists may be called upon for assistance with some of these decisions.

Handling and dispensing of human breast milk in NICU and newborn nursery settings

As breastfeeding has been promoted and collection of breast milk has increased in NICUs, there are increased opportunities for misadministration events. These occur in the NICUs, in the general newborn nursery, or even the general pediatric ward of a hospital. Estimates of the incidence of breast milk administration errors range from one error for every 10,000 feeding opportunities[22] to 0.7 errors per month in one NICU study conducted over a 10-year period.[23]

Errors can occur for multiple reasons, such as when there are infants whose mothers have the same surnames and no other identification name labelling is used. Point-of-care bar code scanners as checkpoint systems have been implemented in many facilities for medication administration and as general identification measures. These can be used to promote accurate breast milk administration by giving bar-coded labels to mothers to label their expressed milk bottles for storage, and by setting an institutional expectation that all breast milk will be scanned before administration, similar to medications.[24] However, human error still occurs with these systems, especially when commitment to the culture of safety and quality improvement measures is not reinforced over time, or when understaffing in a busy, critical care environment occurs.[25]

Donor Breast Milk

Many NICUs provide donor breast milk from professional milk banks. Recent studies have demonstrated the benefits of providing donor milk to preterm infants in preventing acute and long-term adverse events for these fragile newborns.[26-28] Human milk banks are required to have strict screening processes in place for donor mothers, as well as handling and storage procedures. Some of these handling and dispensing procedures can be adapted to the inpatient hospital setting, such as automated bar code labeling, and handling only by dedicated human milk technicians.

Breast milk volunteer donors are screened for eligibility by interview and serological testing for HIV, HTLV 1/2, hepatitis B, hepatitis C, and syphilis. Specific guidelines for the collection of expressed milk are provided, and milk is delivered to the milk bank frozen. Generally, milk is pooled from several donors to create uniform nutritional properties. Holder pasteurization (62°C for 30 minutes) is performed on all banked breast milk. Bacteriological screening is performed on samples of batches. Human milk banks dispense primarily to neonatal intensive care units for use in preterm infants, with contracted arrangements.[3,24] If an infant is given a donor feeding with human milk fortifiers or other additives that were intended for another baby, this is a misadministration event, but it generally does not pose a serious risk to the recipient and should not require an infectious disease transmission evaluation, as the milk banking donation process has already screened the donor to be free of the usual concerns for infection risk.

Suggested Approaches

Every healthcare facility that provides care to children should have policies that outline recommended practices for collection, storage, and administration of breast milk. Proper handling is necessary to prevent overgrowth of bacteria that are normally present, or secondary contamination. In general, expressed breast milk should be stored in glass or food-grade plastic containers with tight-fitting lids, or in plastic bags designed specifically for human milk storage. Each container should be labeled with the infant's full name, medical record number, and the date and time the milk was expressed. Freshly expressed breast milk may be refrigerated safely at 4°C for up to 96 hours, or frozen for up to three months. Thawed breast milk must be kept refrigerated and used within 24 hours. Temperature of the refrigerators and freezers used for breast milk storage should be monitored. Parents should not have access to milk that does not belong to their infant.

Disclosure of the misadministration incident

While exposure to another woman's milk can cause a great deal of anxiety and may result in a lack of confidence in the parents toward the institution's overall care of the newborn, the actual infectious risk to the baby is very low.[3] Nevertheless, administration of breast milk to the incorrect infant is generally treated like other blood and body fluid exposures.[3–5] Example of hospital policy for management of breast milk administrations in Box 7.1.

As soon as the error is discovered, the parents should be informed of the misadministration in a private setting. Disclosure is generally best performed by a senior nurse manager or physician. Families can be reassured about the extremely low risk of any infectious transmission.

The donor mother should be informed and asked to undergo testing for HBV, HCV, and HIV. Prenatal screens can be reviewed, but a current test should be considered to assess for any change in serostatus if a mother was previously seronegative. To the extent feasible, confidentiality of both mothers must be maintained. This may be difficult if the recipient mother is the one who identifies that a bottle of milk labeled with another infant's name has been fed to her baby. The recipient mother should be counseled that the risk to her baby is extremely low; she should be asked to undergo tests for HBV, HCV, and HIV to provide a baseline risk assessment for her own neonate.

Any declinations by either party should be well documented. The hospital staff member who provides disclosure and counseling generally takes responsibility for providing each mother with her own test results. Testing on neonates should be discouraged, as this does not inform staff about any ongoing theoretical transmission risk. If the donor mother refuses testing, further follow-up testing on an infant may be considered on an individual basis.

Appropriate information about the incident should be given to the infant's pediatrician and mother's obstetrical provider in case additional follow-up is needed. Cost of any testing for the mothers is generally covered by the institution as part of the Risk Management and mitigation-of-error policy. Ongoing psychosocial support for the families and staff should be offered. Discussions with the families are documented per each institution's policy, along with consent for testing, or declinations. Communication with the affected families should emphasize that a thorough review will be done with the healthcare personnel involved with the incident, and that the information learned will be used to prevent future events.

Prevention of future errors and exposures

Many human process errors can be the cause of a breast milk misadministration in the hospital setting. These often

BOX 7.1 EXAMPLE OF HOSPITAL POLICY FOR MANAGEMENT OF BREAST MILK ADMINISTRATIONS

Newborns, infants, or children who receive the incorrect expressed human milk shall be evaluated for body fluid exposure.

Purpose

The purpose of this policy is to provide a guideline for clinicians to use in the practice setting for decision making in the event that a newborn, infant, or child receives the incorrect expressed human milk.

Scope

This policy pertains to any *NAME of HOSPITAL* newborn, infant, or child (inpatient and outpatient circumstances) who receives the incorrect expressed human milk. This policy also applies to the source mother whose expressed breast milk is fed to the wrong infant, and the recipient's mother.

Procedure

Nursing's Responsibilities Once an incident of an incorrect feeding of expressed human milk has been established

1. Notify the unit manager or designee.
2. Notify the pediatrician/primary care physician of the infant exposed if not in the NICU.
3. Initiate the post-exposure protocol.
4. Notify the OB/GYN physician of both mothers involved to assure appropriate follow-up for the mother's testing, if necessary.
5. Notify the mothers involved in the incident (accompanied by a physician), individually, in a private setting.

   The attending physician or designee will discuss the incident with both mothers, using the informed HIV consent.

   The source mother and recipient mother, or their legal guardian will be asked to consent for the drawing of HIV and other labs as appropriate.
6. Pediatric Infectious Diseases on-call physician is available for questions regarding appropriate testing of source and recipient babies' mothers, or concerns about post-exposure prophylaxis counseling and testing.
7. Complete a **patient safety** surveillance report, which will trigger Risk Management (and Division of Health Care Quality, if your institution decides that is appropriate).

   The attending physician, Nurse Manager, and other involved personnel will immediately conduct a root cause analysis (RCA) to address process and opportunities for quality improvement. Document this process per your institutional guidelines.

Documentation

1. Document conversation with the mothers in each child's medical record.
2. Document the route of the exposure, and the circumstances of the exposure in the involved newborn/infant/child's chart. Do NOT document names or identification of persons involved. (*For suggested documentation [you may need to discuss this with your Risk Management department]: example: "Breast milk from another mother [amount] was given at [time]."*)

Post-Exposure Testing

Source exposure profile and infant's mother's profile should include:

- HIV antibody
- Hepatitis B surface antigen
- Hepatitis C antibody
- Other infectious diseases testing, if warranted (based on source mother's medical history)
- Breast milk does not require testing

Post-Exposure Monitoring

1. Infant post-exposure prophylaxis medication is NOT routinely required except for babies who receive milk from a mother who is HIV or HBV antigen–positive. The Pediatric Infectious Disease on-call doctor can assist with the determination of any other testing recommended, such as maternal CMV serology, and the need for prophylaxis.
2. Infant will be monitored and condition documented.
3. Follow-up plan will be documented in the infant's medical record and provided to the parent prior to the infant's discharge.
4. Follow-up testing on the infant is rarely recommended, based on low risk of any infectious transmission; however, it can be offered to the parent(s) on an individual case basis and per the anxiety level of the family.

involve misidentification of the milk bottle, but occasionally a mother is misidentified. A recent report describes a baby being given to the wrong mother for a breastfeeding.[29] A study that evaluated the time of day when errors occurred found that more than 75% of breast milk misadministration errors happened during evening and night shifts, and almost 60% took place after 6:00 PM.[30] Other types of errors with breast milk misadministration are rare but potentially more serious, such as mistaken intravenous administration of breast milk. [31,32]

Root cause analysis (RCA) should be pursued for every case so that measures can be implemented to prevent future occurrences. Following any incident, review of current policies and procedures is indicated, along with reeducation of all staff involved with breast milk collection, distribution, and feedings. Potential causal factors, including but not limited to overcrowding, short staffing, and adherence to checking procedure steps, should be addressed. Staffing ratios for nurses and patient care technicians should be analyzed to determine if hiring additional personnel could mitigate repeated errors. Hospitals with large nursery services have reviewed cost analyses of quality errors, including breast milk misadministration incidents, and have determined that hiring human milk technicians to assist with storage, labelling, handling, and dispensing of expressed human breast milk may be cost-effective over time, improve quality, and enhance family satisfaction.[33] Promotion of breast milk administration safety to families upon admission of their newborn to a NICU setting contributes to families' confidence in the services provided to their fragile newborn.

Approach to the Clinical Scenario

In the scenario described at the beginning of the chapter, the NICU team should be advised that the error should be acknowledged by the staff member who becomes aware of the misadministration as soon as possible, and senior staff should be alerted. The pediatrician or neonatologist for the baby should be notified. Counseling of the recipient infant's parents will incude a discussion of potential risks. Fortunately, risks to the infant from a single misadministered feed are very low, including risk of transmissions of infections such as HIV, HBV and HCV.

The incident should be reported to the nursing administrator on duty, as well as the hospital epidemiology and infection control and hospital Risk Management departments. Standard error reporting should be performed, as per individual institutional policy.

Private and confidential conversations to inform each family should be done as soon as possible. Counseling about the nature of the exposure and the presumed low risk of transmission of infectious agents should be provided, and recommendations for testing of each mother should be provided and affirmed.

Information about notification of results should be provided to mothers in initial conversations. Documentation can be placed in the infant's medical record, with an emphasis on recommendations for testing. Any concerns about documentation may be discussed with an institution's Risk Management team. Many institutions have a policy about incident documentation.

Having an institutional policy to refer to in these instances allows for a rational approach with the staff, and provides a framework for documenting errors, and a standardized response for informing families of the error, in the context of a low-risk, but high-anxiety, incident. Every institution should review its policy at regular intervals and should have a process for performance improvement and immediate root cause analysis when breast milk misadministration events occur. Root cause analysis should be performed with every incident.

Unresolved Issues

The unresolved issues regarding misadministration of human breast milk in an institutional setting include best practices for handling storage, labelling, and administering in different settings. Comparative data from similar birthing hospitals with NICU and nursery settings could be analyzed to assist with determining best practice. As more technological solutions are developed for milk banking and distributing collected milk, additional efforts to reduce human error, labelling, and scanning machine fatigue in providers will need to be assessed. Yearly competency training should be developed for health care staff who are tasked with the duties of feeding this vulnerable population.

References

1. American Academy of Pediatrics. Policy statement. Breastfeeding and the use of human milk. *Pediatrics*. 2012;129(3):e827–e841.
2. American Academy of Pediatrics, American Public Health Association, National Resource Center for Health and Safety in Child Care and Early Education. *Caring for our children: national health and safety performance standards; guidelines for early care and education programs, 3rd ed*. Elk Grove Village, IL: American Academy of Pediatrics; Washington, DC: American Public Health Association; 2011.
3. Warner BB, Sapsford A. Misappropriated human milk: fantasy, fear, and fact regarding infectious risk. *Newborn Infant Nurs Rev*. 2004;4:56–61.
4. Doherty D. Mother's milk, but whose mother? Commentary, Agency for Healthcare Research and Quality, 2010. https://psnet.ahrq.gov/webmm/case/228/mothers-milk-but-whose-mother. Accessed October 30, 2018.
5. Centers for Disease Control and Prevention. What to do if an infant or child is fed another woman's breast milk. Available at: http://www.cdc.gov/breastfeeding/recommendations/other_mothers_milk.htm. Accessed October 30, 2018.
6. Gaillard P, Fowler MG, Dabis F, et al. Use of antiretroviral drugs to prevent HIV-1 transmission through breast-feeding: from animal studies to randomized clinical trials. *J Acquir Immune Defic Syndr*. 2004;35(2):178–187.

7. Committee on Pediatric AIDS. Infant feeding and transmission of human immunodeficiency virus in the United States. *Pediatrics*. 2013;131(2):391–396.
8. Academy of Pediatrics. Hepatitis B. In: Kimberlin DW, Brady MT, Jackson MA, Long SS, eds. *Red Book: 2015 report of the Committee on Infectious Diseases*. 30th ed. Elk Grove Village, IL: American Academy of Pediatrics; 2015: 400–423.
9. Shi Z, Yang Y, Wang H, et al. Breastfeeding of newborns by mothers carrying hepatitis B virus: a meta-analysis and systematic review. *Arch Pediatr Adolesc Med*. 2011;165(9):837–846.
10. Academy of Pediatrics. Hepatitis C. In: Kimberlin DW, Brady MT, Jackson MA, Long SS, eds. *Red Book: 2015 report of the Committee on Infectious Diseases*. 30th ed. Elk Grove Village, IL: American Academy of Pediatrics; 2015: 423–430.
11. Nelson CT, Demmler GJ. Cytomegalovirus infection in the pregnant mother, fetus, and newborn infant. *Clin Perinatol*. 1997;24:151–160.
12. Marshall GS, Stout GG. Cytomegalovirus seroprevalence among women of childbearing age during a 10 year period. *Am J Perinatol*. 2005;22(7):371–376.
13. Minamishima I, Ueda K, Minematsu T, et al. Role of breast milk in acquisition of cytomegalovirus. *Microbio Immunol*. 1994;38:549–552.
14. Josephson CD, Caliendo AM, Easley KA, et al. Blood transfusion and breast milk transmission of cytomegalovirus in very low-birth-weight infants. *JAMA Pediatrics*, 2014;168(11):1054–1062.
15. Lawrence RM. Cytomegalovirus in human breast milk: risk to the premature infant. *Breastfeed Med*. 2006;Summer 1(2):99–107.
16. Kurath S, Halwachs-Baumann G, Müller W, Resch B. Transmission of cytomegalovirus via breast milk to the prematurely born infant: a systematic review. *Clinical Microbiology and Infection*. 2010;16(8):1172–1178.
17. Carneiro-Proietti ABF, Amaranto-Dimasio CF, Leal-Horiguchi RHC, et al. Mother-to-child transmission of human T-cell lymphotropic viruses-1/2: what we know, and what are the gaps in understanding and preventing this route of infection. *J Peds Infect Dis Soc*. 2014;3:S24–S29.
18. Hinckley AF, O'Leary DR, Hayes EB. Transmission of West Nile virus through human breast milk seems to be rare. *Pediatrics*. 2007;119(3):e666–e671.
19. Centers for Disease Control and Prevention. Zika virus transmission in infants and children. Available at: https://www.cdc.gov/pregnancy/zika/testing-follow-up/infants-children.html. Accessed October 30, 2018.
20. Schanler RJ, Fraley JK, Lau C, Hurst NM, Horvath L, Rossmann SN. Breastmilk cultures and infection in extremely premature infants. *J Perinatol*. 2011;31(5):335–338.
21. Riordan J, Wambach K. *Breastfeeding and human lactation*. 4th ed. Sudbury, MA: Jones and Bartlett Publishers; 2010.
22. Drenckpohl D, Bowers L, Cooper H. Use of the Six Sigma methodology to reduce incidence of breast milk administration errors in the NICU. *Neonat NetW*. 2007;26(3):161–166.
23. Wolford SR, Smith C, Harrison MLL. A retrospective two year study of breast milk error prevention in the neonatal intensive care unit. *Neonat Intens Care*. 2013;226(2):41–42.

24. Lawrence RA, Lawrence RM. *Breastfeeding: a guide for the medical profession*. 8th ed. Philadelphia, PA: Elsevier Mosby; 2016. Appendix F, 794–796.
25. Dougherty D, Nash A. Bar coding from breast to baby: a comprehensive breast milk management system for the NICU. *Neonat Netw*. 2009;28(5):321–328.
26. Corpeleijn WE, de Waard M, Christmann V, et al. Effect of donor milk on severe infections and mortality in very low-birth-weight infants. The early nutrition study randomized clinical trial. *JAMA Pediatr*. 2016;170(7):654–661.
27. O'Connor DL, Gibbins S, Kiss A, et al. Effect of supplemental donor human milk compared with preterm formula on neurodevelopment of very low-birth-weight infants at 18 month: a randomized clinical trial. *JAMA*. 2016;316(18):1897–1905.
28. Human Milk Banking Association of North America. Best practice for expressing, storing and handling human milk in hospitals, homes and child care settings. 2011 3rd Ed.
29. Sauer CW, Marc-Aurele K. Parent misidentification leading to the breastfeeding of the wrong baby in a neonatal intensive care unit. *Am J Case Rep*. 2016;17:574–579.
30. Zeilhofer UB, Frey B, Zandee J, et al. The role of critical incident monitoring in detection and prevention of human breast milk confusions. *Eur J Pediatr*. 2009;168(10):1277–1279.
31. Doring M, Brenner B, Handgretinger R, et al. Inadvertent intravenous administration of maternal breast milk to a six week old infant: a case report and review of the literature. *BMC Res Notes*. 2014;7:17.
32. Ryan CA, Mohammed I, Murphy B. Normal neurologic and developmental outcome after an accidental intravenous infusion of expressed breast milk in a neonate. *Pediatrics*. 2006;117(1):236–238.
33. Oza-Frank R, Kachoria R, Dail J, et al. A quality improvement project to decrease human milk errors in the NICU. *Pediatrics*. 2017;139(2):e20154451.

8 | Management of Hospital Visitors

PREETI MEHROTRA AND ANDI L. SHANE

Background

Family Centered Care

Family-centered care (FCC) is an approach to health care based on the understanding that the family is a child's primary source of strength and support.[1] It is endorsed and respected by all members of the healthcare team to the fullest extent, when possible. The traditional paradigm of FCC relies on the physical presence of a familiar person, who is not a member of the healthcare team, to provide both comfort and care to children during illness and medical procedures and to be involved in clinical decision-making on the behalf of a child.

Visitors

Visitors are individuals who are not patients and are not members of the healthcare team. Visitors may be parents and guardians who are bedside caregivers as well as other individuals who are familiar to the patient. They may have had varying levels of interaction with, and potentially exposures to, the patient, both prior to and during the provision of healthcare.

Parents and Guardians

Although parents and guardians are traditionally defined as visitors, their close and continued contact with a child-patient places them at risk for acquiring and/or transmitting an infectious pathogen from their ill child. They may have also had the same community-based exposures as the child, placing them at similar risk for infection. FCC may have an integral role in the delivery of care where language barriers or limited health literacy may contribute to challenging social determinants of health.

Policies and Practices

Policies and practices regarding management of visitors vary by hospital system. Current guidance from the Society for Healthcare Epidemiology of America (SHEA) suggests that practices should be based on (a) the pathogen suspected or confirmed, (b) the underlying medical condition of the patient and the visitor, and (c) the endemicity of that pathogen in the hospital and surrounding community—distinguishing between outbreak and non-outbreak settings.[2]

Pediatric infection prevention strategies should strive to balance FCC with policies that minimize the risk of acquiring or transmitting pathogens. Usual practices may require modification when considering the care of a child with high-consequence pathogens such as pulmonary tuberculosis, hemorrhagic fever, or a novel respiratory virus.[3] In addition, the tenets of FCC may need to be modified when children are managed in high-risk units, including intensive care, oncology, transplant, and high-level isolation units.

Clinical Scenario

You are caring for a three-year-old hospitalized child with culture-proven *E. coli* O157:H7 hemolytic uremic syndrome. The child is incontinent, with bloody diarrhea. Several family members arrive to visit the patient.

Questions

Should isolation precautions be required for visitors? If so, what types of precautions are indicated, and for how long? Do these precautions differ between household contacts and non-household visitors? When should visitor restrictions be considered?

Key Challenges

Challenges related to the physical presence of visitors are twofold: (1) the visitor may be a vector of an organism, posing risk of transmission to the patient, healthcare team, and other patients and families in the hospital environment; and (2) the visitor may be exposed to pathogens in the healthcare environment. Outbreaks of severe acute respiratory syndrome (SARS),[4] pertussis,[5] and influenza[6] occurring in hospital settings have involved visitors. Healthcare facilities must balance the benefits associated with the involvement of visitors and FCC with the potential for acquisition and transmission of pathogens in the hospital environment. This often requires an individual assessment of pathogen characteristics and the population at risk.

In order to address these issues, many hospital systems have instituted transmission-based precautions, whereby isolation of the patient is based on symptoms. As an example, an incontinent three-year-old child with diarrhea such as the one in the clinical scenario just described would be placed into contact isolation. Based on the possible contact with the incontinent child's stool, healthcare personnel would be instructed to wear personal protective equipment (PPE) consisting of disposable gloves and a disposable gown when entering the patient's environment or providing care to the patient. Some hospital systems may require any person entering the room, including family members and visitors, to wear PPE. This requirement could extend for the duration of the stool incontinence, or until one or more negative stool diagnostic test results are obtained. As there is no standardized guidance, approaches to transmission-based precautions may vary between hospital systems and even among different entities within a hospital system.

Guidance regarding isolation precautions may be approached from two perspectives: (1) guidance to protect the visitor/parent from being exposed to the patient's pathogens, and (2) guidance to protect the patient and healthcare team from the visitor/parent's potential pathogens. Protecting the visitor/parent from being exposed to the patient's pathogens is challenging to implement and control, and in most situations is not recommended. While the Centers for Disease Control and Prevention (CDC) and Occupational Safety and Health Administration (OSHA) offer guidance for the use of PPE by healthcare personnel, there is no evidence-based guidance for the use of PPE by visitors. A disadvantage of requiring PPE use by parents/visitors is the burden of supply and procurement, and the increased cost to the healthcare system.[2] In addition to supply and cost implications, proper donning and doffing of PPE require dedicated education and practice, as well as ensuring the availability of PPE to fit a range of body sizes, including those of child visitors. The challenge of acceptance of a family member or visitor in PPE by a child may refute the provision of FCC. Finally, the variability of settings and resources in each of these settings makes the provision of standardized PPE challenging for healthcare personnel, and including a requirement for PPE use by visitors in some settings where PPE supplies are already limited would not be practical. All persons, regardless of the isolation precautions, symptoms, or pathogen,[7] should practice hand hygiene, the mainstay of infection prevention. As many facilities face challenges related to PPE compliance among healthcare personnel, efforts to protect visitors and patients are optimally directed toward hand hygiene compliance, as opposed to a focus on visitor PPE compliance.[8]

Ill visitors, including family members, may represent a risk for transmission of an organism in the healthcare environment, either related or unrelated to a patient's condition. Some systems have implemented visitor screening in which visitors are questioned about current or past symptoms or diagnoses. Other systems have implemented temperature monitoring in addition to symptom screening as a requirement for entry into select units. In addition, some systems may implement various forms of symptom screening or temperature monitoring during seasonal periods or outbreak settings. While experts agree that symptomatic visitors should not be permitted in the patient care environment, defining symptomatic and patient care environments may be difficult. Additionally, implementation and enforcement of policies is challenging.[2]

Ideally, screening would occur at the entrance of the healthcare facility rather than at the points of patient care, in order to avoid inadvertent exposures in communal areas where patients and other family members may be present. Symptom screening at the point of entry requires that the screening process be simple and straightforward, both for the screeners who will be completing and interpreting assessments and for the visitor respondents. When possible, graphics, rather than words, may facilitate comprehension. As screening frequently relies on self-report, emphasizing the importance of visitors' deferring visits while symptomatic may facilitate desired self-exclusion. In situations where self-exclusion does not occur or a visitor does not comply with the screening process, an administrator, such as a clinical supervisor or a member of the infection prevention team, may be best suited to explain and enforce policies. Strategies such as replacement of a symptomatic parent with an asymptomatic parent or guardian or a hospital volunteer may serve as a temporizing measure allowing the symptomatic parent/visitor to recuperate away from the healthcare facility. This may be especially important for patients with chronic care needs who require long-term hospitalizations. Incorporation of technology to optimize video-exchanges between hospitalized children and their symptomatic family members facilitates interaction and communication without a need for physical presence. Endorsing uniform policies with very rare exceptions is crucial to ensure success with implementation and acceptance by members of the healthcare team and by families.

Age-based visitor restriction policies have not been shown to uniformly meet the goals of reducing the introduction and transmission of respiratory and gastrointestinal pathogens into the healthcare environment by family members.[2] Age-based restrictions are difficult to uniformly enforce, as ages of child visitors may not be accurately reported. In addition, the developmental stage of the child is likely to be a more important factor than chronological age when considering the risk for transmission of most pathogens. Age-based restriction policies have been inappropriately instituted to limit the number of visitors at bedsides; systems who wish to limit visitor numbers should simply limit the number of visitors, without reliance on age-based restrictions that are generally not effective in reducing the risk for transmission of pathogens. Variation in visitor restriction policies, especially aged-based restrictions, may create challenges related to enforcement, when a patient is transferred to a unit where a different policy may be in place.

Visitor restrictions and the use of PPE by essential visitors may be mandated by the risk of pathogen transmission and resulting infection, such as when a visitor exposure to an infected patient may have dire consequences, for example with a highly transmissible viral hemorrhagic fever organism or a high-consequence respiratory pathogen. In other more common situations, such as when a child is being evaluated for tuberculosis disease with an unidentified source, most experts would recommend restriction of visitors while the patient undergoes evaluation.[9,10] In situations where an essential caregiver must be present, most systems will permit visitor presence by one or two essential asymptomatic caregivers, while evaluations of the patient and contacts are ongoing. When the pathogen of concern is *Mycobacterium tuberculosis*, the essential caregivers may be required to wear surgical masks when not present in the patient's airborne infection isolation room.[9,10] Non-essential visitors should not be permitted to visit, until a diagnosis has been made or excluded, both to protect the visitor and to minimize the risk of further transmission.

During an outbreak or exposure situation, it is also reasonable that a temporary modification of visitor restrictions and isolation procedures may be needed on a particular unit or in an area until transmission is halted or the risk subsides. During the SARS epidemic, several hospitals instituted screening of visitors and employees. Symptom-based questionnaires and temperature assessments were conducted to limit symptomatic visitors and transmission in the healthcare environment.[11–13] Modification of visitor restrictions during a possible or ongoing community outbreak were implemented in many systems during the 2014 Ebola virus disease outbreak in West Africa. Affirmative responses to country-specific travel screening questionnaires frequently resulted in isolation of symptomatic, and sometimes asymptomatic, travelers and their accompanying family members until additional evaluations could be completed. For some hospital systems, this evaluation involved the activation of a unit dedicated to the care of a child with a high consequence pathogen as well as the involvement of public health partners.[3]

Seasonal-based visitor restrictions during periods of increased respiratory virus circulation such as the annual respiratory syncytial virus (RSV) or influenza season may prompt the institution of both seasonal and age-based visitor restrictions.[14–16] A single-center retrospective chart review found that there was a reduction in RSV-infected hospitalized infants in a neonatal intensive care unit from approximately 7% during the 2001–2006 RSV seasons to approximately 2% during the 2007–2010 RSV seasons, after siblings under 13 years of age were not permitted to visit ($p < 0.0001$) during the 2007–2010 seasons.[17] Additionally, there was a reduction in symptomatic infants from 23 (6%) during permissive sibling visitation to 2 (0.04%) during sibling exclusion ($p < 0.001$).[17] While studies may support seasonal and aged-based visitor restrictions in a neonatal care unit, many factors could have contributed to the decline in RSV-infected and symptomatic hospitalized neonates, independent of the seasonal and age-based visitor restrictions.[14–17]

With respect to gastrointestinal (GI) illnesses, current guidance from the CDC recommends the institution of visitor restrictions in the setting of institutional norovirus outbreaks.[18–20] This strategy may require the exclusion of all non-essential visitors and symptomatic parents until no new infections have been reported and visitors and parents have been asymptomatic for more than 24 hours.[18–20] Hand hygiene, a mainstay of infection prevention, should be emphasized with all staff and visitors.[2,7]

To further characterize the visitor restriction policies in North American children's hospital systems, an Emerging Infections Network (EIN) survey was disseminated in 2016 to EIN members who provide care to children. Of the respondents, 104 (61%) reported that their primary inpatient facility implements pediatric visitor restrictions, and that the respondent was familiar with at least some of the details of this policy. Restrictions based on symptoms were more common (reported by 97%) than restrictions based on age (74%) or outbreaks (75%). Symptom-based restrictions were usually in effect all year (70%) versus seasonally only (26%). The timing of seasonal visitor restrictions was determined by the local epidemiology of influenza (76%). The survey elucidated variations in the content of visitor-screening assessments, and responsibilities related to completion, enforcement, and communication of policies.[21]

Suggested Approaches

Visitor restrictions are a central focus of pediatric infection prevention, as these policies must be balanced with the tenets of FCC. Approaches often result in several strategies being implemented simultaneously; therefore, efficacy data related to an individual effort and its contribution to pre-specified outcomes and control are limited.

However, the following strategies have *not* been found to be universally beneficial:

1. Age-based visitor restrictions that are instituted to limit the total number of visitors at the bedside;
2. Routine wearing of PPE by parents/guardians or other visitors.

In contrast, the following strategies may be beneficial:

1. Consistent policies regarding visitor restrictions that are known and endorsed uniformly by healthcare staff. These should be widely disseminated using different strategies such as written materials, signage, and screening, and they should be a part of new-employee trainee orientation and annual accreditation;
2. Minimizing exceptions to policies, except in extenuating circumstances, with clear descriptions of situations that may be subject to exceptions as well as those authorized to make the exceptions;
3. Consistent communication to families and visitors to postpone visitation when symptomatic;
4. Visitor screening tools may be efficacious as an adjunct to symptom self-screening. Residential facilities, often viewed as "home away from home" and where screening may be less likely to be implemented consistently, may benefit from visitor screening tools.[22]

An example is as seen in Handout 8.1.

HANDOUT 8.1 Example Visitor Questionnaire

Please answer YES or NO to all of the questions below.
Have you had any of the following:

YES	NO	Fever higher than 100.4°F (38.0°C) in the past 2 days?
YES	NO	Vomiting in the past 2 days?
YES	NO	Stiff neck or headache with a fever in the past 2 days?
YES	NO	Diarrhea in the past 2 days?
YES	NO	Current skin lesions that are "weepy" (fluid or pus-filled)?
YES	NO	ANY current skin rash?
YES	NO	Current cold or flu symptoms (runny nose, cough, congestion)?
YES	NO	Exposure to tuberculosis (TB) in the past 2 months?
YES	NO	Exposure to any of the following within the past 3 weeks: __Chicken pox __Household member with head lice __Measles __Mumps __Whooping cough

Contact the Charge Nurse or Attending Physician to discuss any "yes" answer above, prior to allowing entry.

Chicken Pox Status:

YES NO Have you had chicken pox or shingles before?
YES NO Have you been vaccinated against chicken pox (varicella)?

[Adapted from Appendix A of cited guidelines][22]

5. Focus on consistent and frequent use of hand hygiene. Every person should perform hand hygiene upon entering and exiting a patient's room and prior to contact with the patient and his/her environment. Hand hygiene is the foundation of infection prevention and plays a critical role in the prevention of pathogen transmission.[7] All visitors should be educated on the importance of frequent hand hygiene, and staff should demonstrate key opportunities to practice hand hygiene by example. The available options and proper techniques for performing hand hygiene should be demonstrated.[23] Alcohol hand-hygiene dispensers as well as sinks with running water, soap, and paper towels should be readily accessible.[7]
6. Utilize audio and visual interaction systems as a substitute for in-person contact between patient and family members if personal interaction represents a risk for infection transmission. The institution of creative models that transcend the "parent in the room" and

utilize advances in technology to provide telemedicine and "virtual support" may optimize FCC.[24] Ancillary healthcare staff, including Child Life, chaplain services, and volunteers, can provide temporary care, substituting for a parent or guardian when parental presence may not be possible.[24]

Approach to the Clinical Scenario

Limited data exist, and hospitals differ in their approaches to the clinical scenario described earlier in the chapter. Little evidence exists to support the notion that PPE use protects visitors, and many hospitals would not require visitors to use PPE routinely.[2] For visitors of patients infected with enteric pathogens, guidance does suggest the use of contact isolation precautions. The cited rationale is as follows:

> The prevalence of some of these pathogens in the community is either unknown or thought to be low; acquisition of these pathogens can be potentially harmful to visitors. For parents/guardians/visitors with extended stay in a patient's room, including overnight visitation, isolation precautions may not be practical. The risk of infection for parents/guardians/visitors is likely reduced if they practice good hand hygiene, and any additional benefit of wearing gowns and gloves in these scenarios of prolonged exposure is unclear.[2]

In this scenario, and in others, a focus on hand hygiene is essential.[2,7] Precautions should not necessarily differ between household contacts and non-household visitors, as household exposure may not correlate with transmission risk, if another exposure, such as a foodborne exposure in this setting, occurred outside the home; for example, at a community-based event.

Visitor restrictions should be considered when the risk to the patient, or to those in the hospital environment, outweighs the benefits of an in-person interaction. Strategies to provide interaction via technology may be considered as an alternative to in-person interaction.

Unresolved Issues

As previously noted, concomitant implementation of several measures related to visitor restriction policies has made measurement of the effectiveness of individual interventions challenging. However, there are some issues that remain outstanding:

1. The 2015 American Academy of Pediatrics (AAP) *Red Book* states, "Siblings who are visiting should have received all recommended immunizations for their age. Before and during influenza season, siblings who visit should have received influenza vaccine."[25]

The ability to monitor, enforce, and in some situations provide immunizations to visitors varies considerably between hospital systems. While adherence to the preceding guidance is optimal, the logistics of universal implementation and challenges related to resource allocation usually mean that families are questioned regarding immunization status, but responses may be limited in their applicability.

2. SHEA guidance states,

"In special situations, in which patients acquire new transmissible infections after admission to the hospital, protection of parent/guardian/visitor by the use of isolation precautions may be considered. Examples of such scenarios could include parents of children with *hospital onset* of *C. difficile* infection or colonization/infection with extensively antibiotic-resistant gram-negative bacilli (e.g., *Klebsiella pneumoniae* carbapenemase-producing bacteria). If parents or other visitors are assisting healthcare personnel with providing care, standard precautions should be utilized, including the use of gowns and gloves, if contact with blood, body fluids, or non-intact skin is anticipated."[2]

Implementation and enforceability may need to be considered individually by hospital system. Such scenarios could serve as an opportunity for educating families about hospital-acquired infections and actions to prevent transmission, including the universal adoption of hand hygiene, the foundation of prevention.

References

1. American Academy of Pediatrics. Family centered care: the pediatrician's role. *Pediatrics.* 2003;112(3):691–696.
2. Munoz-Price L, Banach DB, Bearman, G, et al. SHEA expert guidance: isolation precautions for visitors. *Infect Control Hosp Epidemiol.* 2015 July;36(7):747–758.

3. Davies HD, Byington CL. American Academy of Pediatrics Committee on Infectious Diseases: parental presence during treatment of Ebola or other highly consequential infection. *Pediatrics.* 2016 Sept;138(3):e20161891.
4. Centers for Disease Control and Prevention. Update: severe acute respiratory syndrome—worldwide and United States. *MMWR.* 2003;52:664–665.
5. Leekha S, Thompson RL, Sampathkumar P. Epidemiology and control of pertussis outbreaks in a tertiary care center and the resource consumption associated with these outbreaks. *Infect Control Hosp Epidemiol.* 2009;30(5):467–473.
6. Sagrera X, Ginovart G, Raspall F, et al. Outbreaks of influenza A virus infection in neonatal intensive care units. *Pediatr Infect Dis J.* 2002;21:196–200.
7. Ellingson K, Haas JP, Aiello AE, et al. Strategies to prevent healthcare-associated infections through hand hygiene. *Infect Control Hosp Epidemiol.* 2014;35(8):937–960.
8. Morgan DJ, Murthy R, Munoz-Price LS, et al. Reconsidering contact precautions for endemic methicillin-resistant *Staphylococcus aureus* and vancomycin resistant *Enterococcus*. *Infect Control Hosp Epidemiol.* 2015;36(10):1163–1172.
9. Kellerman SE, Simonds D, Banerjee S, Towsley J, Stover BH, Jarvis W. APIC and CDC survey of *Mycobacterium tuberculosis* isolation and control practices in hospitals caring for children. Part 1: Patient and family isolation policies and procedures. *Am J Infect Control.* 1998;26:478–482.
10. Kellerman SE, Saiman L, San Gabriel P, Besser R, Jarvis WR. Observational study of the use of infection control interventions for *Mycobacterium tuberculosis* in pediatric facilities. *Pediatr Infect Dis J.* 2001;20:566–570.
11. Beck M, Antle BJ, Berlin D, et al. Wearing masks in a pediatric hospital: developing practical guidelines. *Can J Public Health.* 2004;95:256–257.
12. Dwosh HA, Hong HLH, Austgarden D, et al. Identification and containment of an outbreak of SARS in a community hospital. *CMAJ.* 2003;168(11):1415–1420.
13. Tan WM, Chlebicka NL, Tan BH. Attitudes of patients, visitors and healthcare workers at a tertiary hospital towards influenza A (H1N1) response measures. *Ann Acad Med Sing.* 2010;39:303–304. 16.
14. Gupta M, Pursley DM. A survey of infection control practices for influenza in mother and newborn units in US hospitals. *Am J Obstet Gynecol.* 2011;204:S77–S83.
15. Christie CD, Glover AM, Willke MJ, Marx ML, Reising SF, Hutchinson NM. Containment of pertussis in the regional pediatric hospital during the Greater Cincinnati epidemic of 1993. *Infect Control Hosp Epidemiol.* 1995;16:556–563.
16. Fanella ST, Pinto MA, Bridger NA, et al. Pandemic (H1N1) 2009 influenza in hospitalized children in Manitoba: nosocomial transmission and lessons learned from the first wave. *Infect Control Hosp Epidemiol.* 2011;32(5):435–438.
17. Peluso AM, Harnish BA, Miller NS, et al. Effect of young sibling visitation on respiratory syncytial virus activity in a NICU. *J Perinatol.* 2015;35(8):627–630.
18. MacCannell, T, Umscheid CA, Agarwal RK, et al. Guideline for the prevention and control of norovirus gastroenteritis outbreaks in healthcare settings. *Centers for Disease Control and Prevention. Norovirus Guidelines.* 2011;32:939–969.
19. Johnston CP, Qiu H, Ticehurst JR, et al. Outbreak management and implications of a nosocomial norovirus outbreak. *Clin Infect Dis.* 2007;45(5):534–540.

20. Cheng FW, Leung TF, Lai RW, Chan PK, Hon EK, Ng PC. Rapid control of norovirus gastroenteritis outbreak in an acute paediatric ward. *Acta Paediatr.* 2006;95(5):581–586.
21. Pong A, Faltamo M, Beekmann S, et al. Visitor restriction policies and practices in children's hospitals in North America: results of an Emerging Infections Network Survey. *Infect Control Hosp Epidemiol.* 2018;39:968–971.
22. Guzman-Cottrill JA, Ravin KA, Bryant KA, et al. Infection prevention and control in residential facilities for pediatric patients and their families. *Infect Control Hosp Epidemiol.* 2013 Oct;34(10):1003–1041.
23. World Health Organization. Five moments of hand hygiene: tools for training and education. Available at: http://www.who.int/gpsc/5may/tools/training_education/en/ . Accessed October 25, 2018.
24. Mehrotra P, Shane AL, Milstone AM. Family-centered care and high-consequence pathogens: thinking outside the room. *JAMA Pediatr.* 2015;169(11):985–986.
25. American Academy of Pediatrics. Sibling visitation. In Kimberlin, DW (Ed.). *Red Book: 2015 report of the Committee of Infectious Disease*. Elk Grove Village, IL: American Academy of Pediatrics Red Book; 2015.

9 | Hospital-Based Playrooms, Classrooms, and Pet Therapy

JANE M. GOULD

Background

Play is an essential part of childhood and a fundamental developmental process that helps children make sense of their world. The tools of play are toys. A unique feature of most pediatric hospitals is that they provide opportunities for both inpatients and outpatients to participate in play with developmentally appropriate toys during their medical care. Reasons for play in hospitalized pediatric patients may include providing mechanisms to educate a child about their particular medical condition, providing stress reduction during frightening procedures, assisting in the development of coping strategies, and attempting to maintain a sense of normalcy during long hospitalizations. Play can occur in a patient's hospital room or in a playroom with peers, both of which are typically supervised by Play Therapy/Child Life staff. Additionally, surgical and outpatient departments may also provide specific toys and play opportunities for their particular specialty. Although toys and playroom environments provide a vital psychosocial and quality-of-life function, they are known to contribute to the transmission of infectious agents.[1–5]

Infection prevention and control (IPC) personnel at pediatric hospitals have the unique responsibility to train all Play Therapy/Child Life staff and members of all hospital departments that provide toys in basic infection prevention education, provide policies and procedures to ensure that toys and playroom environments are clean and safe, and provide compliance monitoring tools for infection prevention policies pertaining to play therapy.

Clinical Scenario One

A new playroom recently opened in a children's hospital, supported by a gift from a hospital benefactor. The Grand Opening of the playroom was attended by children from several hospital wards, and their siblings. In less than 48 hours, three children develop fever, vomiting, and diarrhea. The hospital's infection preventionist asks if this could be an outbreak related to the playroom event.

Questions

Should there be limitations on which patients can visit a hospital playroom? What are the best practices for toy cleaning?

Key Challenges

One of the key challenges for a hospital play therapy program is providing developmentally appropriate toys and activities for the various ages and cognitive levels of patients, while ensuring that the play environment and toys are clean and sanitized appropriately. Consideration must be given to the fact that young children usually put toys in their mouths. Additionally, there are special patient populations within pediatrics that are at high risk of acquiring hospital-associated infections. Patients with cystic fibrosis (CF), sickle cell anemia, and compromised immune systems present increased challenges with regard to providing a safe play environment. Patients who are colonized or infected with multidrug-resistant organisms (MDROs) and cared for using isolation precautions will need special accommodation for play therapy. Although there are conflicting studies in the literature, pediatric patients who require isolation precautions can sometimes feel socially isolated, especially if the hospitalization is prolonged. This makes play therapy sessions all the more vital to the overall well-being of the patient. Most often, patients in isolation precautions will require play therapy in their hospital rooms. The personal protective equipment (PPE) worn by healthcare personnel to enter isolation rooms, especially if masking is required, can be frightening to pediatric patients. An alternative approach that some facilities use is to allow patients in isolation to participate in private play sessions in the playroom, and when they are finished, the Child Life staff will clean the used table, chairs, and toys.

Another challenge is how best to approach the issue of siblings and or parents/caregivers who may want to attend play therapy sessions with the patient in the playroom. These additional persons may represent potential infectious risk to other patients and should be screened carefully for illness before being allowed to enter the playroom.

Suggested Approaches

The physical design of the playroom should provide enough space, with good ventilation and lighting for safe play. The play surfaces, walls, and floors should be easily cleanable with a hospital-grade disinfectant. There should be adequate supplies of readily available hospital-grade cleaning supplies kept for quick cleanups in the event of accidents. These should be stored in cabinets that are not accessible to patients. Typically, a hospital's Environmental Services staff is responsible for cleaning the surfaces in the playroom at the end of the day. Toys are cleaned by the Play Therapy/ Child Life staff who have been trained in proper cleaning procedures. Environmental Services usually cleans large spills and soilings if they should occur during the course of the playroom activities. Aquariums and tank animals such as reptiles and amphibians should be kept out of playrooms, as these pose some risk of transmitting infectious diseases to patients. Additionally, there should be readily available hand sanitizers and sinks for all patients and staff to ensure appropriate hand hygiene.

Staffing of the playroom should be appropriate for the number and developmental level of the patients attending the play session. All staff should participate in mandatory annual infection prevention education provided via online learning or face-to-face presentations; documentation of course completion should be maintained in the Play Therapy/Child Life department. All staff should be educated on the importance of hand hygiene and when to perform it, as well as the potential need for PPE in order to comply with standard precautions. Hand hygiene should be performed upon room entry by patients, families, and staff. Additionally, hand hygiene should be performed before and after every patient contact. Gloves should be worn when there is the possibility of contact with blood or bodily fluids, secretions, excretions (with the exception of sweat), non-intact skin, or mucous membranes. Disposable gowns should be worn if soiling of clothing is possible, and masks, face-shields, and goggles should be worn when performing activities that may produce aerosols or splashing of blood, body fluids, secretions, and/or excretions as one might experience if cleaning large accidental soilings in the playroom, or if Child Life staff are assisting during procedures performed elsewhere in the hospital to help with patient pain-control and anxiety.

All playroom staff should be vaccinated according to the hospital policy for healthcare personnel, including annual influenza vaccination. They should have documentation of annual compliance with the hospital's tuberculosis (TB) prevention program, typically either an annual tuberculin skin testing (TST) or gamma interferon release assay (IGRA), or symptom screening if already TST- or IGRA-positive. They should also complete annual infection prevention education. The staff should be screened daily for contagious illness and not be allowed to work in the hospital if they are ill. There are numerous reports of viral outbreaks associated with patients who attended hospital playrooms.[1,3,6,7]

The hospital should have policies and procedures in place for the appropriate care of toys, play mats, computers, tablets, and play stations. An example of an infection prevention policy for Play Therapy/Child Life can be found in Handout 9.1. The choice of toys and electronic devices should take into consideration the ease with which the various items can be sanitized. Protective cases for electronic devices can be used to make them easier to disinfect. Game boards can be laminated for cleaning and disinfecting purposes. Proper cleaning and sanitization of the toys and playroom environment requires the use of an Environmental Protection Agency (EPA) registered hospital-grade disinfectant with the correct dilution and contact time necessary for the product to work properly. All toys must be cleaned after each use and if obviously soiled. Toys that are returned from patient rooms should be cleaned before being put back into circulation. An example of a policy pertaining to the proper care of toys to prevent cross contamination can be found in Handout 9.2.

Proper selection of patients appropriate for playroom visits must include considering the patient's underlying disease condition, whether the patient is in any type of isolation, issues of contagiousness, and whether secretions/excretions can be controlled. It may be helpful to engage the unit nursing or Child Life staff to screen patients for playroom eligibility to avoid potential transmission of infectious agents and patient disappointment if turned away at the door. Patients who require isolation are generally not allowed in the playroom. Play therapy staff should follow all isolation precautions listed on the patient's door when conducting play sessions in a patient's room. In general, CF patients are restricted from contact with other cystic fibrosis patients.[8] CF patients colonized or infected with MDROs are not permitted to attend the playroom. Those who are not colonized with an MDRO may go to the playroom with a mask on during specific assigned times, but they are not allowed in the playroom with each other, in order to reduce the transmission of microorganisms. Oncology

HANDOUT 9.1 Example of a Child Life Infection Prevention Policy

Section: Infection Prevention Manual	Policies & Procedures ------------------------ Number:
Title: **Infection Prevention Program for Child Life Services**	Effective Date: ------------------------ Reviewed Date:

I. Policy

The Child Life Staff will be educated on practices that prevent infections and will participate in activities with hospital staff to prevent the spread of infection.

II. Procedure

A. Patient Contact

1. *Hand Hygiene*. Hand hygiene is to be performed before and after every patient contact. All Child Life staff are expected to be meticulous in their hand hygiene technique (Infection Prevention [IP] Policy # _______: Infection Prevention Policy and Procedures).
2. *Standard Precautions*. All Child Life staff are required to utilize Standard Precautions for all patients. Gloves should be worn when there exists the possibility of coming into contact with blood or body fluids, secretions, excretions (with the exception of sweat), non-intact skin, or mucous membranes. Disposable gowns should be worn if soiling of clothing is possible. Additional personnel protective equipment (PPE), i.e., masks, face shields, goggles, should be donned as needed when performing activities that may produce aerosols or splashing of blood, body fluids, secretions, and/or excretions.
3. *Isolation*.
   a. Children who require isolation will not be allowed in the playrooms.
   b. Child Life Specialists caring for hospitalized children who are in isolation will carefully follow (***insert hospital name here***) isolation guidelines (IP Policy #______: Isolation Guidelines) for proper isolation of patients with possible transmissible diseases.
   c. All Child Life staff are expected to read and carefully follow isolation precautions posted on the patient's door. If there are questions regarding the precautions, the patient's nurse is to be consulted. Additional questions, or those concerning communicability of a patient's illness, must be consulted with the infection preventionist or hospital epidemiologist.
   d. Patients with cystic fibrosis (CF) will adhere to the specific Child Life Policy (**Appendix 1,** this chapter) as well as the CF Isolation Policy (IP Policy # ______).

e. Siblings of patient in isolation are not permitted in the playroom (Child Life Policy # ______: Children Other Than Patients in Playrooms).

f. Child Life will maintain a daily log of patients who visited the playroom.

B. Child Life Services' Specific Procedures

1. *Toy Receiving and Distribution.*
   a. Used stuffed toys may not be accepted from outside donors.
   b. Patients in isolation will receive books that they may take home with them upon discharge.
   c. Before lending parents a book or toy for their child, the Child Life Specialist shall ascertain whether or not the child is in isolation and will make a decision as to appropriateness of that toy or book for the child. Only books with wipe-able, shiny surfaces or made of vinyl are recommended for lending.
   d. Fabric toys and stuffed animals are not used by the Child Life program.
2. *Cleaning of Toys.*
   a. Playroom toys must be cleaned with hospital-approved disinfectant after each use and if obviously soiled.
   b. All toys returned from rooms are cleaned before being put back in circulation.
   c. Infant toys are washed daily after each play session.
   d. Keyboards, TV, video center, remote controls, and other equipment are wiped down between patient use.
   e. Mats are wiped off after use by each patient.
3. *Admission of Children Other Than Patients to the Playroom.* (Refer to Child Life Policy #_____.)
   a. All visitors to the playroom must complete a health screen (**Appendix 2,** this chapter) conducted by a Child Life Specialist in order to exclude visitors who may be suffering from or carrying contagious infectious illnesses.
   b. For visitors of patients with extended stays in the hospital, the health screening will be performed at least once each week and as needed if the Child Life Specialist believes there is a change in the status of the visitor.
4. *Pet Visitation.* Pet visitation will be allowed as per Child Life Services Pet Visitation Program Child Life Policy # _____. Family pet visitation is **NOT** permitted. Exceptions may be made under extraordinary circumstances and only with approval of the Hospital Epidemiologist and/or designee. Pet Therapy Program will adhere to IP Pet Therapy Policy #________.

III. Education Program

A. Orientation. All Child Life staff must attend a mandatory orientation upon initiation of employment. This program gives basic information on Infection Prevention and Employee Health issues. Opportunity is given for the new employee to ask question of the infection preventionist and/or Employee Health.

B. Yearly In-services. All Child Life staff will participate in mandatory yearly IP in services (will be assigned annually via online learning). Opportunity is given for questions to be asked of the infection preventionist at any time. Documentation of completion will be kept in the department.

C. Need-Based In-services. All Child Life staff will participate in need-based in services provided for the department. Opportunity is given for questions to be asked of the infection preventionist. Documentation of attendance will be kept in the department.

IV. Employee Health

A. **Upon Employment.** All new employees are requested to fill out a health-screening form including issues pertaining to IP. Appropriate serological and tuberculosis testing is performed according to Employee Health Infection Prevention Policy (IP Policy # __: Employee Health Infection Prevention Policies).

B. **Sickness.** Child Life staff with skin, respiratory, gastrointestinal, or other contagious diseases will not work until they are cleared by their supervisor or Employee Health.

Appendix 1

POLICY: Children Other Than Patients in Playroom

Hospital Name:

Policy No.:

Original Date:

Last Revision Date:

Children other than patients are allowed in the playrooms if they are visiting a patient and are cleared medically.

PROCEDURE

Siblings and other visitors of patients, who have clearance to visit, may come to the playroom.

A **Visitor Health Screen (Appendix 2**, this chapter) must be done on each visitor who enters the playroom. The form will be completed by the parent/guardian with the help of Child Life, if needed, before the visitor is allowed in the playroom. The form will be updated daily. All forms will be stored in a folder in the playroom.

- If the patient is on isolation, his/her visitors will not be allowed in the playroom. Special circumstances will be considered—consult with IPC team.
- If visitors are not able to follow the playroom policies and/or become disruptive, they may be asked to leave.
- If the playroom becomes unsafe because of the number of visitors, they may be asked to leave.
- Staff may not leave their own children in the playrooms for supervised care. The Child Life staff must focus on patients' needs.

Appendix 2

(Insert Hospital Name)

CHILD LIFE SERVICES

VISITOR HEALTH SCREEN

Patient Name: ______________________________________ Room # ________

Visitor Name: ______________________________________ Date: ________

To provide the safest environment possible for our patients and visitors, we must ensure that no one visiting the playroom is suffering from or is carrying any contagious infectious illnesses. Please take a moment to answer the following questions regarding the health status of the visitor to the playroom. This information will be kept confidential and located in the Child Life office.

Child Life Services, in cooperation with the Infection Prevention Program, reserves the right to exclude a visitor from the playroom if the visitor demonstrates any of the following signs and/or symptoms of illness or answers "yes" to any questions. If you have concerns or questions, please feel free to contact the infection preventionist at (***insert phone number***).

Does the visitor have any or been exposed to any of the following in the past week:

	YES	NO
Fever	____	____
Cough	____	____
Sore throat	____	____
Cold or Runny nose	____	____
Diarrhea	____	____
Nausea/Vomiting	____	____
Eye drainage/Pink eye	____	____
Rash	____	____

HANDOUT 9.2 Example of a Toy and Play Equipment Policy

Section: **Infection Prevention Manual**	Policies & Procedures ------------------------ Number:
Title: **Toy and Play Equipment Policy: Preventing Cross-Contamination of Toys and Play Equipment**	Effective Date: ------------------------ Reviewed Date:

I Policy Goals

1. To ensure that patients and siblings have access to clean and safe play equipment, toys, and other supplies provided within patient care areas.
2. To prevent the transmission of infectious organisms from one patient to another.
3. To ensure proper procedures for cleaning and disinfecting toys and equipment.
4. To consistently maintain infection control practices to be followed by Child Life staff, nursing staff, physician office staff, students, and volunteers, and other designated persons (e.g., EVS, or others, depending on specific Unit and Area).

II Responsible Department

All patient care departments.

III General Care of Toys and Equipment

A. Toy Safety and Appropriateness

1. Provide toys and other play equipment for patients that are appropriate for the child's developmental age. Information is available through the Child Life program.
2. Evaluate toys for safety to minimize risk of sharp objects, brittle plastic, glass items, toxic items, choking hazard, pinching hazards, and other safety concerns.
3. Avoid soft, stuffed, or water-retaining toys, and toys that are difficult to clean and dry. Avoid battery-operated and electrical toys that cannot be easily cleaned or immersed in water.
4. Infants, toddlers, and children who put toys in their mouths should not share toys.
5. Avoid providing toys with inappropriate content for the pediatric population; e.g., sexually provocative toys, war/weapon toys, violence, obscene language, movie ratings, etc.

B. Toy Cleaning

1. Toys provided for patient use will be made of materials that can be easily sanitized; e.g., plastic, vinyl, treated woods, and metals. Battery-operated and electrical toys that cannot be easily cleaned or immersed should be avoided. Teaching mannequins, dolls, etc., used for teaching or medical play should be disassembled and cleaned after use.
2. Toy cleaning is the responsibility of all departments housing their own toys.
3. The Child Life Department will deliver, pick up, and clean toys that originate from their department. The Department will follow IP Policy # __ Infection Prevention Program for the Child Life Department that addresses cleaning, receiving, and distribution of toys.
4. The Child Life staff will provide training and supervision for toy cleaning procedures to Child Life students, volunteers, and Child Life staff.

5. Toy cleaning in-services, training, and guidelines are available to hospital staff through the Child Life Program.
6. Clean toys should be clearly separated from dirty ones. Each area will have a specified "soiled toy" container.
7. Segregate toys potentially contaminated with *C. difficile* into a red bag and then place bag into soiled toy container.
8. Hospital-approved disinfectant will be used for cleaning toys. Toys will be cleaned between patients using the hospital-approved disinfectant and following the product's directions and contact time. Items that may go into the mouth should be rinsed with water after disinfection and dried thoroughly. **The contact time is 2 minutes for Sani Cloths:** *i.e., the toy being cleaned must stay wet with the Sani Cloth disinfectant for 2 minutes to be effective. Always read the manufacturer's instructions on the disinfectant to be sure of correct usage.*
9. Toys that are dropped on the floor, found on tabletops, etc., should be assumed to be dirty and disinfected before use.
10. Toys used within the playrooms or waiting areas will be cleaned at the end of each playroom session.
11. Child Life department may substitute dishwasher cleaning for dishwasher-safe toys.
12. General hand hygiene practices will be followed according to established hospital IP policies (refer to IP policy #__).
13. The infection preventionists are available for consultation as needed.

C. Patient Transfer or Discharge

1. If a patient is transferred to another room, the toys provided at the bedside must remain with the patient or be removed for proper cleaning and placed in the soiled toy container for cleaning.
2. At discharge or transfer to another unit, toys must be placed in the soiled toy container. Each unit will have a specified area and procedure for the return of soiled toys; e.g., specified bags, closed bins, etc.

D. TV/Video Game Units

1. TV/video game units will be disinfected, using a hospital-approved disinfectant, between each use when taken to patient rooms by Child Life department, nursing staff, physical therapy, or occupational therapy.
2. Particular attention should be paid to any handheld game controller or remote control unit.
3. Cleaning TV/video game units should be assigned to personnel in departments housing game units/remote controls.
4. Department housed units; e.g., waiting rooms, physician office areas, will be disinfected daily by the department.
5. The units will be unplugged prior to cleaning to prevent risk of electrical shock.

E. Large Toys/Play Equipment: Wagons, Riding Toys, Strollers, Walkers, Swings, Playpens, Play Mats, High Chairs, etc.

1. The staff person initiating use of large toys/play equipment is responsible for cleaning the equipment before and after use with a hospital-approved disinfectant.
2. Linens shall be placed in large toys as appropriate prior to patient use for comfort and IP measures. Linens will be placed in soiled linen bins following each use by patients.

F. Donated Toy Items

1. Donated toys received from the community will be screened for safety and appropriateness by the Child Life staff.
2. Toys received in the original packaging (new toys) may be used as deemed appropriate by the Child Life staff.

patients without MDROs can be allowed to attend the playroom individually with a Play Therapy/Child Life staff member, and only toys, games, and videos that can be cleaned and disinfected should be used. Oncology patients undergoing conditioning or who are recipients of a hematopoietic stem cell transplant (HSCT) usually have their play restricted to the HSCT unit or their room.

Siblings and parents/caregivers of patients in isolation are generally not permitted in the playroom. If hospitals allow siblings and parents/caregivers of patients to attend the playroom, they should also be screened for potential contagious illness and not be allowed to attend the playroom if ill.[8] It is recommended that play therapy programs document their illness-screening of siblings and other visitors, as well as maintain a log of these visitors for potential notification if an infectious exposure should occur. An example of a sibling/visitor screening tool can be found in Appendix 2 of Handout 9.1.

All patients who attend the playroom should be logged in a tracking tool for easy identification in the event of a potential outbreak, to facilitate identification of patients at risk. Typically, this database is maintained in Play Therapy/Child Life department, and it can be a handwritten log or an electronic database. The log should contain two patient identifiers and the date, time, and playroom location of the session; this is especially important if the hospital has more than one playroom. The database should be updated daily. Each play therapy session, whether conducted in the playroom or in the patient's room, should also be documented in the electronic medical record for each patient.

Approach to the Clinical Scenario One

This clinical scenario most likely represents an outbreak related to the Grand Opening event of the new playroom that was attended by patients from several wards, and their siblings. The question is posed regarding limitations on which patients are permitted to visit a hospital playroom. The answer most definitely is "Yes, there should be limitations on which patients and their parents/caregivers or siblings can visit."

- All patients and their siblings and parents/caregivers should be screened for illness and not be allowed to visit a playroom if they have symptoms of a contagious illness.

- All hospital staff should be screened for illness before entering the playroom. Patients with underlying conditions that increase their susceptibility to infections, and patients colonized or infected with MDROs, should not be permitted to attend.
- Play Therapy/Child Life department should maintain a record of all patients (and, ideally, their visitors) who attend events such as this Grand Opening. This allows for rapid identification of persons potentially exposed if outbreaks occur.
- A thorough review of how the playroom environment and toys were cleaned and sanitized is warranted.
- Available toys should be made of substances that allow for disinfection. The best practices for toy cleaning involve using a dishwasher to sanitize the toy if it is dishwasher-safe, or an EPA-registered hospital-grade disinfectant used with the correct dilution and contact time, followed by rinsing in water if the toy is to be used by young children who are likely to put toys in their mouths.
- It is recommended to laminate game boards so that they can be easily disinfected with hospital-approved disinfectant wipes.
- All tablets, video game consoles, and computer keyboards should have protective coverings or cases to allow for disinfectant wiping.
- A system should be in place to separate clean from dirty toys, and to delineate who is responsible for cleaning both the toys and the play environment. Additionally, some facilities have designed their playrooms with consideration of patient separation and use small tables (accommodating three to four persons) to allow families to stay separated from one another. Positioning clean electronics and storage boxes with clean toys in such a way as to surround the play table will keep toys readily available to the patient and their family and prevent accidental usage of dirty toys.

Unresolved Issues

Unresolved issues include how best to provide play therapy for certain patient groups, such as those colonized or infected with MDROs, and those with underlying disease states that put them at high risk for hospital-associated infections. The latter group includes oncology and transplant patients. These patients typically have longer hospital stays and would benefit from group play therapy if it could be accomplished without risk. There is currently no evidence to support group play therapy for these patients, though.

An additional unresolved issue regarding the playroom environment is how best to ensure that adequate cleaning and disinfection of toys and the playroom environment is being accomplished. The Centers for Disease Control and Prevention (CDC) recommend that hospital environmental cleaning and disinfection be monitored and evaluated with educational feedback given to environmental services (EVS) staff.[4] Methods for conducting these evaluations can include direct practice observations, swab cultures, agar slide cultures, fluorescent gel markers, or the ATP (adenosine triphosphate) monitoring system. This system measures ATP surface contamination after cleaning by using a luciferase assay where relative light units are detected with a hand-held luminometer to generate real-time feedback to EVS staff. Of these methods, direct observation, fluorescent gel markers, and the ATP system have been shown in studies to be useful for individual teaching and have been shown to be effective in programmatic improvement.[4]

Pet Therapy: Background

Pet therapy programs are very common in pediatric hospitals. According to a survey conducted by the Society for Healthcare Epidemiology of America, 89% of all U.S. healthcare facilities have animal-assisted activities, 95% allow service animals, but only 40% allow personal pet visitation.[9] Some of the benefits of pet therapy include distraction from pain and loneliness, reduction in feelings of anxiety and depression, and increased patient physical and social activity. The most common uses of animals in health care include animal-assisted activities, service animals, and personal pets. Healthcare facilities may also use animals for research purposes or for therapeutic reasons (e.g., leeches and fly larvae). These will not be discussed in this chapter. The CDC and Healthcare Infection Control Practices Advisory Committee define animal-assisted activities (for specific treatment programs, educational purposes, and recreational and social purposes designed to enhance a patient's quality of life) as pet therapy conducted with animal handlers who are specifically trained for animal-assisted activities. In the United States, "service animals" are specifically defined in the Americans with Disabilities Act (ADA). "Personal pet visitation" is defined as a personal pet being brought into the hospital to interact with that individual patient.

Expert guidance from professional societies suggests that only dogs be used for animal-assisted activities. Cats should be excluded due to the inability to reliably train them to provide safe patient experiences.[9] In general, reptiles, amphibians, birds, primates, ferrets, or rodents should also not be allowed to visit. Exceptions may be made for end-of-life patients who want to see their personal pet and are in single-patient rooms. Dogs and their handlers should be formally trained and certified by organizations such as Pet Partners, Therapy Dogs Incorporated, or Therapy Dogs International.[9] Components of a formal training course for therapy dog handlers are listed in Box 9.1.

Pet therapy dog exposures can result in transmission of infectious diseases to patients (Table 9.1). Infectious organisms can be transmitted via direct contact (bites) or indirect contact, fecal-oral contact, via droplets, or vector-borne where the vector is transmitted from the dog to a human. Additionally, Lefebvre et al. demonstrated that dogs have higher rates of acquisition of methicillin-resistant *Staphylococcus aureus* (MRSA) and *Clostridioides difficile* (4.7 and 2.4 times as high, respectively) if they visited healthcare facilities, compared with rates among dogs involved in other animal-assisted interventions.[10] Dogs who licked patients or accepted treats from patients were more likely to be positive for both MRSA and *C. difficile*.[10] Dog diet was monitored in this study because of the potential confounding effect on pathogen acquisition of the consumption of raw foods of animal origin. Other studies have demonstrated that dogs that consume pig ear treats or raw bones are at increased risk of shedding antimicrobial-resistant strains of *E. coli* and *Salmonella* species.[11] Therefore, pet therapy dogs should be considered as potential sources of healthcare-associated pathogens when evaluating patients for possible

BOX 9.1 REQUIRED EDUCATIONAL MODULES FOR ANIMAL-ASSISTED HANDLERS

Zoonotic Diseases

- Standard precautions, including hand hygiene before and after patient contact.
- Proper cleaning and disinfection of surfaces contaminated by animal excrement.
- Proper disposal of animal waste.
- Visual inspection for ectoparasites.
- Animal body language to identify animal with physical discomfort, stress, fear, or aggression.
- Identification of appropriate hospital contacts in event of an accident or injury.

TABLE 9.1 Selected Disease/Microorganisms Transmitted by Dogs Stratified by Transmission Route

TRANSMISSION ROUTE	SELECTED DISEASES/MICROORGANISMS
Direct contact (bites)	Rabies virus, *Capnocytophaga canimorsus, Pasteurella* spp., *Staphylococcus aureus* (MSSA, MRSA), *Streptococcus* spp.
Direct or indirect contact	Flea bites, mites (*Cheyletiellidae, Sarcoptidae*), *Malassezia pachydermatis, Microsporum canis, Trichophyton mentagrophytes, Staphylococcus aureus* (MSSA, MRSA)
Fecal-oral	*Campylobacter* spp., *Salmonella* spp., *Giardia duodenalis*
Droplet	*Chlamydophila psittaci*
Vector-borne	Ticks (passively carried from dog to human): Rocky Mountain spotted fever (*Rickettsia ricksettsii*), Ehrlichiosis (*Ehrlichia* spp.); Fleas (*Dipylidium caninum, Bartonella henselae*)

healthcare-associated infections and should be prevented from licking patients, accepting treats from patients, and sitting directly on patients' beds without a barrier.

The role of the IPC Department includes ensuring animal handler education and compliance with infection prevention policies pertaining to pet therapy. The department that directly oversees animal-assisted activities, typically the Volunteer or Child Life department, should educate handlers on the hospital's human resource (HR) policies. It is recommended that handlers sign an agreement to comply with all of the hospital's IPC and HR policies.[9] Handlers should be vaccinated according to hospital policy for healthcare personnel.

Additionally, infection preventionists should be involved with determining what locations in the hospital are appropriate for animal-assisted care. Intensive care units, isolation rooms, neonatal and newborn nurseries, and areas of patient treatment that may result in pain for the patient and likely animal distress should be avoided. Hospitals may elect to not allow pet therapy animals in rooms of immunocompromised patients.

"Service animals" are defined under the 1990 U.S. ADA as "dogs that are individually trained to do work or perform tasks for people with disabilities."[12] The statute provides a limited exception for miniature horses if these animals satisfy the definition of a service animal, are housetrained, and do not create safety concerns. Service animals are considered "working animals," not pets.[12] An animal whose only function is comfort or emotional support is not considered a service animal. Legal protection extends only to persons with "disabilities" defined as a physical or mental impairment that substantially limits one or more major life activities, and not to all patients with medical or psychological conditions.[9] According to the ADA, the hospital staff is limited as to the inquiries they are permitted to make, and they may not require documentation about a patient's disability or the animal's training, but they are permitted to ask if the animal is a service animal that is required because of a disability, and what work the animal is trained to perform. Restriction of access to service animals is permitted in situations where the public's health may be compromised, but allergies or fear of the animal by the hospital staff or other patients generally are not acceptable reasons for denying access.[9]

It is recommended that each healthcare facility have a policy regarding admittance of service animals that should be compliant with the ADA as well as any other state or local regulations. Components of a service animal policy are listed in Box 9.2. Situations in which a service animal may be excluded from the healthcare facility can be found in Box 9.3. If the service animal must be restricted from accompanying the patient, reasonable accommodation should be made for the person with the disability to function without the service animal. Hospital areas from which service animals should be prohibited are listed in Box 9.4. The policy should also state that it is the patient or their caregiver's responsibility to ensure the health and care of the service animal while it is in the hospital.

Personal pet visitation to an individual patient involves an animal that is not a service animal or an animal in the pet therapy program. It is important to remember that pets and their owners do not undergo the same training and scrutiny that service or pet therapy animals and their handlers undergo (no formal training of owner/handler; personal pets have not been temperament tested and do not undergo extensive health assessment or exclusion practices). Additionally, because it is difficult to ensure that the personal pet will only encounter that particular individual patient and not healthcare personnel, other patients, or hospital visitors, it should, in general, be prohibited.[9] Exceptions can be considered, such as visitation of a terminally ill patient or a patient who has been hospitalized for a prolonged period of time, if the healthcare team believes that the visit could improve the patient's physical or mental health.

Hospitals that permit a single pet visitation should have a written policy that includes the following: approval from IPC as well as patient's nurse and physician documented in the patient's medical record, with details about the pet as well as the person responsible for the pet's transport and

BOX 9.2 COMPONENTS OF A HOSPITAL POLICY ON SERVICE ANIMALS

- Definition of "service animals" consistent with the ADA.
- Statement that only dogs and miniature horses are recognized as service animals under federal law. Factors used to determine if a miniature horse can be permitted include: must be house-trained, under the handler's control; and whether horse's type, height, and weight can be safely accommodated and will not compromise the safety requirements of the hospital.
- Statement that service animals are not pets and should not be approached, bothered, or petted.
- Statement that the care of the animal is the responsibility of the patient or caregiver/parent (e.g., feeding, exercising, toileting).
- Notification of IPC that an inpatient has a service animal, which should be followed by a discussion to ensure the animal complies with hospital policies.
- Requirement that all service animals be house-trained.
- List of prohibited locations and reasons for that exclusion (if exclusion is based solely on risk to the animal, the patient/caregiver should be consulted).
- Statement that hospital is not liable for costs associated with a hospital-associated infection in the service animal.
- Address the situation of a service animal accompanying a hospital visitor to a patient room (should be allowed, provided visitation is in accordance with hospital's service animal policy and visiting hours and regulations).
- Statement of who is assigned to enforce the policy (e.g., Legal Dept.).

BOX 9.3 SERVICE ANIMAL EXCLUSIONS

- Exhibits aggressive behavior such as scratching, snarling, teeth baring, or biting.
- Excessively noisy (e.g., howling, crying, or whining).
- Unable to contain bodily excretions (not house-trained or has vomiting or diarrhea).
- Infectious or ill (until evaluated by veterinarian, and handler must provide certification that animal does not pose an increased risk to patients and staff).

BOX 9.4 PROHIBITED HOSPITAL AREAS FOR SERVICE ANIMALS

- Invasive procedure areas where sterility is required (e.g., operating rooms, recovery rooms, cardiac catheterization suites, endoscopy suites).
- Units where a patient is immunocompromised or at high risk for infection†
- Rooms of patients in droplet, contact or airborne isolation†
- Food and medication preparation areas (e.g., kitchen, infant formula room, pharmacies).
- Areas that pose exposure risk to animals (e.g. radiation exposure or risk from magnetic resonance imaging to animals with metal tags, collars or implants); risks discussed with patient/caregiver who ultimately assumes full responsibility for any harm to the service animals

†Exceptions possible where the animal does not pose a direct threat and the animal's presence would not require a fundamental change in hospital's policies, practices or procedures.

care. Visitation should be restricted to dogs that are typically at least one year of age and house-trained. Exceptions can be made for a dog less than one year of age, considering the benefits and risks to that individual patient.[9] It is recommended that a hospital give the pet owner written information regarding the visit specifying the following: approved date, time, and location of the visit; maximum duration of one hour; acceptable and unacceptable practices, similar to pet therapy visits. The owner is responsible for supervising the pet at all times, preventing other human contact with the pet, promptly cleaning up any excrement, supervising the visitation process, and reporting any events (e.g., bites or scratches) to the healthcare team. Many hospitals would not permit personal pet visitation if the patient is on contact or droplet isolation, in a critical care unit, has recently undergone solid organ or stem cell transplant, has other immunocompromising conditions, or whose cognitive status would prevent a safe interaction with the pet, unless the patient will only be permitted to see and not touch the pet. Exceptions can be made by IPC and the healthcare team based upon risks and benefits to the particular patient.[9] Recommendations for a safe personal pet visit are outlined in Box 9.5.

Pets of healthcare personnel should not be allowed into the hospital unless they are part of the formal pet therapy program or have been approved for visitation with a patient who is a family member.[9] Due to the risk of infectious disease outbreaks, petting zoos and farm animals should be prohibited from visiting healthcare facilities. In general, aquariums in

BOX 9.5 RECOMMENDATIONS FOR A SAFE PERSONAL PET VISIT

- Choose an appropriate visit site (ideally outside, or if not possible, a private room; if visit must be in a multi-bed room, permission from roommate or their caregiver as well as roommate's physician must be obtained).
- Pet should be taken directly to the visit site, avoiding areas of heavy hospital traffic.
- Transporter should prevent the pet from coming in contact with other patients or healthcare personnel.
- Pet should be transported in a carrier or on a leash that is less than 2 m (6 ft.) in length.
- Pet should not be allowed to roam freely during the visit.
- Pet should not be fed, given treats, or provided with water during visit.
- Pet that is disruptive or aggressive (barking, snarling, biting) should be immediately removed.
- Pet should not have the ability to interfere with catheters, tubing, or medical devices.
- Patients should perform hand hygiene before and after pet contact.
- Use a clean additional bed sheet to cover the bed surface, which should be removed and laundered after the visit.

hospitals should not be allowed, due to risks of infection, but if a hospital chooses to have an aquarium, it should be covered, not accessible to patients, maintained by professional staff, and not placed in clinical areas or in an area with immunocompromised patients. Due to increased infection risks, reptiles and amphibians should not be kept in hospitals.[9]

Clinical Scenario Two

A local zoo has offered to develop an outreach program to entertain hospital patients and their families. The zoo representative proposes to show several small animals that children can pet.

Questions

What animals should be allowed to visit hospitalized children? Are there different principles that govern pets participating in a therapy program versus personal pets? If animals are allowed to visit, what measures will help prevent the spread of zoonotic infections?

Key Challenges

The developmental stage of the patient should be taken into consideration prior to scheduling a pet therapy session. Patients must be able to follow directions for a safe animal visit. Patients should be screened for fear of dogs prior to the visit. Verbal or written consent should be obtained from the patient or parent/caregiver, and preferably from the patient's physician as well.[9] This can be documented in the patient's medical record. Verbal permission should also be obtained from other people (or their caregivers) in the hospital room. The animal handler should notify the patient's nurse or physician prior to the visit. The handler should also direct the visit to prevent patients from touching the animal in inappropriate body sites such as the mouth, nose, and perianal areas. The visit should be conducted in a way to prevent the animal from being handled in a manner that might frighten or harm the animal or the patient.

Typically, animal therapy visits are limited to a maximum of one hour to reduce animal fatigue and potential adverse events.[9] The patient should be approached from the side that is free of any invasive devices: avoiding catheter insertion sites, medical devices, breaks in skin, bandage materials, or other compromised body sites.[9]

Transporting the animal to the pet therapy session can present a challenge. Before the animal enters an elevator, the handler or the accompanying hospital staff member should ask the other passengers for permission, and the handler should not enter if any passenger expresses apprehension or reluctance. The animal must be controlled at all times, usually on a leash, unless transported in a carrier. Some hospitals require the dog to wear a T-shirt to identify itself as an animal belonging to the pet therapy program and to reduce shedding. It is recommended that some form of identification be clearly visible and readily recognizable on the pet therapy animals.[9]

Visits should be terminated if the animal bites or intentionally scratches the patient, and the animal should be permanently withdrawn from the program. If it is determined that the handler's behavior contributed to the incident, then the handler's program participation should be terminated until the program manager has addressed the situation.[9] Visits should also be terminated if the animal develops vomiting or diarrhea, and the animal should be withdrawn from visitation until symptom-free and for a minimum of one week.[9] Protecting patients from infectious agents potentially transmitted by therapy animals is especially important for those with chronic illnesses who have an increased susceptibility to infection. These include, but are not limited to, patients with immunocompromising conditions, cystic fibrosis (CF), and sickle cell disease. The Cystic Fibrosis Foundation recommends that people with CF participate in animal-assisted ("pet") therapy in accordance with institutional policies. To date, there are no reports of transmission of potential pathogens from pet therapy or service animals to people with CF.[8]

Suggested Approaches

Hospitals with a pet therapy program should have a policy that explains best practices for a safe experience for both the animal and the patient. An example of a pet therapy infection prevention policy can be found in Handout 9.3. The proper selection of patients who would benefit from pet therapy is vital to the success of the program. All patients should be screened for colonization/infection with organisms that might be transmitted to the animal, for allergies to dogs, and to see whether the patient would like a visit from the dog. An example of a patient screening reminder card can be found in Appendix 1 of Handout 9.3.

In addition, hospitals should maintain a database of all the animals in the program indicating whether they have been appropriately vaccinated, have been tested for communicable diseases, and have been trained to be pet therapy animals. Likewise, the handler of the animal must also be appropriately vaccinated, screened for illness, and properly trained and certified in animal-assisted activities. Training should include annual infection prevention education, fire safety, and employee health education, as well as annual training on the infection prevention pet therapy policy. An example of a pet therapy data collection/risk assessment tool can be found in Handout 9.4. This database can be maintained by the department that oversees the pet therapy program, as well as the IPC department.

Hospitals should utilize a tracking tool to monitor which animal visited a particular patient on any day, in case the animal later shows signs of infection/infestation that may be communicable to humans. The tool should list the date of the visit, two patient identifiers, patient room number, and whether patient had physical contact with the animal. Some hospitals have the Play Therapy/Child Life department generate a daily list of potential patients who might benefit from pet therapy. When the pet therapists/animal handlers visit, they obtain the patient list and individually inquire with the nursing and/or medical staff, as well as parent/caregiver, whether

HANDOUT 9.3 Example of a Pet Therapy Infection Prevention Policy

Title: Pet Therapy Infection Prevention Policy	**Effective Date:** ------------------------ **Reviewed Date:**
Section: Infection Prevention Policy Manual	**Policies & Procedures** ------------------------ **Number:**

I. Policy Goals

To provide the benefits of an animal therapy program while protecting our patients, employees, and visitors from infectious complications, allergies, and injuries associated with animals in healthcare settings.

II. Procedure

A. Scope:

All hospital staff will comply with the guidelines set forth in this policy and will notify family and/or patients of these guidelines when appropriate. This policy pertains to *pet therapy animals only and does not apply to service animals.*

B. Definitions:

1. **Pet therapy animals—animals that have been trained and certified as pet therapy animals by a nationally recognized organization to provide psychological benefit and stimulation to patients.**
2. **Service animals—animals trained and certified to provide assistance in daily life activities for physically disabled individuals.**

C. Animals Permitted:

1. **Only certified pet therapy dogs will be permitted to enter the hospital.**
2. **Animals must be certified through Pet Partners (formerly Delta Society) Therapy Dogs International, Pet Therapy International, or other recognized organization.**
3. **Dogs are the only animals permitted under the pet therapy program.**
4. **No family or personal pets are permitted in the hospital building or other campus buildings *(see Section I: Exceptions).***
5. **Zoo animals (other than dogs) are not permitted.**

D. Infection Prevention and Animal Health Screening Requirements for Animals:

1. **Animals must be healthy and free of illness.**
2. **All animals must be up to date on immunizations and have documentation for:**
    - **Rabies vaccine**
    - **Leptospirosis vaccine**

- Hepatitis A virus vaccine
- Parvovirus vaccine

3. All animals must undergo annual screening for:
   - Heartworms
   - Stool pathogens: *Campylobacter jejuni*, *Giardia* spp., *Shigella* spp., and *Salmonella* spp.
4. (*Insert Hospital Name*) Microbiology Lab will offer stool screening one time per year at no cost to the animal handler. If results are positive, the animal will not be permitted into the program. If the owner wishes to pursue admission of this animal to the pet therapy program, they must go to their veterinarian to evaluate clearing of the organism and repeat testing of the animal at their own expense.
5. Trainers must visually inspect animals for ticks and fleas, open wounds, and any other sign of illness prior to visits. Dogs found to have any of the above will be excluded from visiting.
6. Any animal appearing ill will be excluded from visitation until well.
7. Excluded animals need veterinarian certification of health prior to reentry into the program.
8. Trainers must maintain documentation of all certifications and health information regarding their animal and must make this information available to (*Insert Hospital Name*).
9. Documentation of veterinarian visits and health records will also be maintained in the Volunteer Department.

E. Infection Prevention and Trainer/Handler Requirements:
1. Animal trainers will be educated on proper IP practices, including standard precautions, personal protective equipment, and handwashing, upon starting as a volunteer.
2. Animal trainers are subject to the same health screening and requirements as all hospital employees and volunteers (*Insert Employee Health Infection Prevention Policy #*).
3. Animal trainers will not visit if they have a respiratory, gastrointestinal, or skin infection, or other possible infectious illness.
4. Trainers will be responsible for reminding patients to wash their hands immediately after touching animals.
5. A log of which patients were visited by the pet therapy animal will be maintained in the Volunteer Department.

F. Animal Visitation Requirements:
1. All animals will be bathed prior to visiting the hospital.
2. Animals must wear a T-shirt or other cover to reduce shedding of hair and dander.
3. Animals will be leashed the entire time they are inside the hospital.
4. In the event that the animal eliminates (defecates, urinates, etc.) within the hospital, Trainer will notify patient's nurse or other available staff to immediately cover/contain the area. Environmental Services will be called immediately for appropriate clean-up and disinfection.
5. No animals will enter the cafeteria or kitchen areas at any time.

6. Animals will not be permitted to enter the NICU, OTU, BU, ICU, CCU, SCU, Dialysis Unit, Recovery Room, or any neutropenic patient's room.
7. Animals will not be permitted to enter rooms of patients in isolation.
8. Animals will not be permitted to enter the following outpatient clinics: Hematology/Oncology, Nephrology, Rheumatology, Pulmonology/Allergy, and Immunology.
9. (*Insert Hospital Name*) reserves the right to exclude any animal from visiting the hospital if the animal appears to pose a threat to patients and/or visitors in the hospital or behaves in an inappropriate manner.

G. Patient Screening for Animal Visitation:

1. All patients will be screened for allergies and/or other contraindications for contact with animals prior to visiting with the animal.
2. Patient screening will be conducted by the animal's trainer and parent/patient in coordination with nursing staff as needed.
3. Each patient will be screened for the presence of allergies, etc. using the attached questionnaire (**Appendix 1**, this chapter).

H. Program Enforcement and Monitoring:

1. Documentation of all animal certifications and health information will be maintained in the Volunteer Department.
2. Documentation of Trainer health information will be maintained in Employee Health.
3. The Volunteer Department will be the primary point of contact for enforcement and monitoring of compliance.
4. Infection Prevention, Administration, and Risk Management will participate in enforcement and monitoring.
5. In the event of an incident (allergy, bite, etc.), an incident form will be completed by Child Life or Volunteer departments.

I. Exceptions:

1. Exceptions to this policy will be considered on a case-by-case basis in extraordinary circumstances and must be approved by the hospital epidemiologist or designee.
2. A multidisciplinary team consisting of Infection Prevention, Child Life, Medical Staff, and Risk Management will assess each request for an exception and determine the appropriateness and/or means for granting the exception.
3. Administrator on-call will be contacted as needed to assist in the determination of an appropriate exception.
4. Family pets are not permitted unless an exception is granted as stated before.
5. Any personal pet approved as an exception must be current with immunizations, be healthy and free of pathogens as described in Section D.
6. Documentation of most recent veterinarian visit/results will be required.
7. Location of visits taking place for exceptions and personal pets will be decided by the multidisciplinary team specified herein to provide the safest environment for other patients/visitors/employees in the hospital.
8. Family pets approved for visitation will be escorted to and from the location of the visit by a hospital staff member.

Insert Hospital Name
Pet Therapy Program
Patient Screening Reminder Card

Animal Trainer must screen each patient prior to visiting with the animal by asking the following questions of the patient/parent and/or nurse as appropriate:

1. Are you allergic to dogs?
2. Is there any reason for a dog not to be in contact with you or the patient?
3. Would you like a visit from my dog?

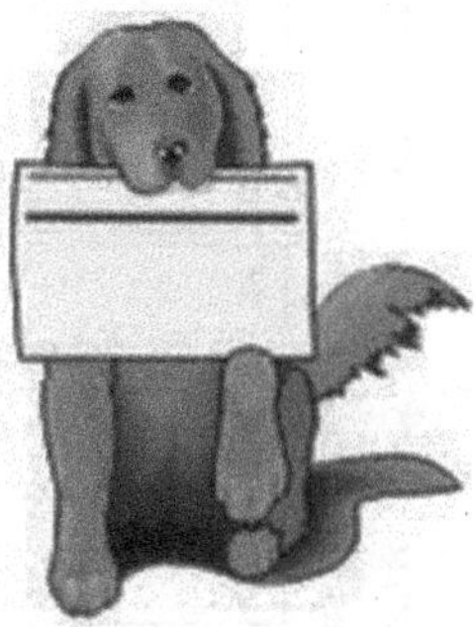

an animal visit is appropriate. If the patient was visited by the animal, the therapist places a check mark at the patient's name on the list. At the end of therapist's shift, the marked list is handed back to the Child Life/Volunteer department for them to keep in their daily tracking log book.

Approach to the Clinical Scenario Two

This clinical scenario of a petting zoo offering to entertain patients and their parents/caregivers in a hospital should be avoided due to infectious risks. The animals that are considered safe to visit hospitalized children are pet therapy dogs. Typically, service animals for a particular patient are dogs or miniature horses. Personal pet visitation is limited to dogs. There

HANDOUT 9.4 Example of a Pet Therapy Data Collection Tool

Example of a Pet Therapy Data Collection Tool

Place Hospital Name Here

Infection Control Risk Assessment/Data Collection Tool

Child Life/Volunteer/Employee Health Departments

Title: Pet Therapy/Infection Control (IC)

Place Hospital Name Here

File Review

Instructions: For each Therapy Dog and Trainer, complete each section by marking: Compliant {**C**} or Non-Compliant {**N/C**}, and the **initials** of the reviewer. Return the completed Quality Improvement form to Infection Prevention.

Month/Yr. of review:	**#1**	**#2**	**#3**	**#4**	**#5**	**#6**	**#7**	**#8**	**#9**	**#10**								**Total**	**% Compliant**
Pet Certification: Therapy dog must be certified through the Delta Society, Therapy Dogs International, Pet Therapy International, or other recognized organization. **Therapy Dog file has documentation of the following:**																			
File contains proof of: **Therapy** **Dog certification**																			
Annual veterinarian **certificate of health**																			

Rabies (***Place State Code # Here***) A dog over 3 months of age shall be vaccinated to maintain immunity against rabies by the administration of a USDA-licensed vaccine, including vaccines producing immunity lasting 3 years, in accordance with instructions prescribed by the manufacturer.

(1) A dog vaccinated when under 1 year of age shall be revaccinated no later than 1 year later.

(2) A dog vaccinated when over 1 year of age with a vaccine producing immunity lasting 3 years shall be revaccinated no later than 3 years later and at least every 3 years thereafter.

(3) A dog vaccinated with a vaccine producing immunity lasting less than 3 years shall be revaccinated no later than 1 year later.

Immunizations: Therapy Dog file has documentation of the following:

• **Rabies**- compliant with ***State Code #***																			
• **Leptospirosis** vaccine																			
• **Hepatitis A** vaccine																			
• **Parvovirus** vaccine																			

Infection Control Risk Assessment/Data Collection Tool

Child Life/Volunteer/Employee Health Departments____________________________________

Title: Pet Therapy/Infection Prevention____________________________________

Place Hospital Name Here

File Review

Month/Yr. of review:	#1	#2	#3	#4	#5	#6	#7	#8										Total	% Compliant
Annual heartworm screen																			
Annual screen for stool pathogens: *Campylobacter jejuni* *Giardia* spp. *Shigella* spp. *Salmonella* spp.																			
Annual flea / tick program																			
Trainer/Handler information:																			
• **Annual Fire, Safety, IP, and Employee Health training**																			
• **Documentation of health screening and requirements: Employee Health Infection Prevention Policy # (*place policy number here*)**																			
• **Documentation of education: IP Pet Therapy Infection Prevention Policy # (*place policy number here*)**																			

Infection Control Risk Assessment/Data Collection Tool

Child Life/Volunteer/Employee Health Departments

Title: Pet Therapy/Infection Control Month/Yr. of review: ____________________

Place Hospital Name Here

File Review

Pet/Trainer/Handler Information

ID #	Trainer /Handler Name (Please Print)	Pet's Name	Compliant Yes/No	Deficiency noted:	Trainer/Handler Notified of Any Deficiency (Date/ Initial)	Comments
#1						
#2						
#3						
#4						
#5						

are different principles that govern animals participating in a pet therapy programs versus personal pets, which have been outlined in this chapter.

If a hospital chooses to have a pet therapy program, important measures that would prevent the spread of zoonotic infections and ensure a safe experience for the patient and the animal include guaranteeing that the dog is healthy, appropriated vaccinated, and properly trained and certified. Additionally, the program should ensure that the handler is healthy, appropriately vaccinated, trained, and certified. Compliance with infection prevention practices with regard to the pet therapy program should be monitored. Especially important is hand hygiene, which should be performed before and after animal contact. Lastly, the choice of patients must be appropriate for a pet therapy session.

Unresolved Issues

Patients, their families, and some healthcare personnel continue to advocate for animals other than dogs for animal-assisted programs. The safety of other animals, particularly those commonly kept as pets, is sometimes debated, and the rationale for excluding them must be explained. Cats, for example, have an increased risk of allergenicity and are difficult to train appropriately.

Another unresolved issue is how to handle service animals that are not dogs. Most often, dogs, and occasionally miniature horses, are the preferred animals to be trained as service animals. Situations where patients might have a service animal that is not the typically accepted animal species will need to be treated on a case-by-case basis, remaining cognizant of the ADA requirements and while following all hospital infection prevention best practices.

Another unresolved issue is whether pet therapy dogs should be screened for MDROs and *C. difficile.* Because dogs participating in pet therapy may visit multiple hospitals and healthcare facilities, they may acquire pathogens from one facility and transmit those to patients at another facility. Currently, it is not routinely recommended to screen pet therapy dogs for MDROs or *C. difficile* colonization.

References

1. Avila-Aguero ML, German G, Paris MM, Herrera JF, Safe Toys Study Group. Toys in a pediatric hospital: are they a bacterial source? *Am J Infect Control.* 20014;32(5):287–290.

2. Akhter J, al-Hajjar S, Myint S, Qadri SM. Viral contamination of environmental surfaces on a general paediatric ward and playroom in a major referral centre in Riyadh. *Eur J Epidemiol.* 1995;11(5):587–590.
3. Fanella ST, Pinto MA, Bridger NA, et al. Pandemic (H1N1) 2009 influenza in hospitalized children in Manitoba: nosocomial transmission and lesson learned from the first wave. *Infect Control Hosp Epidemiol.* 2011;32(5):435–443.
4. Guh A, Carling P. Options for evaluating environmental cleaning. December 2010. Available at: www.cdc.gov/hai/toolkits/evaluating-environmental-cleaning.html. Accessed October 22, 2018
5. Ibfelt T, Engelund EH, Schultz AC, Andersen LP. Effect of cleaning and disinfection of toys on infectious diseases and microorganisms in daycare nurseries. *J Hosp Infect.* 2015;89(2):109–115.
6. Desai R, Pannaraj PS, Agopian J, Sugar CA, Liu GY, Miller LG. Survival and transmission of community-associated methicillin-resistant *Staphylococcus aureus* from fomites. *Am J Infect Control.* 2011;39(3):219–225.
7. Rogers M, Weinstock DM, Eagan J, Kiehn T, Armstrong D, Sepkowitz KA. Rotavirus outbreak on a pediatric oncology floor: possible association with toys. *Am J Infect Control.* 2000;28(5):378–380.
8. Saiman L, Siegel J, LiPuma J, et al. Cystic Fibrosis Foundation guideline. *Infect Control Hosp Epidemiol.* 2014;35(Suppl1):S1–S67.
9. Murthy R, Bearman G, Brown S, et al. Animals in healthcare facilities: recommendations to minimize potential risks. *Infect Control Hosp Epidemiol.* 2015;495–516.
10. Lefebvre S, Reid-Smith RJ, Waltner-Toews D, Weese SJ. Incidence of acquisition of methicillin resistant *Staphylococcus aureus, Clostridium difficile*, and other healthcare-associated pathogens by dogs that participate in animal-assisted interventions. *J Am Vet Med Assoc.* 2009;234:1404–1417.
11. Lefebvre SL, Reid-Smith R, Boerlin P, et al. Evaluation of the risks of shedding salmonellae and other potential pathogens by therapy dogs fed raw diets. *Zoonoses Public Health.* 2008;55:470–480.
12. ADA: Americans with Disabilities Act of 1990. Pub.L.No. 101-336, 104 Stat 328. http://www.dol.gov/dol/topic/disability/ada.htm. Accessed January 16, 2019.

10 | Pertussis and Influenza Cocooning Immunization Strategies

MEERA VARMAN, SARAH TURNER PIETRUSZKA, AND KAREN LEHAN

Background

Cocooning

A parental immunization strategy called "cocooning" is a concept endorsed by the Advisory Committee for Immunization Practices (ACIP), the American Academy of Pediatrics (AAP), and the American Academy of Family Physicians (AAFP),[1–5] specifically for vaccination against influenza and pertussis. The concept refers to immunizing close contacts (parents, family members, and caregivers) of infants and high-risk children, decreasing exposure to these diseases. In 2013, the ACIP revised the tetanus toxoid, reduced diphtheria toxoid, and acellular pertussis vaccine (Tdap) recommendation to vaccinate all pregnant women between 27 and 36 weeks during every pregnancy.[6]

Immunizing any anticipated close contacts of infants and high-risk children two weeks prior to meeting the infant is a way of limiting pathogen exposure. Maternal prenatal vaccination is now the standard; however, siblings and adult contacts are often the sources of infection. Thus, protection may include not only the vaccination of mothers but also of fathers, grandparents, and siblings, extended-family members, daycare staff, healthcare personnel, and other caregivers around the infant. Administration of increased vaccination may seem to be costly. However, cost savings were confirmed by a Dutch study finding cost-effectiveness from a payer's perspective, as well as societal cost savings.[7] A computer simulation suggests that the number needed to vaccinate to prevent one infant from acquiring pertussis (and therefore the cost of vaccination) was lower with a cocooning approach than a vaccination strategy that would implement increased vaccinations and boosters amongst all adolescents and adults.[8] However, this approach (focusing on all adolescents and adults) ignores the morbidity and mortality associated with non-infantile pertussis, which is not insignificant. Pediatric healthcare facilities across the country have created novel vaccine cocooning programs in order to improve household vaccine uptake.

Clinical Scenarios

A child with relapsed leukemia is admitted to the hospital for chemotherapy. She is expected to remain in the hospital for at least two weeks. At the same time, seasonal influenza activity has dramatically increased in your community. The child's mother asks if she can receive a flu vaccine while in the hospital, at low or no cost. The mother does not want to leave the hospital while her daughter is hospitalized.

Questions

What are the barriers to adult immunizations, specifically focused on the parents and adult caregivers of pediatric patients? What strategies can overcome these barriers? Is it feasible for pediatric healthcare facilities to provide immunizations to adult caregivers of pediatric patients?

Key Challenges

Several challenges have been identified as barriers to cocooning infants against influenza and pertussis. These include vaccine cost, staff time, and healthcare staff and parental lack of knowledge about cocooning by vaccination. In addition, concern for medical liability can be a barrier at some facilities. Past patient experience, inadequate vaccine safety information, and healthcare personnel trust can also be determinants for vaccine acceptance. However, several U.S. children's hospitals have successful cocooning programs.

Suggested Approaches

Both Tdap and influenza vaccination for caregivers or close contacts of infants under six months of age can be provided both in ambulatory and inpatient settings. Some healthcare facilities have already established programs for cocooning. In 2011, a survey of 53 U.S. children's hospitals found that 22 hospitals had free vaccine programs for household members[9]; the programs' approaches varied widely across the responding facilities.

Outpatient Setting

- Improved access to care, reminder recall methods, and standing orders can enhance immunization rates.[10] The reminder recalls, either by phone calls by staff, by postcards, or by automated electronic text messages, can be used in outpatient settings.
- Office hours for vaccination should be made more flexible, including after-hours and weekends to accommodate working parents.
- Informational sheets, consisting of vaccination clinic locations and contact information where free vaccines are available such as local health departments and federally qualified health centers (FQHC), can be developed and distributed.
- If funding is not available for cocooning in pediatric ambulatory settings, information should be given about where vaccines can be provided without any cost to patients.
- Two-way communication of the electronic health records (EHR) system should bring the updated vaccination data to a centralized location.
- An AFIX (Assessment, Feedback, Incentives, and Exchange) program can be utilized in collaboration with the local health department to increase vaccination in an outpatient setting.[11]
- Internists and family practitioners should increase their awareness so that the mention to them of a pregnant family member or new grandchild becomes a stimulus for vaccination education and administration.
- The AAP's "Immunizing Parents and Other Close Family Contacts in the Pediatric Office Setting" provides the benefits of immunizing parents, with additional helpful suggestions.[12]

Hospital Setting

Organizational Factors

Support for the implementation of immunization, in either outpatient or inpatient settings, must come from the hospital administration. Support from the hospital administration is vital for a coordinated implementation approach and to enact changes in the system to accommodate the immunization program.

- When a system-wide policy change is planned, staff education is required hospital-wide, including, but not limited to, nursing staff, trainees, and all medical staff.
- Information technology staff support is also vital to the success of the program, to ensure proper documentation of the vaccines that are administered.
- Organizations can provide incentives to staff for increasing vaccination efforts and immunization rates.

Vaccination Locations

If staffing of vaccination programs is a concern, a centralized location can be planned. The following are possible locations to provide cocooning immunizations, as described in the previously mentioned U.S. children's hospital survey[9]:

- Pediatric intensive care and neonatal intensive care units
- Inpatient wards
- Labor and delivery, post-partum units
- Centralized free vaccine clinics
- Ambulatory pediatric clinics
- Outpatient pharmacies
- Hospital lobbies

Funding for Cocooning Programs

Funding for cocooning vaccination programs can be a challenge. Vaccine costs have successfully been budgeted in the following departments and organizations:

- Hospital operational budgets
- Pharmacy departments
- Hospital foundations
- Local health department grant programs
- Federal public health grant programs
- Occupational Health departments
- Hospital volunteer programs
- Corporate sponsorships

One group reported, however, that retail-pharmacy vaccination vouchers given during newborn visits were not successful in promoting cocooning.[13]

Immunization Information System (IIS)

Immunization information systems (IIS) (also known as immunization registries) capture the vaccination records given at different facilities, if all the facilities use the IIS and upload the necessary vaccination information in the appropriate timeframe. There is a cost associated with bridging immunization registries to the hospital-based EHR system:

- Staff time is also required for updating the vaccines administered in the facility into the registry on a regular basis.
- Barcode readers can be used to update the immunizations given at the clinic by the staff.
- Updated ACIP recommended vaccine schedules, if made available in the IIS or in the EHR system, enable the healthcare personnel to assess the delayed vaccination status of patients.
- Reminders and recalls can be generated from the IIS. Centralized reminders from the state health department can be sent to patients.

Trainees

The Accreditation Council for Graduate Medical Education (ACGME) requires advocacy activities to be incorporated in residency training to improve fulfillment of community health objectives. Thus, a cocooning program could fulfill this requirement.

- Under the leadership of residents, students from different disciplines can join the efforts to improve cocooning vaccination.
- Students from medicine, pharmacy, nursing, physician assistant programs, and others can volunteer to administer vaccines, educate families, and enter data into the immunization registry.[14]
- Vaccine educational materials can be developed by healthcare trainees to address vaccine safety concerns of parents. This approach provides medical trainee education as well.
- A multifaceted project involving data collection, analysis, and surveys can lead to immunization research and scholarly activities for medical trainees.

- An active role by residents and students will foster leadership skills, ownership of the project, and creation of learning-implementation tools to improve the current system and understand the barriers to vaccination.
- Residents can improve access to vaccines by changing policies in their healthcare system and improving vaccine delivery systems.

Staff and Parent Education

- Healthcare staff working with infants must be familiar with the current immunization recommendations.
- Nurses can be targeted as educators for new mothers.
- When patients are being referred from other hospitals or primary care physicians, before a patient is evaluated by the medical team, the nursing staff can review the patient's immunization records and advocate for recommended vaccinations.
- Vaccine schedules can be printed out and posted in patient care areas as a constant reminder for the staff.
- Educational binders containing Vaccine Information Statements (VIS), consent forms, ordering instructions, and other logistical details with annual updates can be provided at the immunization locations.
- All educational guidelines and vaccine information should be made available in the hospital intranet system as well.
- Vaccine education sessions for parents and posters promoting vaccination in different languages can be posted in labor and delivery rooms, postpartum and child care areas, lobbies, prenatal clinics, newborn nursery, and breastfeeding areas. Additional education can be provided if needed, by trained medical personnel.[15]

Pharmacy Role

- Pharmacies play a vital role in immunizations for both outpatients and inpatients. Hospitals may implement a policy for pharmacists to routinely review the patient immunization records prior to discharge.
- If there is an easily transferable EHR along with a centralized IIS, analyzing immunization records becomes feasible.
- Prior to each patient discharge, immunizations should be updated.

Electronic Health Records (EHR)

- Collaborative work with information technology to build vaccine reminders and flags to prompt that vaccines that are due would assist the healthcare personnel and pharmacists in providing the immunizations during prenatal and postpartum care.
- If new ACIP recommendations are announced for any vaccines, these recommendations should be incorporated into the EHR system without undue delay. This prevents potential missed opportunities to vaccinate.

Approach to the Clinical Scenario

There are several potential approaches to successfully providing influenza vaccine to a patient's mother in the hospital. If the parent is also a registered patient within her child's healthcare system, a pediatric healthcare team member (physician, nurse, or medical assistant) could vaccinate the mother as an ambulatory encounter, with documentation in the health record and billing per the usual protocol. If an onsite ambulatory pharmacy exists on the hospital grounds, and hospital policy allows pharmacists to give injections, the parent could receive the influenza vaccination at the pharmacy without leaving the hospital. Finally, partnering closely with your local and state public health immunization programs can frequently identify novel methods of supporting cocooning in the inpatient pediatric setting.

Unresolved Issues

How to pay for the costs of cocooning programs when one or more family caregivers is not a registered patient in a healthcare system remains a challenge for many facilities. Creating a durable and transparent immunization record for an individual not registered in a healthcare system, such as the parent of an child on an inpatient unit, may be problematic states without robust IIS.

References

1. Centers for Disease Control and Prevention. Prevention and control of seasonal influenza with vaccines: recommendations of the Advisory Committee on Immunization Practices—United States, 2017–18 influenza season. *MMWR*. 2017;66(2):1–20.

2. American Academy of Pediatrics. Committee on Infectious Diseases. Policy statement: recommendations for prevention and control of influenza in children, 2017–18. *Pediatrics.* 2017;140(4):1–20.
3. American Academy of Family Physicians. 2017. Prevention and control of seasonal influenza with vaccines. Available from: http://www.aafp.org/online/en/home/clinical/immunizationres/influenza/expansionofinfluenza.html. Accessed January 16, 2019.
4. Centers for Disease Control and Prevention. Preventing tetanus, diphtheria, and pertussis among adults: use of tetanus toxoid, reduced diphtheria toxoid, and acellular pertussis vaccine. *MMWR.* 2006;55(RR-17):1–33.
5. American Academy of Pediatrics. Committee on Infectious Diseases. Policy statement: prevention of pertussis among adolescents: recommendations for use of tetanus toxoid, reduced diphtheria toxoid, and acellular pertussis (Tdap) vaccine. *Pediatrics.* 2006;117:965–978.
6. Centers for Disease Control and Prevention. Updated recommendations for use of tetanus toxoid, reduced diphtheria toxoid, and acellular pertussis vaccine (Tdap) in pregnant women—Advisory Committee on Immunization Practices (ACIP), 2012. *MMWR.* 2013;62:131–135.
7. Westra TA, de Vries R, Tamminga JJ, et al. Cost- effectiveness analysis of various pertussis vaccination strategies primarily aimed at protecting infants in the Netherlands. *Clin Ther.* 2010;32(8):1479–1495.
8. Van Rie A, Hethcote HW. Adolescent and adult pertussis vaccination: computer simulations of five new strategies. *Vaccine.* 2004;22(23–24):3154–3165.
9. Guzman-Cottrill JA, Phillipi CA, Dolan SA, et al. Free vaccine programs to cocoon high-risk infants and children against influenza and pertussis. *Am J Infect Control.* 40(2012):872–876.
10. http://www.immunize.org/standing-orders/. Accessed October 26, 2018.
11. https://www.cdc.gov/vaccines/programs/afix/index.html. Accessed October 26, 2018.
12. Lessin HR, Edwards KM, the Committee on Practice and Ambulatory Medicine, Committee on Infectious Diseases. Immunizing parents and other close family contacts in the pediatric office setting. *Pediatrics.* 2012;129:e247–e253.
13. Buttenheim AM, Fiks AG, Burson II RC, et al. A behavioral economics intervention to increase pertussis vaccination among infant caregivers: a randomized feasibility trial. *Vaccine.* 2016;34(6):839–845.
14. Shepard JE, Douglas AE, Phillipi CA, et al. Free Vaccines for Parents program: a novel (and successful) pediatric resident advocacy project. *Acad Pediatr.* 2015;15(5):476–479.
15. Healy CM, Rench MA, Baker CJ. Implementation of cocooning against pertussis in a high-risk population. *Clin Infect Dis.* 2011;52(2):157–162.

11 | Infection Prevention in Ambulatory and Emergency Department Settings

W. MATTHEW LINAM, MICHELE D. HONEYCUTT, AND VINI VIJAYAN

Background

There has been an expansion of healthcare delivery to children into a variety of outpatient settings, including outpatient clinics, urgent care clinics, emergency departments, and ambulatory surgery centers. In 2013, there were almost 1 billion outpatient office visits, including 102 million pediatric visits.[1] A major area of growth has been ambulatory procedures. In 2006, there were an estimated 53 million ambulatory procedures performed. Between 1996 and 2006, there was a 300% increase in the rate of procedures performed in freestanding ambulatory surgery centers, but it is unknown how much of this increase involved children.[2] Despite limited data, healthcare-associated infections (HAIs) do occur in outpatient settings.[3,4] Much of our understanding of HAIs in outpatient settings comes from a variety of outbreaks, including those of measles, pertussis, and tuberculosis.[5–7] Outbreaks of hepatitis B and C have occurred due to lapses in safe injection practices.[8,9]

Similar to inpatient settings, HAIs linked with outpatient care are frequently attributed to a breakdown in basic infection prevention practices and processes. For some, the apparent cause is a lack of the necessary infrastructure. In one measles outbreak in an outpatient pediatric clinic, the building's ventilation design with recirculated air may have contributed to the spread of the infection.[5] In general, the same infection prevention principles used in inpatient settings apply in ambulatory settings, but these locations have their own set of challenges that must be overcome. The goal of this chapter is to describe the basic infrastructure and processes, including strategies for implementation, needed to prevent HAIs in pediatric outpatient settings.

Clinical Scenarios

Scenario 1

A toddler is seen for a follow-up visit in a pediatric ambulatory clinic. Two days earlier, he was seen in the emergency department of the Children's Hospital for a buttocks abscess that was drained and packed. The wound culture is now growing methicillin-resistant *Staphylococcus aureus* (MRSA). A resident physician preparing to examine the child and remove packing from the wound asks about the need for isolation precautions.

Questions

What personal protective equipment (PPE), if any, should be worn for the care of this patient? What type of isolation precautions should be used to prevent transmission?

Scenario 2

A six-year-old child arrives at a pediatric ambulatory clinic to be seen for an ill visit. The child presents with a two-day history of fever, chills, cough, rhinorrhea, and pharyngitis. A nurse asks what can be done to prevent the spread of this respiratory illness from this child to other patients and the clinic staff.

Questions

What measures can be taken to prevent transmission of respiratory illness to other patients and their caregivers? What can the ambulatory clinic staff do to protect themselves from respiratory illnesses? What PPE, if any, should be worn for the care of this patient?

Scenario 3

A 13-month-old infant presents to the emergency department with fever, respiratory symptoms, and a maculopapular rash. The child has not yet received her one-year immunizations and has recently returned from a trip to

India. The triage nurse asks if this could be measles and what needs to be done to protect other patients and the emergency department staff.

Questions

What steps can be taken at the point of entry to minimize exposure to other patients and the emergency department staff? What steps need to be taken during the emergency department visit to prevent exposure?

Key Challenges

General Challenges

Until recently, most available infection prevention resources have focused on the inpatient setting. With the significant expansion of healthcare delivery in the ambulatory settings, infection prevention programs have been working to increase the infrastructure necessary to perform infection prevention activities and surveillance in these areas. Despite this, challenges remain in making this transition into the outpatient setting.

- ***Surveillance:*** In addition to the added time and personnel required to perform surveillance in the outpatient setting, there are challenges in detecting HAIs that occur in ambulatory patients. For example, triggers that are often used to detect surgical site infections (SSIs) in the inpatient setting, such as readmission, diagnostic testing, microbiological cultures or return to the operating room (OR), may not trigger further evaluation in the outpatient setting.[10] Other challenges include monitoring of various key infection prevention practices such as healthcare personnel (HCP) hand hygiene and exam room and device cleaning. Care in outpatient clinics and emergency departments often occurs behind closed doors or curtains, which can make monitoring behaviors like hand hygiene difficult.[11–13]
- ***Infrastructure:*** Design of the healthcare environment in the outpatient setting can also create barriers to effective infection prevention. For example, patients with active tuberculosis or possible contagious tuberculosis should be seen in an airborne isolation room. In addition, pulmonary function tests are often performed in pulmonary clinics. These procedures potentially generate aerosols and should also be performed in negative pressure/airborne isolation rooms. Approved airborne isolation rooms may not be available.

Pediatric-Specific Challenges in Infection Prevention

Unique challenges exist in implementing infection prevention practices in the pediatric and neonatal populations when compared to adults.[14–16]

- Infants and young children have underdeveloped immune systems and have had limited exposure to childhood diseases; hence, they can readily acquire and transmit infections. Additionally, infants and young children may be too young to be completely vaccinated against common vaccine-preventable diseases, thereby placing them at risk of infection.
- Behavioral characteristics such as drooling, frequent mouthing of hands and toys or other objects, and direct contact among children during play are factors that facilitate the transmission of infection. Children may not be developmentally capable of practicing appropriate hygiene, respiratory etiquette, or social distancing. In addition, they frequently harbor and may shed infectious organisms, even if asymptomatic.[17,18] These make children both susceptible to, as well as good transmitters of, disease.
- Ambulatory office procedures such as blood draws and line placements can place HCP at risk of accidental needle sticks, as children tend to be fearful and uncooperative during blood draws and line placements.
- The pediatric ambulatory office environment is different from that of a practice that provides care only to adults. Children are usually accompanied by one or more parents and/or siblings. This increases the number of people in waiting rooms, who can contribute to the spread of infection.
- Toys that are often provided in the pediatric office may be contaminated with respiratory viruses, fecal coliforms, and rotavirus that can pose potential health risks.[19–21] Although the American Academy of Pediatrics (AAP) Committee on Infectious Diseases and Committee on Practice and Ambulatory Medicine have issued recommendations for infection control in physicians' offices, the rate of compliance with these recommendations is unknown.[16]

Suggested Approaches

Several core components form the basis for infection prevention programs in outpatient settings.

Basic Infrastructure for Infection Prevention

Regardless of the location within a healthcare environment, an effective infection prevention program must have some basic infrastructure components, including administrative support, a risk assessment, education of HCP, and surveillance.[22]

- ***Administrative support:*** Leaders, whether of an individual practice, a group of practices, or a hospital, must recognize the importance of infection prevention and occupational health programs and ensure that they have the necessary resources, and that personnel are empowered to carry out their duties. These programs must be adequately staffed by trained individuals capable of performing the necessary day-to-day activities of these programs. Evidence-based policies should be developed and updated regularly to provide guidance to HCP regarding infection prevention processes and behavioral expectations. Resources commonly available in hospital settings (i.e., policies to guide HCP hand hygiene, use of standard and transmission-based precautions, immunization requirements for HCP, processes to clean the patient care area, and processes to clean, sterilize, and disinfect reusable medical equipment [RME]) outline expectations for care in hospital-affiliated emergency departments, but may not exist as formal documents in other ambulatory settings. Appropriate supplies, such as alcohol-based hand rub and PPE, must be readily available at the point of care with processes to quickly identify and replace depleted supplies.
- ***Risk assessment:*** All infection prevention programs should perform an annual risk assessment to determine gaps in practice and areas for improvement. Checklists specific for ambulatory settings, such as those available at the Centers for Disease Control and Prevention (CDC), can provide a basic evaluation of the infection prevention infrastructure, resources, and processes.[22] Review of local prevalence data for certain pathogens (e.g., tuberculosis and pertussis) or outbreaks (e.g., measles and mumps) can provide further insight into what is currently circulating in the community; this information can be used to focus infection prevention resources.
- ***Education of HCP:*** Standardized policies and procedures for all infection prevention processes help to ensure that education and training are consistent over time. All HCP, including contracted employees and volunteers, should be provided with job-specific education and training. Training should focus not only on HCP safety, but also patient

safety. It should be provided at the time of hire and should be repeated at least annually to prevent drift in practice, and whenever there is a change in policy or process. Education alone is not enough, however. Demonstration of HCP competency is necessary to show that HCP are able to perform the necessary infection prevention behaviors and processes. An example of a competency-based checklist is the CDC Infection Prevention Checklist for Outpatient Settings.[22]

- ***Surveillance:*** Surveillance often focuses on outcome data such as overall HAIs or specific HAIs such as SSIs. Outcome measures such as HAI numbers/rates can be used to identify areas for improvement and assess the effectiveness of local efforts to reduce HAIs, and they may be required for reporting to state and federal organizations. Surveillance can also include the tracking of various healthcare processes such as HCP hand hygiene, compliance with transmission-based precautions and effectiveness of environmental cleaning. Tracking processes that measure data over time are necessary to determine HCP adherence to processes and to monitor the effectiveness of interventions designed to improve outcomes.

Determining what outcome and process measures to track over time can be difficult. At a minimum, healthcare facilities should adhere to local, state, and federal requirements for reportable diseases and outbreak reporting. In addition, some facilities are also required to report surveillance data on certain HAIs or processes for accreditation or Medicare certification.[23] For example, an outpatient surgical center may be required to report SSI data as well as data related to perioperative antibiotic prophylaxis. Healthcare facilities should also perform regular audits of infection prevention practices such as hand hygiene, environmental cleaning, device reprocessing, and safe injection practices. The CDC has created standardized checklists to guide audits (see https://www.cdc.gov/hai/settings/outpatient/outpatient-care-guidelines.html).

Surveillance in the outpatient setting is challenging for a number of reasons. Patient encounters are often brief and may only occur sporadically for individual patients. Symptoms of a HAI are likely to develop at home, undetected by healthcare surveillance systems. In addition, if an infection develops, care may be sought elsewhere, preventing the linkage between exposure to an ambulatory care facility, process failures (such as poor hand hygiene practices by clinic staff), and the subsequent development of the HAI. In order to bridge these surveillance gaps that occur in outpatient locations, patients or their caregivers can be engaged to assist with the identification. Patients and caregivers should be educated about signs and symptoms of infection and instructed to contact the initial facility if there is concern for infection.

Infection Prevention Starts at the Door

Outpatient clinics, urgent care facilities, and emergency departments are frequently the first point of contact for patients presenting with signs of a contagious illness. From the time of arrival to when an HCP recognizes the pattern of symptoms as a contagious illness, there are opportunities for multiple other patients, families, and caregivers to be exposed. Shortening this window is imperative to reduce exposure and prevent outbreaks. Unprotected exposure to infections such as pertussis, influenza, and measles have led to HCP illness.[5–7,24] Patients should be screened at the point of entry for symptoms of contagious illness such as respiratory symptoms or fever and rash. This allows for prompt separation from other waiting patients and appropriate isolation.

Recent healthcare outbreaks, such as Middle-Eastern respiratory syndrome (MERS) in South Korea, and Ebola virus exposures of U.S. HCP, have highlighted the need for increased vigilance regarding travelers returning from abroad.[25,26] Patients and their families/caregivers should also be screened at the point of entry for recent foreign travel or travel to an area of an ongoing outbreak. The CDC website provides up-to-date information on countries or locations with ongoing outbreaks of contagious illness.[27] The combination of recent travel to an area where there is ongoing transmission of an epidemiologically significant pathogen and the patient or family member having symptoms of contagious illness should alert HCP to promptly isolate the patient and alert hospital infection prevention staff and public health officials.

Precautions to Prevent Transmission of Infectious Agents

The CDC Healthcare Infection Control and Prevention Advisory Committee (HICPAC) has proposed a two-tiered structure to prevent transmission of infectious agents.[28]

- ***Standard precautions:*** These constitute the primary strategy for preventing transmission of organisms between patients and healthcare workers.
- ***Transmission-based precautions:*** These were designed for the care of patients suspected of or known to be colonized or infected with

epidemiologically important pathogens that can be transmitted by physical contact, or droplet or airborne transmission.

These are described in detail in the Appendix. While standard precautions are recommended for all patient care settings, there are design challenges that make implementation of transmission-based precautions difficult in outpatient settings. Therefore, emphasis should be placed on the implementation of standard precautions. In ambulatory settings, the management of children with potentially contagious illnesses should focus on rapid identification of potentially contagious patients at the point of entry, and prompt movement of the children to a single-patient exam room or cohorting/segregating these patients in a "sick waiting room." Patients with highly contagious illnesses (e.g., tuberculosis and measles) should quickly be discharged back to their home setting or transferring to a facility capable of managing these patients as appropriate.

Hand Hygiene

Hand hygiene remains the most effective and least expensive measure to prevent transmission of pathogenic organisms in the ambulatory setting.[29,30] Adherence to hand hygiene has been shown to reduce the transmission of antimicrobial-resistant organisms, and overall infection rate.[13,31,32] The World Health Organization (WHO), the CDC, and others have issued hand hygiene guidelines specifying when hand hygiene is indicated, how to clean hands, what agents to use, and how to choose the appropriate agent.[33,34]

Proper Hand Hygiene

- Hand washing with non-antimicrobial-containing soap and water.
- Cleaning hands with a waterless alcohol-based hand rub (ABHR), containing 60–95% alcohol.
- Cleaning hands with an antiseptic handwash or antiseptic hand rub preoperatively by surgical personnel to eliminate transient flora and reduce commensal hand flora. This is referred to as surgical antisepsis or surgical hand hygiene.

Use of ABHR is considered the preferred method of hand hygiene and is recommended by the CDC and the WHO in healthcare settings because of its activity against a broad spectrum of pathogens.[33,34] Additionally, use of ABHR can increase compliance with recommended hand hygiene practices as it is convenient, acts rapidly, and facilitates hand hygiene at the patient's bedside. Soap and water should be used when hands are visibly soiled (e.g., dirt, blood, body fluids), before eating, after using the restroom, and after exposure to a patient with known or suspected *Clostridioides difficile* or norovirus in outbreak settings.[33–36]

Despite the critical importance of hand hygiene, hand hygiene compliance among healthcare workers is well below 50%.[37] Compliance in the ambulatory settings is also relatively low and varies from 10% to 30%.[38,39] Shimokura et al. reported a hand hygiene compliance rate of 36% among hemodialysis staff.[40] Similarly, only 18% of HCP at an ophthalmology clinic performed appropriate hand hygiene.[41]

HCP in outpatient settings perceive their hand hygiene performance as much closer to optimal than the reality, and they report several factors that may negatively impact their adherence with recommended practices.[42] Some of these factors include irritation and dryness due to hand washing; inconveniently located sinks or ABHR dispensers; lack of soap, paper towels, or other hand hygiene supplies; not enough time; understaffing or overcrowding; and patient needs taking priority, or the perception that their patient is not infectious.[12,43] Lack of knowledge of guidelines/protocols, forgetfulness, and disagreement with the recommendations were also self-reported factors for poor adherence to hand hygiene.[12,33] It is essential to address these barriers to improve hand hygiene behavior.

Surgical Hand Antisepsis

Surgical hand hygiene (or antisepsis) involves cleaning of the hands and forearms with an antiseptic agent before donning sterile gloves when performing surgical procedures. This is an essential component in the prevention of SSI. Surgical hand preparation should reduce resident skin flora on the hands of the surgical team for the duration of the procedure, thereby reducing the risk of bacteria being released into the surgical field if gloves become punctured or torn during surgery.[44,45] The two most common forms of surgical hand antisepsis are washing hands with antimicrobial soap and water, and alcohol-based hand rubs.

- ***Antimicrobial soaps:*** These are water-based solutions containing antiseptic ingredients such as chlorhexidine-alcohol or povidone iodine. Preoperative skin cleansing with chlorhexidine has been found to be superior to povidone-iodine for preventing SSIs after clean-contaminated surgery.[45] Scrubbing involves wetting the hands and forearms with water, systematically applying an antimicrobial solution using either hands or sponges, rinsing under running water, and then repeating this process for the length of time recommended by the manufacturer, typically 2–5 minutes. Long scrub times (e.g., 10 minutes) are not necessary, and washing with hot water should be avoided, as this may remove the protective fatty acids from the skin.

- ***ABHR products:*** ABHRs containing additional active ingredients are used to perform an "alcohol rub." Surgical teams systematically apply the AHBR solutions to their hands and allow it to dry thoroughly before donning sterile gloves. The time required for surgical alcohol-based hand-rubbing depends on the product used, but most commercially available products recommend a 3-minute exposure.[46]

Although traditionally, surgical hand hygiene was performed by use of antimicrobial soaps and water, ABHR products have shown greater effectiveness in preventing SSIs.[33] ABHR products have a rapid antimicrobial action, wider spectrum of activity, cause less irritation to the hands, and require less time than washing hands, and hence are the favored agent for surgical hand preparation. Brushes are not recommended for surgical hand preparation, and brushless scrubbing is less abrasive and helps in maintaining skin integrity.[47]

Respiratory and Cough Etiquette

Respiratory and cough etiquette were added to Standard Precautions in 2007.[28] These infection prevention measures were designed to control the transmission of respiratory pathogens spread though droplet or airborne routes. Implementation of these infection prevention measures should begin upon entry to the facility/ambulatory settings (e.g., reception and triage areas). These apply to any person, including HCP, with signs of respiratory illness including cough, congestion, rhinorrhea, or increased production of respiratory secretions when entering the ambulatory setting.[48]

- ***Interrupting spread:*** Implementation of measures to prevent the spread of respiratory infections from anyone in a healthcare setting with signs or symptoms of a respiratory illness, beginning at point of entry to the facility and continuing throughout the duration of the visit.
  1. Use of appropriate language and education displayed on posters and signs at entrances asking persons with symptoms of respiratory infection to:

a. Cover their mouth and nose when coughing or sneezing, and coughing or sneezing into the elbow rather than the hand.
b. Use and dispose of tissues.
c. Perform hand hygiene after hands have been in contact with respiratory secretions.

2. Provide tissues and no-touch receptacles for their disposal.
3. Provide resources for performing hand hygiene in or near waiting areas.
4. Offer masks to symptomatic patients upon arrival.
5. A separation of at least 3 feet should be made between symptomatic patients and others in common waiting areas.

- ***Education:*** Educating HCP on the importance of prevention measures when examining and caring for patients with signs and symptoms of a respiratory infection

Personal Protective Equipment (PPE)

The selection of PPE is based on the nature of the interaction between the provider and the patient and potential for exposure to blood, body fluids, or infectious agents. All HCP should be trained on proper selection and use of PPE. It is important that PPE is used effectively, correctly, and at all times where contact with blood and body fluids of patients may occur. HCP should be aware that use of PPE does not replace the need to follow basic infection control measures such as hand hygiene. The CDC has issued recommendations for when and what PPE should be used to prevent exposure to infectious diseases.[28,49]

Recommendations for Use of PPE as Part of Standard Precautions in Ambulatory Settings

Gloves

- Wear gloves (clean, non-sterile) in situations involving potential contact with blood (e.g., during phlebotomy), body fluids, mucous membranes, non-intact skin, or contaminated equipment.
- Wear gloves that fit appropriately (select gloves according to hand size).
- Do not wear the same pair of gloves for the care of more than one patient.
- Do not wash gloves for the purpose of reuse.

- Change gloves between tasks and procedures on the same patient after contact with material that may contain a high concentration of microorganisms.
- Perform hand hygiene before donning and immediately after removing gloves.

Gowns

- Gowns should be used to protect skin and clothing during procedures or activities where contact with blood or body fluids is anticipated.
- Do not wear the same gown for the care of more than one patient.
- Remove gown and perform hand hygiene before leaving the patient's environment (e.g., exam room).

Facemasks (Procedure or Surgical Masks)

- Masks should fully cover the nose and mouth and prevent fluid penetration. Masks should fit snugly over the nose and mouth. For this reason, masks that have a flexible nose piece and can be secured to the head with string ties or elastic are preferred.
- Use mouth, nose, and eye protection during procedures that are likely to generate splashes or sprays of blood or other body fluids.
- Mask should be worn when placing a catheter or injecting material into the spinal canal or subdural space, to protect patients from exposure to infectious agents carried in the mouth or nose of HCP.

Eye Protection

- Goggles provide barrier protection for the eyes; personal prescription lenses do not provide optimal eye protection and should not be used as a substitute for goggles.
- Wear eye protection in the form of goggles alone or goggles with a facemask or face shield to protect the mouth, nose, and eyes from a potential splash or spray of blood, respiratory secretions, or other body fluids.

Respirators

- Respirators are used to prevent transmission by airborne droplet nuclei of infectious agents such as *Mycobacterium tuberculosis.*[50]
- Respirators differ from surgical masks or facemasks. Facemasks are designed to prevent large droplets from entering the nose and mouth

and to catch large droplets that are expelled by the wearer. They do not seal tightly to the wearer's face and do not prevent inhalation of small particles that may be transmitted from a patient by exhalation, coughs, or certain medical procedures. In contrast, respirators seal tightly to the face of the wearer and are designed to prevent inhalation of small particles.

- The most commonly used respirators in healthcare settings are the N95, N99, or N100 particulate respirators. The device has a submicron filter capable of excluding particles that are less than 5 microns in diameter. The annual risk assessment, which should factor in local epidemiology, will help determine the potential for staff exposure to pathogens transmitted by the airborne route (e.g., tuberculosis and measles). HCP who have job-related potential for exposure to someone with a pathogen transmitted by the airborne route should be medically cleared and fit-tested annually for a facial respirator. They should be trained in the proper use of respirators, safe removal and disposal, and medical contraindications to respirator use according to Occupational Safety and Health Administration (OSHA) requirements.[50–52]
- Powered air-purifying respirators (PAPRs) with high-efficiency filters have a battery-powered blower that pulls the air in the room through filters to clean it before delivering it to the breathing zone of the wearer. PAPRs can be used by HCP who are unable to be appropriately fit-tested with a facial respirator.

Safe Injection Practices

Safe injection practices are measures taken to perform injections in safe manner and thereby prevent transmission of infectious diseases between patients or between a patient and an HCP during preparation and administration of parenteral medications or injections. OSHA Bloodborne Pathogens' standard outlines best practices to protect HCP from blood exposure and sharps injuries.[53] Despite this, multiple outbreaks and patient notifications resulting from HCP's failing to adhere to these guidelines continue to be reported.[9,11] More work is needed to improve implementation of best practices for injection safety. The CDC has published recommendations for safe injection practices (Box 11.1).[53,54]

BOX 11.1 RECOMMENDATIONS FOR SAFE INJECTION PRACTICES[60,61]

- Use aseptic technique when preparing and administering medications.
- Cleanse the access diaphragms of medication vials with 70% alcohol before inserting a device or needle into the vial.
- Never administer medications from the same syringe to multiple patients, even if the needle is changed or the injection is administered through an intervening length of intravenous tubing.
- Do not reuse a syringe to enter a medication vial or solution.
- Do not administer medications from single-dose or single-use vials, ampoules, bags or bottles of intravenous solution to more than one patient.
- Do not use fluid infusion or administration sets (e.g., intravenous tubing) for more than one patient.
- Dedicate multi-dose vials to a single patient whenever possible. If multi-dose vials will be used for more than one patient, they should be restricted to a centralized medication area and should not enter the immediate patient treatment area (e.g., operating room, patient room/cubicle).
- Dispose of used syringes and needles at the point of use in a sharps container that is closable, puncture-resistant, and leak-proof.
- Adhere to federal and state requirements for protection of HCP from exposure to bloodborne pathogens.

Transmission-Based Precautions

The effectiveness of transmission-based precautions in the ambulatory care setting is largely unestablished, but outbreaks of measles, tuberculosis, and respiratory infections such as influenza have been attributed to physicians' offices or clinics.[5,6,11,24,55] Procedures need to be developed to limit exposure to other patients, families, and staff. The creation of evidence-based policies outlining the processes to screen for potentially contagious illness, interrupt transmission, and manage potential exposure events can help ensure that processes are followed consistently. Screening patients at the point of entry for symptoms of contagious illness and quickly moving them to a single-patient room are key to limiting exposure. Respiratory hygiene and cough etiquette should also be followed. For patients with symptoms of a respiratory illness, the addition of droplet precautions (wearing a facemask) while in the exam room can further prevent HCP exposure. Most ambulatory settings do not have the infrastructure in place to manage a patient with a highly contagious illness transmitted by airborne droplet nuclei (e.g., tuberculosis, measles, and varicella). Once identified, these patients should be given a mask to wear, if possible, and immediately moved to a single patient room. If one is available, the patient should be placed in an airborne isolation room. HCP should don an appropriately fit-tested N-95 respirator, if available, or a facemask prior to entering the patient room. Although children under 12 years of age with active tuberculosis are often not contagious, caregivers accompanying the child occasionally have active tuberculosis and should be screened for symptoms and given a mask to wear if appropriate. Arrangements should be made to quickly discharge the patient back to the home setting or transfer to a healthcare facility with the capacity to manage the patient in airborne precautions. After discharge, exam rooms occupied by the patient should remain empty with the door closed for at least an hour.

Isolation Precautions and the Care of Patients with Cystic Fibrosis

Infection Prevention and Control Guidelines published by the Cystic Fibrosis Foundation provide detailed recommendations for the care of CF patients in both ambulatory and inpatient settings.[56] These include use of contact precautions for all patients in all settings regardless of pathogen status, mask use by all patients when in common areas in healthcare settings (i.e., waiting rooms), and maintaining at least a 6-foot distance between CF patients in common areas. Additional recommendations appear in Box 11.2.

Care of the Potentially Contaminated Healthcare Environment

Environmental Cleaning

Routine and effective cleaning of the patient care environment is critical to preventing the transmission of potentially pathogenic microorganisms. Cleaning consists of the removal of visible soil and organic contamination from equipment and environmental surfaces by the use of detergents or other cleaning agents. Cleaning must always precede disinfection or sterilization. Disinfection removes virtually all microorganisms but may not remove spores.

The frequent turnover of patient rooms in outpatient clinics and emergency departments creates logistical challenges to cleaning and disinfection. The focus should be on cleaning frequently touched areas of the

BOX 11.2 EXAMPLE MESSAGING FOR CYSTIC FIBROSIS STAFF EDUCATION HANDOUT

CYSTIC FIBROSIS INFECTION PREVENTION

The following infection prevention practices will be use *to protect* our patients with Cystic Fibrosis as recommended by the CDC, and the World Health Organization.

Private Room

- All patients with CF will be placed in a single-patient room, including when in the PICU.
- Siblings with CF may share a semi-private room.
- CF patients should not sit in the waiting area of the ED, OR, pulmonary function lab, etc. They should be immediately escorted to a private area if there will be a wait to be placed in a room.

Contact Precautions

- All patients with CF, regardless of respiratory tract culture results, will be in contact precautions. This requirement is intended to protect the patient, and is not intended to limit the activity of the patient.
- The CDC does not recommend that healthcare personnel routinely wear a mask.
- A mask should be worn by healthcare personnel when droplet precautions are required, or splashes/sprays of respiratory secretions are anticipated.

Mask Use

- All people with CF should wear a mask when in a healthcare setting to reduce the risk of transmission or acquisition of CF pathogens.
- This includes hallways and common areas.

Six-Foot Rule

- All people with CF, regardless of respiratory tract culture results, should be separated by at least 6 feet from other people with CF in all settings in order to reduce the risk of droplet transmission of CF pathogens.
- This does not apply to members of the same household.

Handheld Disposable Nebulizers

- After each use, rinse residual volume with sterile water and wipe mask or mouthpiece with alcohol pad.
- Discard the nebulizer every 24 hours (respiratory therapy will do this).

Infection Prevention Consult

- Please enter an IP consult on all CF patients admitted to the hospital so they can follow up with the patient.

Adapted with permission from an educational sheet created by Nicole Saling, MSN, RN (Norton Children's Hospital, Louisville, KY, 2018).

environment that are most likely to become contaminated (e.g., bedrails and doorknobs). These surfaces and high-touch areas should be cleaned with an Environmental Protection Agency (EPA)-approved disinfectant or detergent/disinfectant after each patient encounter.[57] Other surfaces, such as floors and walls, should be cleaned with an EPA-approved disinfectant or detergent at least once daily, and more often in the event they become contaminated with blood or body fluids. Privacy curtains should be changed and laundered on a regular basis, as determined by the organization, or when visibly soiled.[57]

Toys present another challenge frequently encountered in pediatric settings. They are frequently contaminated by handling and mouthing by small children. In addition, they are often difficult to clean/disinfect in a timely fashion. In general, the use of toys should be minimized. When made available, toys are to be made of smooth, hard surfaces that can be cleaned with an EPA-approved disinfectant or detergent. Toys are to be cleaned at least daily. If mouthed or otherwise contaminated, toys are to be cleaned between each patient use. [20]

Implementation

- ***Policies and procedures:*** The organization should ensure that there are clear policies and procedures that outline the expectations for environmental cleaning and disinfection. These policies and procedures should include:
  - *Assignment of responsibility:* Policies must clearly define who is responsible for cleaning each surface and item of equipment to ensure consistent cleaning.
  - *Cleaning processes:* There must be clear procedures that define what environmental surfaces should be cleaned, how they should be cleaned, and what cleaning product should be used. Recommendations for cleaning and disinfection should follow the manufacturer's instructions for use (MIFU) for both the equipment and the cleaning agents.
  - *Process to clean blood/body fluid spills:* There must be a clear process/procedure for cleaning up blood/body fluid spills that avoids HCP exposure.
- ***Training:*** HCP performing the cleaning and disinfection should receive the appropriate training, and their competencies should be reviewed upon hire and on at least an annual basis.
- ***Monitoring:*** The organization should periodically monitor compliance with cleaning and disinfection practices.

Device Reprocessing

Medical devices and equipment are frequently used in the ambulatory setting. These include everything from blood pressure cuffs to endoscopes and surgical instruments. Depending on their use and potential reuse, there is the potential for transmission of pathogens if they are not cleaned and disinfected/sterilized appropriately. Medical equipment is considered either reusable or single use. Single-use devices (SUD) are considered disposable and are not to be reprocessed for additional use except by entities that have received FDA clearance to do so.[58,59] All RME must be cleaned and stored following the MIFU in order to prevent transmission of infections between patients.

All RME should be cleaned between each patient use. RME must be pre-cleaned/decontaminated, according to the MIFU, to remove organic material at the point of use prior to high-level disinfection (HLD) or sterilization. Failure to do so may reduce the effectiveness of the HLD/sterilization process.[58] The level of cleaning, HLD, or sterilization of RME is determined according to how that equipment is used for patient care. The Spaulding Classification system is followed in order to determine the level of HLD or sterilization needed for RME, based on the risk of transmitting pathogens should the device become contaminated during use (Table 11.1).[58] MIFU for cleaning, HLD, and sterilization agents must be followed, with specific attention to contact times of the agents. It is recommended that organizations establish centralized processes to manage the HLD/sterilization of critical and semi-critical RME due to the high-risk nature of these processes.

Implementation

- ***Location for processing:*** There should be an appropriate location in the facility to perform the cleaning and reprocessing according to the manufacturer's recommendations.
- ***Clear reprocessing instructions:*** There should be clear policies and procedures outlining cleaning and reprocessing instructions for all RME. These should follow MIFU and should be visibly posted at the site of reprocessing.
- ***Training:*** Reprocessing of RME should be performed only by trained HCP. These HCP should trained on MIFU instructions for reprocessing of the RME and the appropriate PPE. Competencies should be demonstrated. Training should occur upon hire, at least annually, and whenever a new device is introduced.

- ***PPE:*** Recommended PPE should be readily available to HCP, and they should be trained in how to use the PPE correctly.

Strategies for Implementation

Historically, the focus of infection prevention has been on the inpatient setting, so HCP may be unaware of the necessity of basic infection prevention processes in the ambulatory environment. In contrast to the hospitals, ambulatory care settings may have less resources or infrastructure dedicated to a comprehensive infection prevention and control program; hence adequate equipment and supplies may not be available. A risk assessment can be very useful in determining the gaps and challenges that are present. This information can be used to develop strategies to

Table 11.1 Spaulding Classification[64]

EQUIPMENT CLASSIFICATION	EXAMPLES	LEVEL OF DISINFECTION/ STERILIZATON	AGENTS FOR DISINFECTION/ STERILIZATION
Non-Critical *Items that come in contact with intact skin but not mucous membranes.*	Stethoscope Blood pressure cuff Computer	Low level *Removes visible soil and decreases microbial burden*	EPA approved cleaner or disinfectant
Semi-Critical *Items that contact mucous membranes or non-intact skin.*	Endoscopes Laryngoscope blades Respiratory Therapy equipment Dental equipment	High Level *Eliminates all microorganisms except for bacterial spores*	hydrogen peroxide peracetic acid glutaraldehyde *ortho*-phthalaldehyde
Critical *Items that enter sterile tissue or the vascular system.*	Surgical instruments Cardiac and urinary catheters Implants Ultrasound probes used in sterile body cavities	Sterilization	steam hydrogen peroxide gas plasma peracetic acid glutaraldehyde *ortho*-phthalaldehyde

improve infection prevention infrastructure and processes within an outpatient setting.

Although most of the available data regarding HCP adherence to recommended infection prevention practices are for the inpatient setting, significant gaps are also likely to be present in the ambulatory setting. Multiple studies have shown that, despite guidelines recommending infection prevention best practices in healthcare settings, HCP behavior often falls short of these recommendations.[37,60] In order to improve this, it is important to understand the reasons that failures occur. HCP often cite lack of awareness of what the recommended processes or behaviors are, and inadequate training on how perform these tasks correctly.[12,33,34] In addition, lack of a standardized process, and infrastructure barriers, such as the absence of hand hygiene supplies at the point of care, can prevent HCP from following best infection prevention practices.

The Institute for Healthcare Improvement has published a white paper to guide improving process reliability in healthcare settings. It recommends the following interventions as effective first steps to improve a process.[61]

- Creating a standardized process
- Increasing awareness about the problem and the new process
- Providing education and training about the new process
- Creating reminders such as signs or checklists
- Providing feedback of adherence data to staff

These basic strategies can be applied to any process. When implemented, these interventions can improve the reliability of a process to 80–90%. In situations where increased reliability is needed or desired, the white paper provides additional interventions that further improve the reliability of a process.[61]

Approach to the Clinical Scenarios

Scenario 1

In the first scenario, the child has a draining wound due to MRSA. He should be placed in a private room. In addition to hand hygiene, the resident should wear gloves and possibly a gown as part of standard precautions.

Scenario 2

In this scenario, patients with respiratory illnesses should be screened and identified upon presentation to the healthcare facility in order to prevent spread of infection to others. The ambulatory clinic staff should provide the patient with a mask and encourage the patient to perform respiratory hygiene and cough etiquette. The patient should be placed in a private room. In addition to hand hygiene, the HCP caring for patients should wear a facemask when they are within 6 feet of the patient. Annual influenza immunization can also help decrease the risk of infection for staff.

Scenario 3

In this scenario, patients should be screened at the point of entry for symptoms of contagious illnesses to minimize exposure to other patients and HCP. This child should not wait in the waiting area but should be placed immediately in a private room, and the door should remain closed. If one is available, the child should be placed in an airborne isolation room. The patient should wear a mask, if old enough to comply. If available, HCP should wear either an N95 or higher respirator or a PAPR. Otherwise, a facemask should be worn. Only HCP who have been fully immunized against measles should care for this patient. The patient should be discharged home or admitted to an airborne isolation room as soon as feasible.

Unresolved Issues

As much of the current body of evidence related to infection prevention has been focused on the inpatient environment, there are gaps in our understanding infection prevention in the ambulatory setting.

Future research efforts should investigate:

- The best way to perform surveillance in the ambulatory setting and the most appropriate surveillance targets
- How to best implement practices such as transmission-based precautions in the outpatient environment
- The impact of various outpatient infection prevention practices on HAI reduction.

References

1. Hing ERP, Palso K. National Ambulatory Medical Care Survey: 2013 State and National Summary Tables. 2013; http://www.cdc.gov/nchs/ahcd/ahcd_products.htm. Accessed January 4, 2017.
2. Cullen KA, Hall MJ, Golosinskiy A. Ambulatory surgery in the United States, 2006. *Natl Health Stat Report.* 2009;11:1–25.
3. Feemster KA, Odeniyi FM, Localio R, Grundmeier RW, Coffin SE, Metlay JP. Surveillance for healthcare-associated influenza-like illness in pediatric clinics: validity of diagnosis codes for case identification. *Infect Control Hosp Epidemiol.* 2016;37(10):1247–1250.
4. Simmering JE, Polgreen LA, Cavanaugh JE, Polgreen PM. Are well-child visits a risk factor for subsequent influenza-like illness visits? *Infect Control Hosp Epidemiol.* 2014;35(3):251–256.
5. Bloch AB, Orenstein WA, Ewing WM, et al. Measles outbreak in a pediatric practice: airborne transmission in an office setting. *Pediatrics.* 1985;75(4):676–683.
6. Askew GL, Finelli L, Hutton M, et al. Mycobacterium tuberculosis transmission from a pediatrician to patients. *Pediatrics.* 1997;100(1):19–23.
7. Kuncio DE, Middleton M, Cooney MG, Ramos M, Coffin SE, Feemster KA. Health care worker exposures to pertussis: missed opportunities for prevention. *Pediatrics.* 2014;133(1):15–21.
8. Thompson ND, Perz JF, Moorman AC, Holmberg SD. Nonhospital health care-associated hepatitis B and C virus transmission: United States, 1998–2008. *Ann Intern Med.* 2009;150(1):33–39.
9. Williams IT, Perz JF, Bell BP. Viral hepatitis transmission in ambulatory health care settings. *Clin Infect Dis.* 2004;38(11):1592–1598.
10. Mangram AJ, Horan TC, Pearson ML, Silver LC, Jarvis WR. Guideline for prevention of surgical site infection, 1999. Hospital Infection Control Practices Advisory Committee. *Infect Control Hosp Epidemiol.* 1999;20(4):250–278; quiz 279–280.
11. Goodman RA, Solomon SL. Transmission of infectious diseases in outpatient health care settings. *JAMA.* 1991;265(18):2377–2381.
12. Larson E, Killien M. Factors influencing handwashing behavior of patient care personnel. *Am J Infect Control.* 1982;10(3):93–99.
13. Lederer JW Jr, Best D, Hendrix V. A comprehensive hand hygiene approach to reducing MRSA health care-associated infections. *Jt Comm J Qual Patient Saf.* 2009;35(4):180–185.
14. Balkhy HH, Zingg W. Update on infection control challenges in special pediatric populations. *Curr Opin Infect Dis.* 2014;27(4):370–378.
15. Sandora TJ. The unique challenge of infection control in pediatric care. 2012. Available at: http://www.medscape.com/viewarticle/763137. Accessed January 5, 2017.
16. Rathore MH, Jackson MA, Committee on Infectious Diseases. Infection prevention and control in pediatric ambulatory settings. *Pediatrics.* 2017;140(5): e20172857.
17. Jarvis WR, Robles B. Nosocomial infections in pediatric patients. *Adv Pediatr Infect Dis.* 1996;12:243–295.

18. Graman PS, Hall CB. Epidemiology and control of nosocomial viral infections. *Infect Dis Clin North Am.* 1989;3(4):815–841.
19. Lobovits AM, Freeman J, Goldmann DA, McIntosh K. Risk of illness after exposure to a pediatric office. *N Engl J Med.* 1985;313(7):425–428.
20. Geyer SA. Guidelines for processing toys. *J Healthc Mater Manage.* 1986;4(3): 52–53.
21. Merriman E, Corwin P, Ikram R. Toys are a potential source of cross-infection in general practitioners' waiting rooms. *Br J Gen Pract.* 2002;52(475):138–140.
22. Centers for Disease Control and Prevention. Infection prevention in ambulatory settings guideline. 2016. Available at: https://www.cdc.gov/infectioncontrol/pdf/outpatient/guidechecklist.pdf. Accessed January 5, 2017.
23. Kawai AT, Calderwood MS, Jin R, et al. Impact of the Centers for Medicare and Medicaid Services hospital-acquired conditions policy on billing rates for 2 targeted healthcare-associated infections. *Infect Control Hosp Epidemiol.* 2015;36(8):871–877.
24. Davis RM, Orenstein WA, Frank JA, Jr., et al. Transmission of measles in medical settings. 1980 through 1984. *JAMA.* 1986;255(10):1295–1298.
25. Yang JS, Park S, Kim YJ, et al. Middle East respiratory syndrome in 3 persons, South Korea, 2015. *Emerg Infect Dis.* 2015;21(11):2084–2087.
26. Rhymer W, Speare R. Countries' response to WHO's travel recommendations during the 2013–2016 Ebola outbreak. *Bull World Health Organ.* 2017;95(1):10–17.
27. Centers for Disease Control and Prevention. CDC Current Outbreak List. 2017. Available at: https://www.cdc.gov/outbreaks/index.html. Accessed April 9, 2017.
28. Siegel JD, Rhinehart E, Jackson M, Chiarello L, Health Care Infection Control Practices Advisory Committee. 2007 Guideline for isolation precautions: preventing transmission of infectious agents in health care settings. *Am J Infect Control.* 2007;35(10 Suppl 2):S65–S164.
29. Semmelweis I. The etiology, concept and prophylaxis of childbed fever. In: Buck CLA, Najera E, Terris M (Eds.). *The challenge of epidemiology*. Washington: PAHO Scientific Publication; 1988: 46–59.
30. Steere AC, Mallison GF. Handwashing practices for the prevention of nosocomial infections. *Ann Intern Med.* 1975;83(5):683–690.
31. Girou E, Legrand P, Soing-Altrach S, et al. Association between hand hygiene compliance and methicillin-resistant *Staphylococcus aureus* prevalence in a French rehabilitation hospital. *Infect Control Hosp Epidemiol.* 2006;27(10):1128–1130.
32. Trick WE, Vernon MO, Welbel SF, et al. Multicenter intervention program to increase adherence to hand hygiene recommendations and glove use and to reduce the incidence of antimicrobial resistance. *Infect Control Hosp Epidemiol.* 2007;28(1):42–49.
33. Boyce JM, Pittet D, Healthcare Infection Control Practices Advisory Committee, Force HICPAC/SHEA/APIC/IDSA Hand Hygiene Task Force. Guideline for hand hygiene in health-care settings. Recommendations of the Healthcare Infection Control Practices Advisory Committee and the HICPAC/SHEA/APIC/IDSA Hand Hygiene Task Force. Society for Healthcare Epidemiology of America/Association for Professionals in Infection Control/Infectious Diseases Society of America. *MMWR Recomm Rep.* 2002;51(RR-16):1–45, quiz CE41–44.

34. World Health Organization. WHO guidelines on hand hygiene in health care. 2009. Available at: http:// whqlibdoc.who.int/publications/2009/9789241597906_eng.pdf. Accessed October 24, 2018.
35. Dubberke ER, Carling P, Carrico R, et al. Strategies to prevent *Clostridium difficile* infections in acute care hospitals: 2014 update. *Infect Control Hosp Epidemiol.* 2014;35(Suppl 2):S48–S65.
36. MacCannell T, Umscheid CA, Agarwal RK, et al. Guideline for the prevention and control of norovirus gastroenteritis outbreaks in healthcare settings. *Infect Control Hosp Epidemiol.* 2011;32(10):939–969.
37. Erasmus V, Brouwer W, van Beeck EF, et al. A qualitative exploration of reasons for poor hand hygiene among hospital workers: lack of positive role models and of convincing evidence that hand hygiene prevents cross-infection. *Infect Control Hosp Epidemiol.* 2009;30(5):415–419.
38. Thompson D, Bowdey L, Brett M, Cheek J. Using medical student observers of infection prevention, hand hygiene, and injection safety in outpatient settings: A cross-sectional survey. *Am J Infect Control.* 2016;44(4):374–380.
39. Arai A, Tanabe M, Nakamura A, et al. Utility of electronic hand hygiene counting devices for measuring physicians' hand hygiene adherence applied to outpatient settings. *Am J Infect Control.* 2016;44(12):1481–1485.
40. Shimokura G, Weber DJ, Miller WC, Wurtzel H, Alter MJ. Factors associated with personal protection equipment use and hand hygiene among hemodialysis staff. *Am J Infect Control.* 2006;34(3):100–107.
41. Mensah E, Murdoch IE, Binstead K, Rotheram C, Franks W. Hand hygiene in routine glaucoma clinics. *Br J Ophthalmol.* 2005;89(11):1541–1542.
42. Squires JE, Linklater S, Grimshaw JM, et al. Understanding practice: factors that influence physician hand hygiene compliance. *Infect Control Hosp Epidemiol.* 2014;35(12):1511–1520.
43. Smiddy MP, O'Connell R, Creedon SA. Systematic qualitative literature review of health care workers' compliance with hand hygiene guidelines. *Am J Infect Control.* 2015;43(3):269–274.
44. Spruce L. Back to basics: hand hygiene and surgical hand antisepsis. *AORN J.* 2013;98(5):449–457; quiz 458–460.
45. Darouiche RO, Wall MJ Jr, Itani KM, et al. Chlorhexidine-alcohol versus povidone-iodine for surgical-site antisepsis. *N Engl J Med.* 2010;362(1):18–26.
46. Rotter ML, Kampf G, Suchomel M, Kundi M. Population kinetics of the skin flora on gloved hands following surgical hand disinfection with 3 propanol-based hand rubs: a prospective, randomized, double-blind trial. *Infect Control Hosp Epidemiol.* 2007;28(3):346–350.
47. Berman M. One hospital's clinical evaluation of brushless scrubbing. *AORN J.* 2004;79(2):349–354, 357–348.
48. Centers for Disease Control and Prevention. Respiratory hygiene/cough etiquette in healthcare settings. 2009. Available at: www.cdc.gov/flu/professionals/infectioncontrol/resphygiene. Accessed November 18, 2016.
49. Centers for Disease Control and Prevention. Guidance for the selection and use of personal protective equipment in healthcare settings. Available at: https://www.cdc.gov/hai/prevent/ppe.html. Accessed January 5, 2017.

50. Jensen PA, Lambert LA, Iademarco MF, Ridzon R, CDC. Guidelines for preventing the transmission of *Mycobacterium tuberculosis* in health-care settings, 2005. *MMWR Recomm Rep.* 2005;54(RR-17):1–141.
51. Occupational Health & Safety Administration. Occupational Safety and Health Standards, subpart I—personal protective equipment. Respiratory protection. 2003. Available at: https://www.osha.gov/pls/oshaweb/owadisp.show_document?p_table=standards&p_id=9696. Accessed January 5, 2017.
52. US Dept. of Labor. Regulations (Standards - 29 CFR) Bloodborne pathogens. 1910.1030. Available at: www.osha.gov/pls/oshaweb/owadisp.show_document?p_table=STANDARDS&p_id=10051. Accessed October 24, 2018.
53. Occupational Health and Safety Administration. Bloodborne pathogens and needlestick prevention. Available at: www. osha.gov/SLTC/bloodbornepathogens/index.html. Accessed November 18, 2016.
54. Marini MA, Giangregorio M, Kraskinski JC. Complying with the Occupational Safety and Health Administration's bloodborne pathogens standard: implementing needleless systems and intravenous safety devices. *Pediatr Emerg Care.* 2004;20(3):209–214.
55. Centers for Disease Control and Prevention. Transmission of hepatitis B and C viruses in outpatient settings—New York, Oklahoma, and Nebraska, 2000–2002. *MMWR.* 2003;52(38):901–906.
56. Saiman L, Siegel JD, LiPuma JJ, et al. Infection prevention and control guideline for cystic fibrosis: 2013 update. *Infect Control Hosp Epidemiol.* 2014;35(Suppl 1):S1–S67.
57. Sehulster L, Chinn RY, Centers for Disease Control and Prevention, HICPAC. Guidelines for environmental infection control in health-care facilities. Recommendations of CDC and the Healthcare Infection Control Practices Advisory Committee (HICPAC). *MMWR Recomm Rep.* 2003;52(RR-10):1–42.
58. Centers for Disease Control and Prevention. Guideline for disinfection and sterilization in healthcare facilities, 2008. Available at: http://www.cdc.gov/hicpac/pdf/guidelines/Disinfection_Nov_2008.pdf. Accessed November 19, 2016.
59. Food and Drug Administration. FDA regulations on reprocessing of single-use devices. 2006. Available at: http://www.fda.gov/MedicalDevices/DeviceRegulationandGuidance/GuidanceDocuments/ucm071434. Accessed November 19, 2016.
60. Anderson DJ, Chen LF, Weber DJ, et al. Enhanced terminal room disinfection and acquisition and infection caused by multidrug-resistant organisms and *Clostridium difficile* (the Benefits of Enhanced Terminal Room Disinfection study): a cluster-randomised, multicentre, crossover study. *Lancet.* 2017;389(10071):805–814.
61. Frankel A, Haraden C, Federico F, Lenoci-Edwards J. *A Framework for Safe, Reliable, and Effective Care.* White Paper. Cambridge, MA: Institute for Healthcare Improvement and Safe & Reliable Healthcare; 2017. (Available on ihi.org).

12 | Pediatric Long-Term Care, Behavioral Health, Residential Facilities, and Similar Settings

CANDACE JOHNSON, MEGHAN MURRAY, OLIVIA JACKSON, AND NATALIE NEU

Background

There are unique infection prevention issues associated with pediatric long-term care facilities, behavioral health units, rehabilitation hospitals, and other residential facilities. All of these facilities provide care to children with complex, chronic medical conditions.[1] These children are at increased risk for healthcare-associated infection due to factors such as age-related vulnerability to infections, especially respiratory viral infections; chronic exposure to indwelling medical devices such as tracheostomies, gastrostomy tubes, and central venous catheters; and frequent close contact with other children and healthcare personnel (HCP) during therapeutic and social activities.[2] Outbreaks of viral respiratory illness are not uncommon in this population and may result in substantial morbidity.[3] Carriage of multidrug-resistant bacteria is well described.[4] In the absence of best practice guidelines specific to this setting, this chapter will highlight specific challenges and practical solutions related to infection prevention.

Any discussion on infection prevention and control (IPC) practices in pediatric long-term care facilities (pLTCFs) must start with a description of the population being served and the setting in which IPC measures are implemented. Residents of pLTCFs fall within the broad grouping of children with special healthcare needs as defined by the Maternal and Child Health Bureau; more specifically, within this category they are the subgroup of the most medically fragile, medically complex children.[5] These are children with chronic, severe health conditions, substantial health service needs, functional limitations, and high health-resource utilization.[6] Emerging epidemiological data describe a population with multiple comorbidities—including developmental, neurological, respiratory, and gastrointestinal conditions—as well as a population that is growing thanks to medical advances and technologies that enable the survival of preterm neonates and children with congenital or acquired conditions previously thought to be incompatible with life.[6,7] While some of these children receive care at home, an increasing number of children reside in pLTCFs. There is no standardized definition for pLTCFs[1]; however, it is commonly agreed that these are facilities that provide comprehensive care for medically complex children. For the purposes of this chapter, these encompass the spectrum of skilled nursing facilities, rehabilitation facilities, behavioral health units, and group homes.[2]

IPC measures in pLTCFs are integral to preventing and managing healthcare-associated infections (HAIs). Studies looking at types of infections in pLTCFs identify respiratory tract infections (RTIs) as the most common type of infection[8,9]; this stands in contrast to adult LTCFs where urinary tract infections often exceed rates of RTIs,[10] and highlights the fact that IPC policies cannot be simply extrapolated from adult facilities to fit pediatric facilities. Residents of pLTCFs are at risk for infections due to both individual factors as well as facility factors that contribute to infection transmission. From an individual standpoint, residents may have multiple features that contribute to an increased susceptibility to infections, such as age-related immune immaturity in young patients, use of invasive devices such as tracheostomy tubes that increase portals of entry of infectious agents, chronic medical conditions such as neurological or movement disorders that increase risk for aspiration, as well as chronic lung disease resulting in decreased physiological reserves.[1,11,12] In addition to the disease transmission risks that are found in acute care facilities, pLTCFs may present additional risks as they seek to create a homelike atmosphere for their residents. To this end, many facilities incorporate shared play, therapy, and dining areas. Some facilities have on-site schools that residents and, in some instances, children with medical complexities from the community attend.[11] These shared settings as well as shared equipment serve as potential points for infection transmission. Furthermore, residents of pLTCFs are in contact with multiple caregivers—such as physicians, nurses, medical assistants, therapists (respiratory, physical, occupational, speech), teachers, teachers' aides—and visitors.[13] In a study on frequency of contact in acute care settings, patients had a median of 5.5 room entries by HCP and visitors in an hour, which could arguably be considered a conservative estimate for residents of pLTCFs.[14]

Given the risk for HAIs in pLTCFs it should come as no surprise that outbreaks have been well described in these facilities. Viral outbreaks have most commonly been reported[15,16,17]; colonization and outbreaks of infections with multidrug-resistant organisms (MDROs) have also been described in this population and have raised concern for transmission of MDROs from pLTCFs to acute care facilities, which has been described in the adult long-term care setting.[4,18,19] That HAI outbreaks have been found to be associated with significant morbidity and increased health-care costs as well serves to further emphasize the importance of IPC measures.[3,15,20]

As in acute care settings, the scope of IPC interventions in pLTCFs is broad, including developing procedures for both admissions and transfers of residents, optimizing hand hygiene, enforcing vaccination policies for residents and staff, and managing outbreaks. This chapter seeks to identify the challenges in developing and implementing IPC measures in pLTCFs and provide strategies for overcoming some of these challenges.

Clinical Scenario

A four-year-old child suffers a high spinal cord injury in a motor vehicle accident, resulting in spastic quadriplegia and ventilator dependence. During this hospitalization, the child becomes colonized with methicillin-resistant *Staphylococcus aureus* (MRSA). After a five-week-hospital stay, the child is transferred to a pLTCF. The nursing director asks about requirements for isolation precautions, including whether the child should be prevented from participating in group activities.

Questions

Are the isolation precautions used in the acute care setting applicable to pediatric residential facilities? Which strategies can minimize the transmission of multidrug-resistant (MDR) organisms in residential facilities while supporting the psychosocial needs of a child? Can infection prevention guidelines for adult LTCFs be adapted for use in pediatrics?

Key Challenges

PLTCFs present unique challenges for IPC. Children residing in pLTCFs are at increased risk for infection before they are even admitted, due to their complex comorbid conditions, multiple device use, and age-related immunological immaturity.[6,7] IPC methods utilized in pLTCFs have been adapted from adult LTCFs or pediatric acute care facilities, but they do not translate well. The disease burden of pLTCF residents varies greatly from their adult counterparts', and they often require greater direct care, as most are dependent on clinical and therapeutic staff for all activities of daily living. The environment in a pLTCF is very different from the acute care setting, as the former focuses on creating a homelike atmosphere for residents.[1] PLTCFs desire to create a living space that not only encourages appropriate child development, but also facilitates interaction between the residents and staff as well as between the residents and their families. However this focus on a homelike environment can lead to the perception that IPC interferes with that goal. Despite the frequent interactions residents have with staff and visitors, it has been shown that IPC is not a priority in these interactions; staff assert that, independent of personal behaviors, residents will become ill as part of the normal developmental process, and also due to the added burden of their comorbidities.[21]

Another challenge for IPC in pLTCFs is the dilemma of how to incorporate these practices into the resident's daily care. To promote the quality of life and developmental needs in pLTCFs, residents participate in many therapeutic groups, attend school, and, when able, engage in play with one another. These direct and indirect interactions among residents lead to an increased opportunity for the spread of infections, especially for respiratory viral infections. Incorporating IPC into these interactions is difficult, as it depends not only on the actions of staff, but at times on the behaviors of the residents. A study evaluating the incorporation of hand hygiene into the workflow of common activities done by direct care staff found it was difficult to achieve widespread adoption by staff,[22] in part due to the unique nature of certain of these activities. For example, school staff reported that residents often share devices used in the classroom. To implement appropriate IPC according to the World Health Organization's recommendations,[23] the school staff would be required to wash their hands after each resident interaction, as well as wash each of the residents' hands and the shared device. Staff reported this was not feasible, as it would require that the majority of class and/or therapeutic time would be spent on IPC and not on the class's intended purpose.

Moreover, residents in pLTCFs receive care from a diverse group of caregivers. In addition to clinical care provided by HCP, nurses, and respiratory therapists, they receive services from occupational, physical, recreational, music, and art therapists, as well as Child Life, teachers, and school aides. While indirect interactions occur on a daily basis with dining services, housekeeping, environmental services, and facilities, due to the homelike environment previously described, residents also have direct contact with these staff. Effective IPC interventions need to encompass all the varied facets of care residents receive.[24]

IPC efforts are further challenged by the lack of standardized HAI case definitions for the pediatric long-term care population. Limited guidelines are available for HAI surveillance in pLTCFs, necessitating the adaptation of recommendations from either adult long-term care or acute pediatric care settings.[8] Standardized HAI case definitions enable the tracking of infections within and across facilities. PLTCFs are part of the continuum of care for their residents; therefore, the infection burden present in other pLTCFs and referring acute care facilities is often reflected in an individual site's epidemiology. Pediatric long-term care–specific HAI case definitions are needed in order to assess the need and impact of IPC interventions. Developing appropriate case definitions for such a varied and complex population is a difficult task, especially since residents are often unable to communicate their symptoms. Diagnostic testing is useful in this context, as it guides appropriate care for the individual and also informs the IPC actions necessary to limit its impact on the rest of the residents, staff, and families. Given testing's utility, case definitions need to incorporate diagnostic testing; however, there is limited evidence of its routine use in this population. PLTCFs are often reimbursed for their services per resident daily rate, leaving limited room in the budget for extensive diagnostic testing.[20] Also, pLTCFs may not have access to certain diagnostic tools, including a chest radiograph, without transferring their residents to an outside facility, laboratory, or clinic.

Lastly, many pLTCFs lack staff designated for IPC. Even in facilities with an infection preventionist (IP), this individual may have competing responsibilities, such as oversight of employee health activities. The role of the IP is comprehensive and includes environmental health, antimicrobial stewardship, surveillance and mitigation of infections and outbreaks, and staff education on appropriate IPC behaviors, as well as the monitoring and evaluation of these activities. Substantial resources are needed, not only for the hiring of an IP, but to aid in the implementation of IPC throughout the pLTCF. Without an IP and appropriate support from the facility, it is difficult to implement appropriate IPC in pLTCFs.

Suggested Approaches

In spite of the challenges outlined in the prior section, IPC measures can and should be implemented in pLTCFs; the following are proposed recommendations for doing so. All pLTCFs should have comprehensive and easily accessible policies and procedures; e.g., an online reference source, for IPC. When developing facility-specific policies, it can be useful to adapt pediatric acute care guidelines; however, it is important to consider the unique challenges faced by HCP implementing IPC in pediatric long-term care. In the absence of strong evidence for IPC in pLTCFs, we here present approaches modified from acute care and adult LTCF IPC policies and procedures and will highlight some suggested policies and procedures and algorithms for IPC in pLTCFs.

Isolation Precautions

In pLTCFs, IPC precaution policies need to include guidelines for standard and transmission-based precautions, such as contact, contact and droplet, droplet, or airborne transmission precautions (Box 12.1). Similar to acute care, all residents at pLTCFs must be on standard precautions, which include appropriate hand hygiene as well as gowns, glove, masks, and eye protection when coming in contact with blood, body fluids, secretions, and excretions.[25,26]

Determining when a resident should be placed on transmission-based precautions is based on the identification of the causative pathogen or in lieu of diagnostic testing, in accordance with the likely route of transmission: for example, contact precautions for a resident with conjunctivitis. Without diagnostic testing, it can be difficult to distinguish among respiratory viral pathogens. For suspected viral respiratory infections, residents should be placed on both contact and droplet precautions. In order to simplify implementation of isolation precautions, pLTCFs may decide to order contact and droplet precautions for all confirmed and suspected respiratory infections. Airborne precautions are required for pathogens that may be transmitted by droplet nuclei such as *Mycobacterium tuberculosis*, varicella-zoster virus, and rubeola virus (measles virus). Airborne precautions require the use of special air-handling and ventilation systems and the use of specific respiratory protection with certified N95 or higher level respirators for HCP.[25] For facilities that do not have the necessary infrastructure to support it, residents requiring airborne precaution should be transferred to acute care.

BOX 12.1 PROPOSED RECOMMENDATIONS FOR ISOLATION PRECAUTIONS IN PEDIATRIC LONG-TERM CARE*

Isolation Precautions for Pediatric Long-Term Care

- Standard (hand hygiene):
  - All residents
  - Gowns, gloves, masks, and/or eye protection as appropriate for potential contact with blood, body fluid, secretions, and excretions
- Contact (hand hygiene, gowns, gloves):
  - Gastrointestinal illness
  - Skin/soft tissue infections
  - Conjunctivitis
- Contact and Droplet (hand hygiene, gowns, gloves, masks, and if close contact, eye protection):
  - All respiratory symptoms
  - Meningitis
- Airborne (hand hygiene, N95 or higher respirator, resident in airborne infection isolation room):
  - Disseminated herpes zoster—e.g., shingles or varicella—in immunocompromised patient
  - Measles
  - Tuberculosis

* Proposed recommendations are based on the Healthcare Infection Control Practices Advisory Committee's 2007 Guidelines for Isolation Precautions (http://www.cdc.gov/hicpac/2007ip/ 2007ip_part4.html).

The goal of maintaining a homelike environment for the residents poses further challenges for implementing transmission-based precautions. As an example, if a resident contracts a skin or soft-tissue infection, placing the child on contact precautions can minimize the risk for transmission, but it also restricts the resident from participating in activities outside of their room. If the site of infection can be covered and the area is not accessed during school or therapeutic sessions, the resident may be able to attend, as there is minimal risk for exposure. Proposed guidelines for isolation precautions, including common viral pathogens, diagnostic testing, incubation periods, and length of isolation, are in Tables 12.1 and 12.2.

TABLE 12.1 Common Viral Respiratory Pathogens for Which Contact and Droplet Precautions Are Recommended In Pediatric Long-Term Care Facilities

VIRUS	SEASON	INCUBATION PERIOD	AVAILABLE TESTING	TREATMENT OR VACCINES	SUGGESTED LENGTH OF ISOLATION FROM SYMPTOM ONSET
Respiratory Syncytial Virus	Winter/ Spring	4–6 days	EIA/DFA/ CX/ PCR	Palivizumab (SYNAGIS®)	24 hrs without fever or 7 days (whichever greater)
Influenza (A & B)	Winter/ Spring	1–4 days	EIA/DFA/ CX/ PCR	Oseltamivir (Tamiflu®) Seasonal vaccine	24 hrs without fever or 7 days (whichever greater)
Human Metapneumovirus	Winter/ Spring	3–5 days	DFA/PCR	Supportive care	24 hrs without fever or 10 days (whichever greater)
Parainfluenza	Type 1: Fall Type 2: Spring Type 3: Spring/ Summer	2–6 days	DFA/CX/ PCR	Supportive care	24 hrs without fever or 7 days (whichever greater)
Enterovirus/ Echovirus	Summer/Fall	3–6 days	PCR	Supportive care	24 hrs without fever or 7 days (whichever greater)
Rhinovirus (Common Cold)	Year round	2–3 days	PCR	Supportive care	24 hrs without fever or 7 days (whichever greater)
Adenovirus	Winter/Spring/ Early Summer	2–14 days	DFA/CX/ PCR	Supportive care	14 days asymptomatic

[1]EIA = enzyme-linked immunosorbent assay; DFA = direct fluorescent antibody test; CX = viral culture; PCR = polymerase chain reaction test

TABLE 12.2 Common Gastrointestinal Pathogens and Other Syndromes for Which Contact Precautions Are Recommended in Pediatric Long-Term Care

GASTROINTESTINAL PATHOGEN	INCUBATION PERIOD	AVAILABLE TESTING	TREATMENT OR VACCINES	SUGGESTED LENGTH OF ISOLATION
Rotavirus	1–3 days	EIA/ELISA	RV5 vaccine or RV1 vaccine (infants), Supportive care	Resolution of symptoms or 10 days after onset (whichever greater)
Norovirus	24–48 hrs	EIA	Supportive care	>72 hrs after resolution of symptoms
Clostridioides difficile	unknown	EIA (3 stools) PCR	Precipitating antibiotic discontinued & antibiotic for *C. difficile* started	>72 hrs after resolution of symptoms
Adenovirus	3–10 days	PCR	Supportive care	After 10 days asymptomatic
Enterovirus	3–6 days	PCR	Supportive care	Duration of illness
By Presentation				
Viral/Bacterial Conjunctivitis	Pathogen-dependent	Viral: DFA/PCR/CX Bacterial: CX	Pathogen dependent	*Suspected bacterial:* 48 hrs or until symptoms resolve *Suspected viral*: Resident placed on *Contact and Droplet*, testing done, discontinue depending on pathogen (Adenovirus most common 14 d, Enterovirus 5 d)
Skin and Soft Tissue Infection	Possible colonization	Bacterial/Fungal CX	Pathogen dependent	If purulent drainage, testing done and resident remains on Contact (i.e., no school if draining and/or not coverable). Discontinue when dry.

[1] EIA/ELISA = enzyme-linked immunosorbent assay; DFA = direct fluorescent antibody test; CX = culture; PCR = polymerase chain reaction test

Immunization Policies: IPC strategies should begin prior to admission to a pLTCF. Requiring completion of a preadmission form and a universal consent for childhood immunizations ensures appropriate capture of medical and vaccination information and sets precedence for acceptance of future vaccines; such records could be completed and/or obtained during an initial tour of the facility by a parent or guardian and facilitated by the pLTCF's admissions' department. Review of these documents by the IP and medical staff before the resident's admission allows for shared knowledge, planning, and prevention of immunization delay. In cases of parental refusal of standard immunizations, facilities may consider requiring parents to sign a Declination of Immunization form. Finally, if there is a school at the facility that is managed by the Board of Education, the facility and the parents of residents attending the school must follow state-mandated policies and procedures for immunizations.

Universal Isolation Upon Facility Admission: In order to minimize the risk of transmission of community-based infections at the time of admission, pLTCFs may choose to apply universal contact and droplet precautions for both new residents as well as transfers back to the facility. New resident admissions, and residents returning from an emergency department visit or unplanned/ nonscheduled acute care stay, could be placed on contact and droplet precautions for a 72-hour observation period to determine if an infectious process is present. Due to the high frequency of outside clinic appointments attended by medically complex residents, it is suggested that these residents should not be subjected to the 72-hour observation period. The observation period could potentially decrease infection transmission to other residents and staff and allow time for staff to identify the residents' baseline medical needs.

Designated Admission Units: Some pLTCFs have designated admissions units as a way to minimize the potential transmission of community-acquired infection transmission from new residents. However, pLTCF admissions units may lead to staff burnout due to an increased workload and the use of isolation precautions during the admission process. Also, admissions units may have the unintended consequence of increased risk of outbreaks due to frequent exposure to residents from outside facilities. PLTCFs need to individualize their IPC policies for admissions and monitor their infections to evaluate the impact of admissions and transmission of infection.

Surveillance

Line Lists, Isolation Precautions, and Staffing

Monitoring residents' health status is necessary due to the high risk for infection transmission in pLTCFs. Infection control surveillance rounds should occur on a daily basis, concentrate on identifying potential resident infections, and aid in the determination of whether resident isolation precautions are necessary. Documentation of infections should occur in a standard formatted line list, and a memo of those on precautions should be circulated daily to all members of the facility (Box 12.2).

During the respiratory viral season, a heightened awareness of infection symptoms and strict adherence to criteria for placing residents on isolation precautions is essential for IPC. To prevent viral respiratory infection outbreaks, it is suggested that a resident be placed on contact and droplet precautions when exhibiting one or more of the following signs and symptoms above a resident's baseline: fever, rhinorrhea, new-onset vomiting, new-onset feeding intolerance, increased secretions, increased oxygen support, cough, and/or wheezing. Additionally, the affected resident's roommates as well as residents in rooms connected by a personal care area or bathroom should be placed on contact and droplet precautions to further contain transmission of infection due to shared caregivers and living spaces. Box 12.3 provides an example of how to educate staff about giving care during an outbreak.

BOX 12.2 TYPICAL COMPONENTS OF A LINE LIST FOR MANAGING INFECTION CONTROL SURVEILLANCE AT A PEDIATRIC LONG-TERM CARE FACILITY

Resident information and characteristics for Surveillance Line List for Infection:

- Demographic characteristics: Name, date of birth, gender, bed location, classroom location, date of onset
- Symptoms: Fever, change in secretions, vomiting, diarrhea, cough, wheezing, change in oxygen requirements, congestion
- Diagnostics: Cultures, pathogen identified
- Outcome: Date precautions initiated, date precautions ended, date transferred to acute care, date returned from acute care
- Other: Tracheostomy, ventilator, influenza vaccine status

BOX 12.3 WORKFLOW FOR THERAPEUTIC STAFF FOR PATIENTS ON ISOLATION PRECAUTIONS

INFECTON CONTROL: Prioritizing Sessions for Residents

See Residents in the Following Order:

1. Unexposed asymptomatic residents in open rooms
2. Exposed asymptomatic residents in open rooms
3. Asymptomatic residents in closed rooms
4. Symptomatic resident in closed room
5. For concerns, call the Infection Control Coordinator or Designee

Special Instructions:

1. Once you see a symptomatic resident, you *cannot* see another resident either in the neighborhood or in school.
2. When a symptomatic resident is cleared by a Nurse Manager for a session, sessions with residents can be divided up as best as possible among disciplines.
3. Each resident must be seen by at least one discipline by the end of each day.
4. Residents who cannot receive therapy sessions due to being symptomatic and on isolation precautions should be entered as sick for that therapy session.
5. It is essential to apply and remove PPE carefully and appropriately.
6. Hand hygiene is to be performed before and after sessions.

Ensuring that all staff and residents are vaccinated against influenza should also be a priority during the respiratory viral season. Some facilities and states (e.g., New York State) have a mandated influenza vaccine policy for HCP requiring either vaccination or donning of masks at the start of the respiratory viral season. In general, it is very important for the pLTCF to monitor and encourage all staff to adhere to the Advisory Committee on Immunization Practices for vaccination, both at hire and annually. Further guidance can be found in the Centers for Disease Control and Prevention's (CDC's) "Toolkit for Long-Term Care Employers" (www.cdc.gov/flu/toolkit/long-term-care/index.htm).

Diagnostic Testing

Testing for infections, especially viral pathogens, is not routine in pLTCFs, but it may help to determine the length and type of precaution required for the ill resident. One approach is to test the resident who first exhibits viral-like symptoms—the index case—with a comprehensive respiratory viral panel (RVP) polymerase chain reaction (PCR) to confirm the type of pathogen present. These tests are routinely used in emergency care, acute care, and some long-term care sites and have been shown to be a useful component of IPC.[15,27,28] Neighboring residents with similar symptoms can be considered suspect cases; appropriate isolation precautions should be instituted and remain in place for the duration recommended for the pathogen identified in the index case (Table 12.1). If the RVP is negative and the resident's symptoms resolve, the IP could consider discontinuation of isolation precautions (Figure 12.1). Although viral direct fluorescent antibody (DFA) testing is significantly cheaper than PCR-based testing, PCR tests are more advantageous due to the rapid turnaround time and its comprehensive identification of numerous viral pathogens.[29] Rhinovirus and enterovirus, both common respiratory viral pathogens in pLTCFs throughout the year, are not detected on a DFA but are easily detected by PCR.

As with respiratory illness, pLTCFs should create specific algorithms to manage gastrointestinal illness (Figure 12.2). Contact precautions should be initiated when a resident has at least two episodes of diarrhea and/or vomiting in 24 hours, with or without fever, or displays vomiting or diarrhea above the resident's baseline pattern. As with respiratory infections, placing the roommates of the symptomatic resident as well as the residents in the adjoining rooms on contact precautions can help confine the infection. Sending stool specimens for *Clostridioides difficile* testing and viral pathogen testing can be used to determine whether treatment is required and/or if contact precautions should be continued (Table 12.2). Caution should be exercised when sending *C. difficile* testing in children under one year of age, as colonization is common in this age group. Negative stool specimen results or improvement in resident symptoms for 72 hours can be used as an indication for contact precaution discontinuation.

Outbreak Management and Unit Closures

During outbreaks (defined in this text as more than one resident positive with the same pathogen or exhibiting similar symptoms) in a pLTCF, it is important to directly communicate with the local Department of Health (DOH). Providing information from infection line lists to the DOH enables them to assess exposures and potential causes of transmission, and allows their participation in decision making to help manage the outbreak. Conversely, it is also beneficial for pLTCFs to be aware of infections in the

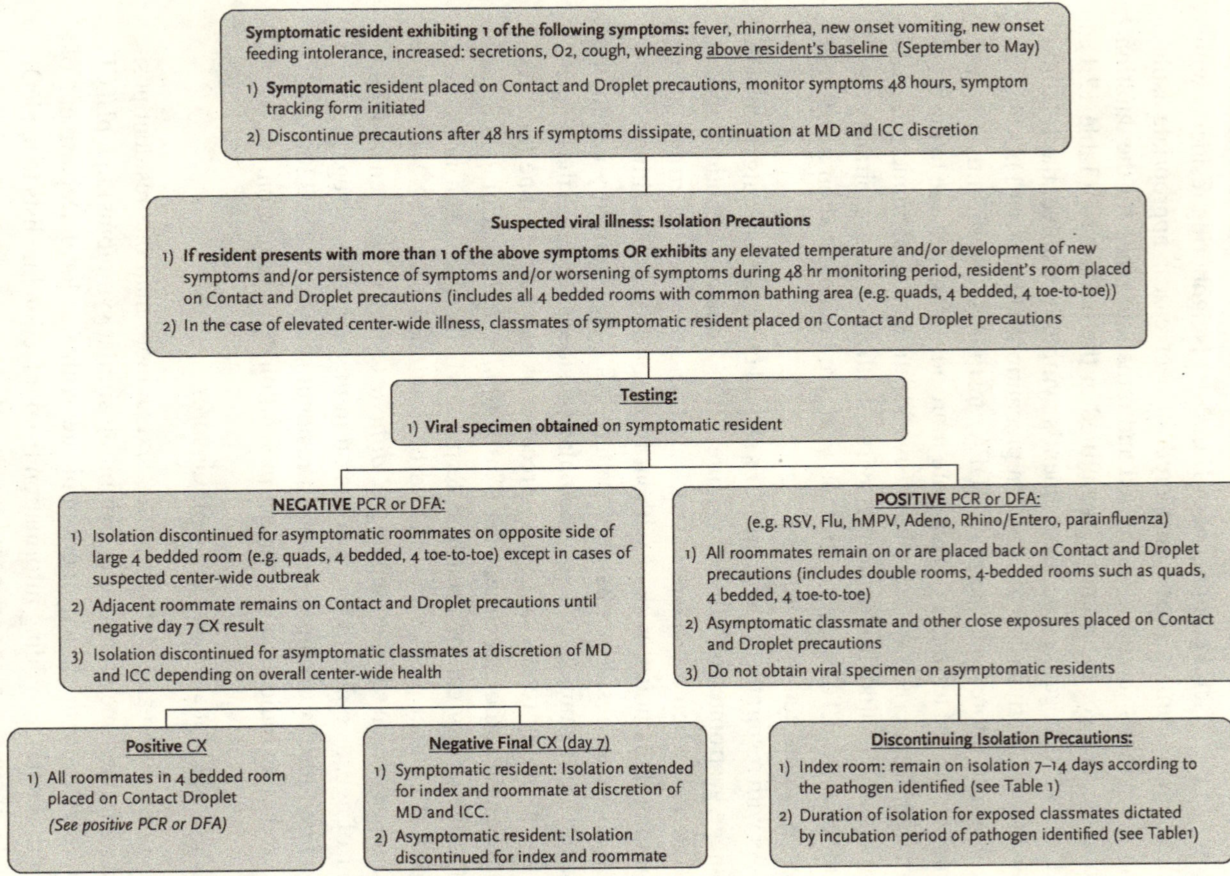

FIGURE 12.1 Proposed guideline for respiratory illness isolation precautions.

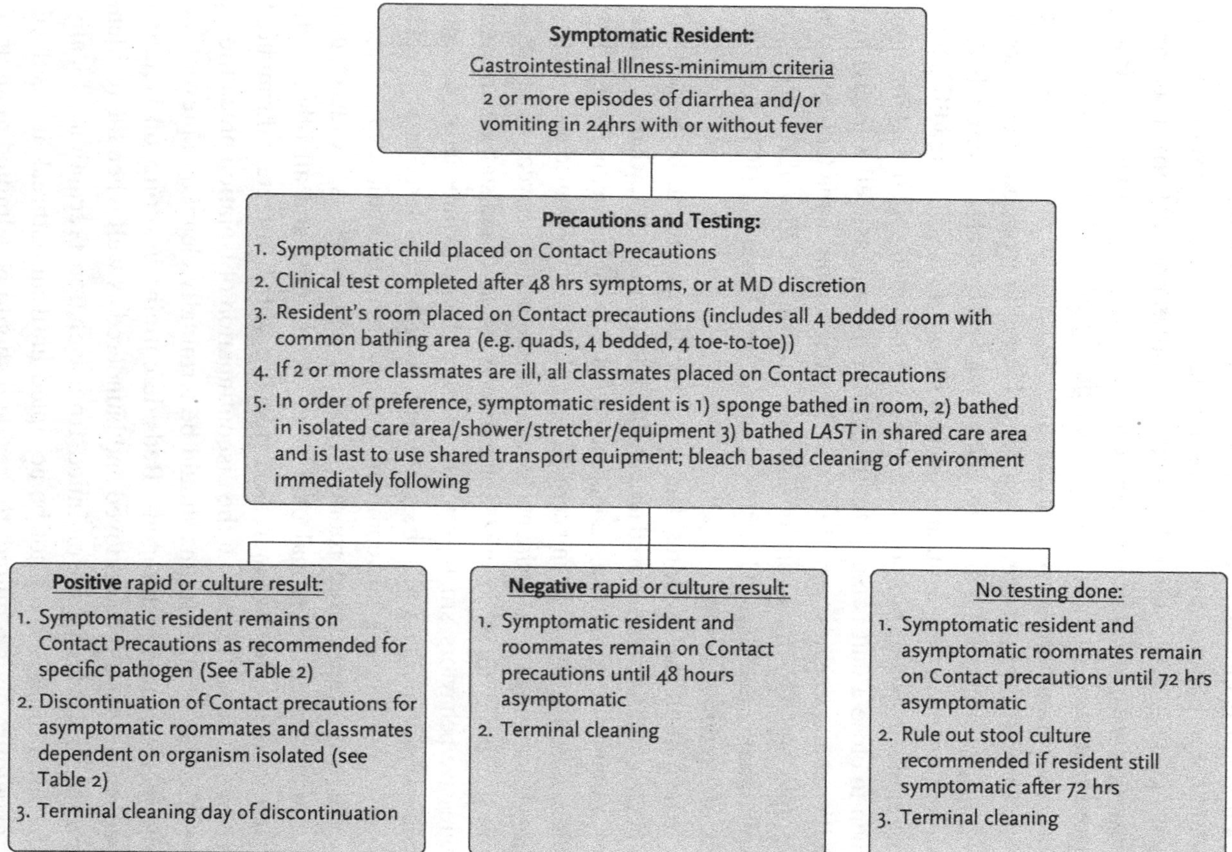

FIGURE 12.2 Proposed guideline for gastrointestinal illness isolation precautions.

community and in other healthcare facilities; a relationship with the DOH will facilitate the sharing of this information.

During an outbreak, unit closure can be an important IPC measure. When a unit is closed, to avoid infection exposures, uninfected residents should not be permitted to enter closed units. Use of floating staff between open and closed units should be avoided to further prevent horizontal transmission; close communication between the staffing department and IP will ensure that nurse staffing is optimized during an outbreak. In instances when exceptions are permitted due to short staffing, staff that work on a closed unit during a previous shift and agree to work additional hours on an open unit should be required to change into clean scrubs before entering the open unit. Laundry services should have scrubs readily available at all times and promote changing scrubs when soiled. Determining when to close a unit is based on the size of the unit as well as individual facility characteristics; e.g., the acuity of the residents in the facility. As an example, a pLTCF may consider closing a unit when 20% of residents are symptomatic, and the IPC team, including the IP and the HCP, deem the risk of infection is high.

When a unit is closed, resident activities do not need to be suspended. While the residents in a closed unit should not attend school, whether on-site or community-based, the residents may receive bedside teaching when their unit is closed. If multiple units are closed, pLTCFs may consider instituting bedside teaching for all residents to prevent interaction between residents in large groups. To allow socialization between residents and staff and prevent regressive behaviors, small group activities with two to three asymptomatic residents within a unit may be permitted. Avoidance of large group events for residents, families, and community members is recommended.

When units are closed, rooms on isolation precautions, elevators, unit community areas, personal care areas, restrooms, and all other high-touch areas should have increased cleaning with disinfectant throughout the day. As in acute care, at the discontinuation of isolation precautions, the affected resident rooms should be terminally cleaned to prevent the potential spread of pathogens. Bedside curtains in rooms on isolation precautions should be removed and laundered as well when the resident or entire room(s) is discontinued from isolation precautions. Ideally, new admissions should not be accepted until an outbreak is resolved. If an admission is required, the resident should be admitted to an unaffected unit. When preparing for a discharge, a resident should be asymptomatic; if symptoms persist, postponing discharge is recommended for the sake of the health of those residing in the outside community.

Environmental Policies

IPC includes comprehensive environmental policies and procedures, including, but not limited to, the appropriate disposal of medical waste, maintaining a clean environment, the proper use and disuse of resident and staff items, and laundry services. Complete environmental rounds conducted on a monthly basis by both a manager or director of Environmental Services and the IP to promote heightened cleaning and disinfection of community area surfaces, medical equipment, and toys, as well as to mitigate breaches in infection control practices, are recommended as best practice. Generating and distributing reports with environmental round findings to nursing, medical, environmental, and rehabilitation management can increase awareness of noncompliance issues with infection control protocols. The need for corrective actions should be determined by the infection control and environmental services managers. Non-punitive direct HCP feedback during environmental rounds can increase education about and compliance with IPC and environmental services policies and procedures. Handout 12.1 is an example of a checklist to standardize environmental rounds.

On-site School and Infection Prevention and Control

Monitoring residents' health status is necessary due to high risk for large exposures in the school setting. If there is a school on site, communication between the pLTCF and the school staff (who may be different from the staff at the pLTCF) is important in order to quickly recognize and isolate residents who are potentially infectious. Classrooms may be comprised of residents from multiple units, creating an environment for the easy spread of infections. Also, residents often participate in school-based group activities where there may be close contact between staff and residents, as well as among residents. A daily care form (Handout 12.2), completed every school day by the classroom staff and reported to the pLTCF medical staff by telephone or as a written document, can be an effective way of communicating any changes in the residents' appetite, voiding and stool patterns, and behavior that may signal the onset of an illness. If nursing staff in the school identify a change in a resident's baseline status, an illness evaluation form (Handout 12.3) including the resident's vital signs and symptoms could assist the pLTCF physician or nurse practitioner when the resident returns to their unit. The HCP and IP could then determine whether isolation precautions are necessary and whether the resident

HANDOUT 12.1 Example of Environmental Rounds Checklist for Pediatric Long-Term Care Facilities

Location/Item	Yes	No	Comments
Medicine Room—Door locked, cart locked, no employee personal items, sharps container, OSHA and spill kits available			
Medicine Refrigerator—Thermometer present, temperatures logged, only meds stored			
Supply Closets—Neat, no items on floor or within 18 inches of ceiling			
Linen Carts—Covered			
Shower Room—Clean, no personal care items, suction canister ready for use			
Tub Room—Clean, no personal care items			
Dining/Play Area—Clean, suction canister available and ready for use			
Pantry—Opened items in refrigerator are labeled, dated, and discarded after 24 hours			
Hall Bathroom—Clean, no odors			
Emergency Carts—Available and ready for use; log completed, not blocked			
Hallway—All hand sanitizer dispensers have shields and are not over electrical outlets; items not blocking fire doors or exits			
Room # ________			
Clean and clutter-free			
Nightlights working			
No items on floors			
No soiled or chipped ceiling tiles			
No uncapped saline or other containers			
Open saline dated for 24 hours			
Closets are clean, neat, no items on floor			
No staff items (e.g., coats, bags) are in room			
Nothing under sink in bathroom			
No excess soap (bar/pump) at bathing sink			
Personal care items labeled			
Laundry bins are covered			
Garbage cans are covered			
All cubicle curtains clean			

No clinical information posted			
Do all mattresses fit tightly around all four sides of the crib?			
If a child in room is on precautions:			
Sign posted at door			
Protective equipment available			
Staff are using protective equipment			

HANDOUT 12.2 Example of School Daily Care Record for Resident at Pediatric Long-Term Care Facility

Student:	Date:	Unit:	Classroom:
	Description: Check appropriate boxes as indicated and/or write comments in the space provided.		
<u>Vomiting</u> Time Name ____ ________ ____ ________	No. of Times ____________ Before meal: Yes ☐ No ☐ After meal: Yes ☐ No ☐ During meal: Yes ☐ No ☐ Large ☐ Medium ☐ Small ☐		
<u>Voiding</u> Time Name ____ ____________ ____ ____________ ____ ____________	Not applicable: ☐ Amount: ____________ (only if on intake/output) Voided: No ☐ Check the boxes below each time the resident voided: ☐ 1 ☐ 2 ☐ 3 ☐ 4 ☐ 5 ☐ 6		
<u>Bowel Movements</u> Time Name ____ ____________ ____ ____________	<u>Check the boxes below to indicate when resident had a BM:</u> ☐ 1 ☐ 2 ☐ 3 ☐ 4 ☐ 5 ☐ 6 <u>Check the boxes that describe the BMs:</u> Soft ☐ Loose ☐ Diarrhea ☐ Large ☐ Medium ☐ Small ☐		
<u>Feedings</u> Time Name ___ ____________ ___ ____________	<u>Solids</u> Time:______ All ☐ (100%) Half ☐ (50%) Most ☐ (75%) Little ☐ (25%) None ☐ (0%) Not applicable ☐	<u>Fluids</u> Time:_____ All ☐ (100%) Half ☐ (50%) Most ☐ (75%) Little ☐ (25%) None ☐ (0 %) Not applicable ☐	<u>Enteral Feeds</u> Time:______ Formula: _____ Amount: _____ Flush: ________ Amount:_____
<u>Seizure Activity</u> Time Name ___ ____________ ___ ____________ *School nurse <u>must</u> report to neighborhood nurse ASAP.	Part(s) of body affected: ____________ Duration of activity: ______ minutes Color Change: Cyanotic ☐ Pale ☐ Difficulty Breathing: Yes ☐ No ☐ Incontinent: Yes ☐ No ☐ Loss of consciousness: Yes ☐ No ☐ School Nurse Notified: Yes ☐ No ☐ Time: ________		

Comments/Other: (Explain Below) Time___ Signature:__________	Any Occurrences: Yes ☐ No ☐ If yes was the occurrence form submitted: Yes ☐ No ☐
Detachable Devices Did the child use a Passy Muir valve? Yes ☐ No ☐ If yes, what is the approximate duration of use: ________________. Orthotics: Does child wear orthotics during school? Yes ☐ No ☐ If yes, please check all that apply: Upper extremity ☐ Lower extremity ☐ Thoracic Lumbar Ssacral Orthosis ☐ Other ____________________	

should return to school. A completed plan of action would close the loop of communication by informing school staff of the HCP's assessment and decision.

Visitor Policies

Visitor policies are another component of providing IPC in pLTCFs. Family, friends, and other visitors can introduce pathogens that are currently circulating in the community. In addition to providing IPC education (e.g., appropriate hand hygiene), pLTCFs may want to consider screening visitors at the entrance to the facility for symptoms of infection, particularly during respiratory viral season. Additional strategies to consider during an outbreak or during respiratory viral season include implementation of a center-wide age-restricted visitor policy (i.e., no visitors under the age of 13 years) and limiting the number of visitors at the bedside. An example of a proposed screening form is included as Handout 12.4. It is important to note that this type of screening tool would ideally be used to educate visitors on appropriate actions to mitigate the spread of disease, such as wearing a mask throughout the visit.

Approach to the Clinical Scenario

PLTCFs are part of the continuum of care that links community, acute care facilities, and post-acute facilities with the management of medically complex pediatric patients. Organisms typically associated with acute care facilities such as MDROs are a concern for all of these facilities, but post–acute care facilities must balance the medical, social,

HANDOUT 12.3 Example of Illness Evaluation Form for Resident at Pediatric Long-Term Care Facility

Illness Evaluation Form

Child's name ______________________________

Unit ______________ Date ______________ Time ______________

School Nursing Evaluation *(to be completed by school nurse)*

(Check all that apply)

☐ Fever, ______ °F
☐ Irritability
☐ Vomit, x______
  ☐ Blood
☐ Increased stooling
  ☐ Loose BM, x_______
  ☐ Diarrhea, x_______

☐ Fatigue
☐ Increased congestion
☐ Skin/wound draining
☐ Erythema
☐ Seizure
☐ Change secretions
☐ Green/yellow
☐ Odor change

Other ______________________________

Physician Evaluation *(to be completed by physician)*

(Check all that apply)

☐ Fever, ______ °F
☐ Irritability
☐ Vomit, x______
  ☐ Blood
☐ Increased stooling
  ☐ Loose BM, x_______
  ☐ Diarrhea, x_______

☐ Fatigue
☐ Increased congestion
☐ Skin/wound draining
☐ Erythema
☐ Seizure
☐ Change secretions
☐ Green/yellow
☐ Odor change

Comments: ______________________________

Plan of Action

☐ Return to school
☐ Stay at home (monitored for further symptoms in residence)

HANDOUT 12.4 Example of a Proposed Screening Form

Date: ________________________________

In the last 24 hours, have you had any of the following symptoms? ☐ Yes ☐ No

If yes, please check below:

☐ "Cold" symptoms	☐ Nasal congestion
☐ Body aches	☐ Nausea
☐ Fever	☐ Vomiting
☐ Cough	☐ Diarrhea
☐ Sore throat	☐ Severe headache
☐ Stomach pain	☐ Muscle pain/weakness
☐ Unexplained bruising/bleeding	☐ Other, specify: ____________________

Have you had your seasonal flu shot? Yes ☐ No ☐

Visitor's Name: ________________________________

Resident's initials and location: ________________________________

Number of Adults: ________________________

Number of Children: ________________________

and therapeutic care of their residents with the need for infection control and prevention, as these policies may have unintended medical and behavioral consequences due to the use of isolation measures. MDROs of concern are MRSA, vancomycin-resistant enterococci (VRE), and drug-resistant Gram-negative organisms such as *Pseudomonas aeruginosa*, *Acinetobacter* spp., and extended spectrum beta-lactamase (ESBL) producing Enterobacteriaceae. Residents of the pLTCFs may be either colonized or infected with these organisms, and making this distinction is often very difficult for HCPs.

Using the acute care IPC guidelines may provide a framework for IPC policies in pLTCFs, but acute care guidelines are not always easily implemented in pLTCFs. For example, patients with a known history of infection or colonization with an MDRO, such as the child described in the clinical scenario, would be placed in contact isolation in an acute care facility. However, pLTCFs provide a homelike atmosphere where the availability of single rooms is often limited; therefore isolation for MDROs for residents with known history of infection or colonization is not possible or recommended. In addition, a policy of cohorting residents with similar colonization may be difficult for pLTCFs, as residents are placed in "bedrooms," and movement around the facility is considered detrimental to the residents' well-being. Current Healthcare Infection Control Practices Advisory Committee (HICPAC) guidelines for long-term care provide flexibility with regard to decisions about placement of residents with infections or colonization with MDROs and allow for decisions to be made on a case-by-case basis balancing need for isolation, risk of infection transmission to residents, and the benefit or risk in terms of behavioral impact to the child.[25]

Potential approaches to minimize infection transmission of MDROs include: prescreening admissions, universal gloving, "modified" protocols such as wearing gloves for the care of those colonized with MRSA, single rooms, cohorting infected residents, and antibiotic stewardship to decrease the further development of resistant organisms. It is uncommon to refuse admission to a facility for patients colonized with MDROs, but some facilities may refuse admission due to lack of single rooms.[30] Likewise, restricting activities for those with MRSA is uncommon, although some centers advocate decolonization procedures for residents with recurrent and chronic MRSA infections.[31] In general, IPC for pLTCFs should focus on reducing the spread of MDROs by identifying residents with MDROs, communicating MDRO status to institutions where residents are being transferred, and assessing compliance with appropriate isolation precautions and hand hygiene.[32]

Many of the adult long-term care policies for IPC can be applicable to pLTCFs, but they need to be adapted to balance the desire for socialization and childhood development. The desire to maintain normal development and socialization during play and school often result in modifications to IPC policies. Notably, children do not maintain three feet of distance between them during play. As with adult long-term care patients, pediatric patients are often colonized with MDROs, but unlike the plentiful adult long-term care literature, little is known about the impact on morbidity and mortality of MDROs in children in pLTCFs. In the adult literature, MDRO colonization significantly increased the risk for MDRO infections.[33] However, recent studies do not show an increase in one-year mortality of those colonized with MDROs.[34] The nursing director in the clinical scenario and other HCPs in pLTCFs should be aware of available adult long-term care policies and procedures, but they must be aware that all of the suggested policies may not be applicable to pediatric settings.

In summary, monitoring, communicating, education (within the facility and with acute care centers), environmental cleaning, and antimicrobial stewardship all play a role in IPC in pLTCFs. The length of stay for patients in pLTCFs and the need to balance precautions with their impact on socialization and development make determining IPC strategies for pLTCFs an ever-evolving process that requires flexibility and patience. Use of adult long-term care guidelines is recommended, but these policies must be adapted to the pediatric setting.

Unresolved Issues

PLTCFs are an ever-growing setting for pediatric health care. These facilities are linked to acute care organizations as well as to the community; thus considerations of issues in acute care, such as MDROs and viral infection outbreaks, are critical for development of policies for IPC in pediatric long-term care. Due to the paucity of research in this unique population, there are several unresolved issues regarding IPC in pediatric long-term care. First is the lack of case definitions for HAIs specifically designed for pediatric long-term care. Second, guidelines are needed to help distinguish between colonization and infection with MDROs and other organisms. Helping HCPs make this distinction may impact antimicrobial use and thus aid with antimicrobial stewardship and infection control policies. More research is needed to understand the prevalence and transmission rates of viral infections and MDROs in pLTCF. Finally, studies are needed to determine the impact of MDROs on the morbidity and mortality in pLTCFs.

Developing best practices with regard to IPC in pLTCFs, setting standards for communication of IPC between acute care and long-term care facilities, and measuring the impact of isolation and precautions on transmission of infections in pLTCFs will provide measurable data to help evaluate our current policies and practices.

References

1. Harris J. Infection control in pediatric extended care facilities. *Infect Control Hosp Epidemiol.* 2006;27:598–603.
2. Murray MT, Cohen B, Neu N, et al. Infection prevention and control practices in pediatric long-term care facilities. *Am J Infect Control.* 2014;42:1233–1234.
3. Murray MT, Pavia M, Jackson O, et al. Health care–associated infection outbreaks in pediatric long-term care facilities. *Am J Infect Control.* 2015;43:756–758.
4. Lidsky K, Hoyen C, Salvator A, Rice LB, Toltzis P. Antibiotic-resistant gram negative organisms in pediatric chronic-care facilities. *Clin Infect Dis.* 2002;34:760–766.

5. U.S. Department of Health and Human Services, Health Resources and Services Administration, Maternal and Child Health Bureau. *The national survey of children with special health care needs chartbook 2009–2010*. Rockville, MD: U.S. Department of Health and Human Services; 2013.
6. Pediatric Complex Care Association. A white paper prepared for Centers for Medicare and Medicaid Services: Children and young adults with medical complexity: serving an emerging population. January 2016. Retrieved from http://pediatriccomplexcare.org/wp-content/uploads/2016/03/PCCA-CMSWhitePaper012716.pdf.
7. Cohen E, Kuo D, Agrawal R, et al. Children with medical complexity: an emerging population for clinical and research initiatives. *Pediatrics*. 2011;127(3):529–538.
8. Murray MT, Neu N, Cohen B, et al. Developing case definitions for health care-associated infections for pediatric long-term care facilities. *Clin Pediatrics*. 2015;54(14):1380–1382.
9. Murray MT, Pavia M, Jackson O, et al. Health care-associated infection outbreaks in pediatric long-term care facilities. *Am J Infect Control*. 2015;43:756–748.
10. Van Buul LW, van der Steen JT, Veenhuizen RB, et al. Antibiotic use and resistance in long term care facilities. *J Am Med Dir Assoc*. 2012;13:568.e1–568.e13.
11. Larson E, Cohen B, Murray M, Saiman L. Challenges in conducting research in pediatric long-term care facilities. *Clin Pediatrics*. 2014;53(11):1041–1046.
12. Centers for Disease Control and Prevention (CDC). Severe influenza among children and young adults with neurologic and neurodevelopmental conditions—Ohio, 2011. *MMWR*. 2012;60:1729–1733.
13. Schweon SJ, Kirk J. A realistic approach towards hand hygiene for long-term care residents and health care personnel. *Am J Infect Control*. 2011;39:336–338.
14. Cohen B, Hyman S, Rosenberg L, Larson E. Frequency of patient contact with health care personnel and visitors: implications for infection prevention. *Jt Comm J Qual Patient Saf*. 2012;38:560–565.
15. Neu N, Plaskett T, Hutcheon G, et al. Epidemiology of human metapneumovirus in a pediatric long-term care facility. *Infect Control Hosp Epidemiol*. 2012;33(6):545–550.
16. Kopel E, Amitai Z, Grotto I, et al. Recurrent outbreak of pandemic (H1N1) 2009 virus infection in a pediatric long-term care facility and the adjacent school. *Clin Infect Dis*. 2010;51(4):481–482.
17. James L, Vernon M, Jones R, et al. Outbreak of human adenovirus type 3 infection in a pediatric long-term care facility—Illinois, 2005. *Clin Infect Dis*. 2007;45(4):416–420.
18. Viau RA, Hujer AM, Marshall SH, et al. "Silent" dissemination of *Klebsiella pneumoniae* isolates bearing *K. pneumoniae* carbapenemase in a long-term care facility for children and young adults in northeast Ohio. *Clin Infect Dis*. 2012;54:1314–1321.
19. Perez F, Endimiani A, Ray AJ, et al. Carbapenem-resistant *Acinetobacter baumannii* and *Klebsiella pneumoniae* across a hospital system: impact of post-acute care facilities on dissemination. *J Antimicrob Chemother*. 2010;65(8):1807–1818.
20. Murray M, Heitkemper E, Jackson O, et al. Direct costs of acute respiratory infections in a pediatric long-term care facility. *Influenza Other Respir Viruses*. 2016;10(1):34–36.

21. Loyland B, Wilmont S, Hessels A, Larson E. Staff knowledge, awareness, perceptions and beliefs about infection prevention in pediatric long-term care facilities. *Nurs Res.* 2016;65:132–141.
22. Carter E, Cohen B, Murray M, Saiman L, Larson E. Using workflow diagrams to address hand hygiene in pediatric long-term care facilities. *J Pediatr Nurs.* 2015;36 (4):e17–e21.
23. Sax H, Allegranzi B, Uckay I, Larson E, Boyce J, Pittet D. "My five moments for hand hygiene": a user-centered design approach to understand, train, monitor and report hand hygiene. *J Hosp Infect.* 2007;67:9–21.
24. Loyland B, Wilmont S, Cohen B, Larson E. Hand-hygiene practices and observed barriers in pediatric long-term care facilities in the New York metropolitan area. *Int J Qual Health Care.* 2016;28:74–80.
25. Siegel JD, Rhinehart E, Jackson M, Chiarello L, Healthcare Infection Control Practices Advisory Committee. 2007. Guideline for isolation precautions: preventing transmission of infectious agents in healthcare settings. Available at: http://www.cdc.gov/ncidod/dhqp/pdf/isolation2007.pdf.
26. Smith P, Bennett G, Bradley S, et al. July 2008 SHEA/APIC Guideline: Infection prevention and control in the long-term care facility. *Am J Infect Control.* 2008;36:504–535.
27. Rogers BB, Shankar P, Jerris R, et al. Impact of rapid respiratory panel test on patient outcomes. *Arch Pathol Lab Med.* 2015. 139;5:636–641.
28. McGrath E, Thomas R, Asmar B, et al. Detection of respiratory co-infections in pediatric patients using a small volume polymerase chain reaction array respiratory panel: more evidence for contact droplet and contact isolation. *Am J Infect Control.* 2013;41;10:868–873.
29. Mahony J, Petrich A, Smieja M. Molecular diagnosis of respiratory virus infections. *Crit Rev Clin Lab Sci.* 2011;48:217–249.
30. Ye Z, Mukamel D, Huan S, Li Y, Temkin-Greener H. Healthcare-associated pathogens and nursing home policies and practices: results from a national survey. *Infect Control Hosp Epidemiol.* 2015;36(7):759–766.
31. Aureden K, Burdsall D, Harris M, Rosenbaum P. Guide to the elimination of methicillin-resistant *Staphylococcus aureus* (MRSA) in the long-term care facility. Washington, DC: Associations for Professionals in Infection Control and Epidemiology; 2009. Accessed June 12, 2014, at http://www.apic.org/Resource_/EliminationGuideForm/08b12595-9f92-4a64-ad41-4afdd0088224/File/APIC-MRSA-in-Long-Term-Care.pdf.
32. Kahvecioglu D, Ramiah K, McMaughan D, et al. Multidrug-resistant organism infections in US nursing homes: a national study of prevalence, onset and transmission across care settings, October 1, 2010–December 31, 2011. *Infect Control Hosp Epidemiol.* 2014;35(Suppl 3):S48–S55.
33. Cassone M, Mody Lona. Colonization with multi-drug resistant organisms in nursing homes: scope, importance and management. *Curr Geriatr Rep.* 2015;4(1):87–95.
34. Schoevaerdts D, Agelas JP, Ingels MG, et al. Health outcomes of older patients colonized by multi-drug resistant bacteria (MDRB): a one-year follow-up study. *Arch Gerontol Geriatr.* 2013;56:231–236.

13 | Antimicrobial Stewardship in Pediatrics

EMILY A. THORELL AND JARED OLSON

Background

The rapid emergence of multidrug-resistant bacteria has become a global public health crisis. As a response to this threat, President Obama issued an executive order on September 18, 2014, entitled "Combating Antibiotic Resistant Bacteria."[1] Shortly thereafter, the U.S. Department of Health and Human Services (HHS) announced the Presidential Advisory Council on Combating Antibiotic-Resistant Bacteria in 2015.[2] One effective strategy used to decrease the emergence of multi-drug-resistant organisms (MDROs) is the antimicrobial stewardship program (ASP): a coordinated healthcare program that seeks to provide optimal antimicrobial treatment to patients to reduce the emergence of MDROs, improve patient outcomes, and decrease cost. The Centers for Medicare and Medicaid Services, in response to the Executive Order, issued "Conditions of Participation" for hospitals to develop programs in accordance with the Centers for Disease Control and Prevention (CDC) recommendations, effective January 1, 2017. The Joint Commission followed suit and announced a new Medication Management standard beginning in 2017.

As antibiotics are the only class of medications where use in one patient can compromise their efficacy in another patient, stewardship is critical to preserving this shared resource. The CDC has focused on improving antimicrobial use for many years. The launch of the "Get Smart for Healthcare" campaign in 2003 had a major objective of reducing antimicrobial use in the community through education of clinicians about their own prescribing habits. The educational materials included treatment guidelines for upper respiratory infections, tools to aid clinicians in addressing patient concerns, educational videos, and the viral prescription pad. In 2006, the CDC released a guideline, "Management of Multi-Drug Resistant Organisms in Healthcare Settings," and brought attention to the necessity of judicious antimicrobial use with these efforts.[3] In 2007, the Infectious Diseases Society of America (IDSA) and the Society for Healthcare Epidemiology of America (SHEA) released guidelines for developing an institutional program to enhance antimicrobial stewardship.[4] Also endorsed by the Pediatric Infectious Diseases Society (PIDS) and the American Academy of Pediatrics (AAP), these guidelines provided an initial framework of basic elements for an antimicrobial stewardship program. In 2009, the CDC and the Institute for Healthcare Improvement (IHI) launched the "Get Smart for Healthcare" campaign to provide a roadmap to aid programs in prioritizing, implementing, and measuring changes in acute care facilities. They developed a conceptual model of key drivers to reduce inappropriate antimicrobial use.[5] This package provides a tool kit of resources to help physicians tailor ASPs to the needs of their own hospitals. In 2012, "A Policy Statement on Antimicrobial Stewardship"[6] was released by SHEA, IDSA, and PIDS; this outlined recommendations for the mandatory implementation of ASP throughout healthcare. In 2014, the CDC recommended that all acute care hospitals implement ASPs in order to meet the urgent need to improve antibiotic use. They released the "Core Elements of Hospital Antibiotic Stewardship Programs" guidance[7] to help hospitals initiate and monitor their programs and summarize the core elements of successful hospital ASPs. IDSA, SHEA, and PIDS released further guidance in 2016 evaluating the wide range of interventions that can be implemented by ASPs.[8] All of these guidelines and campaigns together provide roadmaps for clinicians, administrators, pharmacists, and others interested in starting and maintaining an ASP. Institutional commitment to stewardship is also measured as a quality indicator in metrics used to rank U.S. children's hospitals.[9] ASPs ensure that patients receive the right antibiotic, at the right dose, at the right time, and for the right duration.

Clinical Scenario

A hospital pharmacist is concerned about the use of broad-spectrum antibiotics in the inpatient pediatric units of your hospital. She reports long courses of carbapenems for patients diagnosed with appendicitis and third generation cephalosporins for patients with community-acquired pneumonia. She also notes that clinicians do not "narrow" therapy when microbiological culture and susceptibility reports suggest many antibiotic options.

Questions

What are the most important elements of a successful inpatient ASP? What are important objective metrics to detect the positive impact of a successful ASP?

Key Challenges

Many studies demonstrate large variations in care for common pediatric conditions such as pneumonia, skin and soft tissue infections, appendicitis, and febrile infants,[10–13] even in the setting of national guidelines. Pediatric expertise is critical for both clinicians and pharmacists who are implementing ASPs. This expertise may not be readily available in many settings. Recent regulatory measures do not address the specific needs of the pediatric population, and institutional ASPs in adult facilities may focus their efforts on adult-specific projects. In institutions without pediatric-specific ASPs, clinicians with pediatric training may need to be trained in the principles of antimicrobial stewardship to optimize clinical outcomes of children.

Antibiotic Overuse in Children

Studies have shown that 30–50% of antibiotic use in hospitals is inappropriate.[7] In children, antimicrobials are among the most commonly prescribed drugs in both inpatient and outpatient settings. A recent study from the Pediatric Hospitals Information Systems database showed that variability in antibiotic exposure in hospitalized children ranged from 38% to 72%, despite normalizing the patients for case mix; and that 60% of hospitalized children received at least one course of antibiotics.[12]

Adverse Drug Events

Antibiotics are not benign. Antibiotic pressure selects for MDROs, which are a public health crisis. Unintended consequences of antimicrobials other than increasing MDROs include drug eruptions/allergy, neutropenia, and *Clostridioides difficile.* In children, early antibiotic use has also been associated with diseases such as obesity, inflammatory bowel disease, and juvenile idiopathic arthritis.[14–16] Antibiotics are the most common cause of emergency department visits for adverse drug events in children less than 18 years of age.[17]

Special Populations: Neonatal Intensive Care and Immunocompromised Hosts

Special populations within pediatrics are important targets for ASPs, although tailored approaches may be required.

Neonatal Intensive Care Units (NICU)

NICUs provide unique challenges to ASPs, as a high proportion of infants receive antibiotics at any given time.[18] Antibiotic use has been associated with development of MDROs[19] and invasive candidiasis.[20] In these fragile patients, antibiotic use is prevalent as the signs and symptoms of sepsis in neonates and infants are non-specific and can mimic other common conditions. Adequate volumes of blood for cultures may not be feasible given the small size of the patients, which leads clinicians to doubt the validity of blood culture results due to concern for poor sampling. Distinguishing between colonization and infection is difficult, given that common commensals such as coagulase-negative staphylococci may cause disease in this population.[21] Although challenges exist, opportunities to optimize antimicrobial use are present in the NICU. One study examined antimicrobial use in 127 NICUs across California in 2013 and found a 40-fold variation in antibiotic prescribing practices in all the NICUs, despite similar burdens of proven infection, necrotizing enterocolitis, surgical volume, and mortality.[22] In addition to wide variability in NICU antimicrobial use, mounting evidence suggests that inappropriate antibiotic use leads to worse outcomes; each empiric antimicrobial treatment day increases the odds of necrotizing enterocolitis and death for extremely low birthweight infants.[23] The principles of antimicrobial stewardship apply to NICUs despite the lack of clear treatment guidelines for many conditions.[8]

Immunocompromised Host

Antimicrobial stewardship efforts in the immunocompromised host can be one of the more difficult endeavors; however, targeted ASPs remain important as the risk of MDROs is high in this population. Antifungal use is high, and concerns about fungal resistance are growing. The CDC listed fluconazole-resistant *Candida* species among the pathogens posing a serious threat to human health. Prior exposure to both fluconazole and echinocandins has been associated with reduced susceptibility to these agents,[24] as has subtherapeutic dosing of fluconazole.[25]

A recent survey of pediatric ASP practitioners summarized goals and barriers to ASP interventions specifically in the immunocompromised population.[26] Similar to other populations, the most common goal of ASPs was to reduce the time to antimicrobial de-escalation. The most important barrier identified by the ASP practitioner was the perception that oncology clinicians are more motivated by fear of rare adverse outcomes than long-term risks of antimicrobial use.

Suggested Approaches

There are many tools available to help initiate an antimicrobial stewardship program. The following approach is based on the Summary of Core Elements of Hospital Antibiotic Stewardship Programs from the CDC.[7] All bulleted lists that follow are taken directly from this document and can be accessed on the CDC website (www.cdc.gov/getsmart/healthcare/implementation/core-elements.html). The associated checklist (Handout 13.1) can be used to systematically assess these core elements and actions to ensure optimization of the antimicrobial prescribing practices in hospitals. It can be useful for both those beginning a program and those evaluating interventions. Each topic will be covered in this chapter, with a pediatric perspective.

Summary of Core Elements of Hospital Antibiotic Stewardship Programs

The following are the core elements of hospital ASPs, which will each be discussed in more detail later in this chapter.

- *Leadership Commitment:* Dedicating necessary human, financial, and information technology resources.
- *Accountability:* Appointing a single leader responsible for program outcomes. Experience with successful programs shows that a physician leader is effective.[4]
- *Drug Expertise:* Appointing a single pharmacist leader responsible for working to improve antibiotic use.

HANDOUT 13.1 Checklist for Core Elements of Hospital Antibiotic Stewardship Programs

Checklist for Core Elements of Hospital Antibiotic Stewardship Programs

The following checklist is a companion to *Core Elements of Hospital Antibiotic Stewardship Programs.* This checklist should be used to systematically assess key elements and actions to ensure optimal antibiotic prescribing and limit overuse and misuse of antibiotics in hospitals. CDC recommends that all hospitals implement an Antibiotic Stewardship Program.

Facilities using this checklist should involve one or more knowledgeable staff to determine if the following principles and actions to improve antibiotic use are in place. The elements in this checklist have been shown in previous studies to be helpful in improving antibiotic use, though not all of the elements might be feasible in all hospitals.

LEADERSHIP SUPPORT		ESTABLISHED AT FACILITY	
A.	Does your facility have a formal, written statement of support from leadership that supports efforts to improve antibiotic use (antibiotic stewardship)?	☐Yes	☐No
B.	Does your facility receive any budgeted financial support for antibiotic stewardship activities (e.g., support for salary, training, or IT support)?	☐Yes	☐No

ACCOUNTABILITY			
A.	Is there a physician leader responsible for program outcomes of stewardship activities at your facility?	☐Yes	☐No

DRUG EXPERTISE			
A.	Is there a pharmacist leader responsible for working to improve antibiotic use at your facility?	☐Yes	☐No

KEY SUPPORT FOR THE ANTIBIOTIC STEWARDSHIP PROGRAM ***Does any of the staff below work with the stewardship leaders to improve antibiotic use?***			
B.	Clinicians	☐Yes	☐No
C.	Infection Prevention and Healthcare Epidemiology	☐Yes	☐No
D.	Quality Improvement	☐Yes	☐No
E.	Microbiology (Laboratory)	☐Yes	☐No
F.	Information Technology (IT)	☐Yes	☐No
G.	Nursing	☐Yes	☐No

ACTIONS TO SUPPORT OPTIMAL ANTIBIOTIC USE			
POLICIES		**POLICY ESTABLISHED**	
A.	Does your facility have a policy that requires prescribers to document in the medical record or during order entry a dose, duration, and indication for all antibiotic prescriptions?	☐Yes	☐No
B.	Does your facility have facility-specific treatment recommendations, based on national guidelines and local susceptibility, to assist with antibiotic selection for common clinical conditions?	☐Yes	☐No

SPECIFIC INTERVENTIONS TO IMPROVE ANTIBIOTIC USE *Are the following actions to improve antibiotic prescribing conducted in your facility?*			
BROAD INTERVENTIONS		**ACTION PERFORMED**	
C.	Is there a formal procedure for all clinicians to review the appropriateness of all antibiotics 48 hours after the initial orders (e.g., antibiotic timeout)?	☐Yes	☐No
D.	Do specified antibiotic agents need to be approved by a physician or pharmacist prior to dispensing (i.e., pre-authorization) at your facility?	☐Yes	☐No
E.	Does a physician or pharmacist review courses of therapy for specified antibiotic agents (i.e., prospective audit with feedback) at your facility?	☐Yes	☐No

PHARMACY-DRIVEN INTERVENTIONS *Are the following actions implemented in your facility?*		ACTION PERFORMED	
F.	Automatic changes from intravenous to oral antibiotic therapy in appropriate situations?	☐Yes	☐No
G.	Dose adjustments in cases of organ dysfunction?	☐Yes	☐No
H.	Dose optimization (pharmacokinetics/ pharmacodynamics) to optimize the treatment of organisms with reduced susceptibility?	☐Yes	☐No
I.	Automatic alerts in situations where therapy might be unnecessarily duplicative?	☐Yes	☐No
J.	Time-sensitive automatic stop orders for specified antibiotic prescriptions?	☐Yes	☐No

DIAGNOSIS AND INFECTION-SPECIFIC INTERVENTIONS ***Does your facility have specific interventions in place to ensure optimal use of antibiotics to treat the following common infections?***		**ACTION PERFORMED**	
K.	Community-acquired pneumonia	☐Yes	☐No
L.	Urinary tract infection	☐Yes	☐No
M.	Skin and soft tissue infections	☐Yes	☐No
N.	Surgical prophylaxis	☐Yes	☐No
O.	Empiric treatment of methicillin-resistant *Staphylococcus aureus* (MRSA)	☐Yes	☐No
P.	Non-*C. difficile* infection (CDI) antibiotics in new cases of CDI	☐Yes	☐No
Q.	Culture-proven invasive (e.g., bloodstream) infections	☐Yes	☐No

PROCESS MEASURES		**MEASURE PERFORMED**	
A.	Does your stewardship program monitor adherence to a documentation policy (dose, duration, and indication)?	☐Yes	☐No
B.	Does your stewardship program monitor adherence to facility-specific treatment recommendations?	☐Yes	☐No
C.	Does your stewardship program monitor compliance with one of more of the specific interventions in place?	☐Yes	☐No

ANTIBIOTIC USE AND OUTCOME MEASURES		**MEASURE PERFORMED**	
D.	Does your facility track rates of *C. difficile* infection?	☐Yes	☐No
E.	Does your facility produce an antibiogram (cumulative antibiotic susceptibility report)?	☐Yes	☐No

Does your facility monitor antibiotic use (consumption) at the unit and/or facility-wide level by one of the following metrics:		**MEASURE PERFORMED**	
F.	By counts of antibiotic(s) administered to patients per day (Days of Therapy; DOT)?	☐Yes	☐No
G.	By number of grams of antibiotics used (Defined Daily Dose, DDD)?	☐Yes	☐o
H.	By direct expenditure for antibiotics (purchasing costs)?	☐Yes	☐No

Reporting Information to Staff on Improving Antibiotic Use and Resistance			
A.	Does your stewardship program share facility-specific reports on antibiotic use with prescribers?	☐Yes	☐No
B.	Has a current antibiogram been distributed to prescribers at your facility?	☐Yes	☐No
C.	Do prescribers ever receive direct, personalized communication about how they can improve their antibiotic prescribing?	☐Yes	☐No

Education			
A.	Does your stewardship program provide education to clinicians and other relevant staff on improving antibiotic prescribing?	☐Yes	☐No

- *Action:* Implementing at least one recommended action, such as systemic evaluation of ongoing treatment need after a set period of initial treatment (e.g., "antibiotic time out" after 48 hours).
- *Tracking:* Monitoring antibiotic prescribing and resistance patterns.
- *Reporting:* Regular reporting information on antibiotic use and resistance to doctors, nurses, and relevant staff.
- *Education:* Educating clinicians about resistance and optimal prescribing.

Leadership Commitment

Clear support from hospital leadership is necessary for the success of any ASP, as dedication of human, financial, and information technology resources is critical for success. This can take many forms, including:

- Formal statements that the facility supports efforts to improve and monitor antibiotic use
- Stewardship-related duties incorporated in job descriptions and annual performance reviews

- Ensuring staff from relevant departments are given sufficient time to contribute to stewardship activities
- Supporting training and education
- Ensuring participation from the many groups that can support stewardship activities

As regulatory mechanisms and quality measures are now in force to require stewardship programs, the commitment to ASPs should be in place. In 2014, 38 of 42 children's hospitals that are members of the Children's Hospital Association responded to a survey about their stewardship practices.[27] At that time, 38% had formal programs, and 36% were in the process of implementation. The median number of total full-time equivalents (FTE) was 0.63 (range 0.1–1.8) per program. Physician FTE had a median of 0.25 (range 0.1–0.5), and pharmacist median FTE was 0.5 (range 0.1–1.5). Only one program had data analyst support at that time, which was a surprising finding, given the critical nature of data to an ASP. In a separate study, the hospitals with dedicated stewardship programs had a larger decline in overall antibiotic use after the release of the 2007 IDSA guideline than those without ASPs.[28]

ASPs can pay for themselves through savings both in antimicrobial expenditures and in indirect costs such as administration fees and nursing time. Programs have been shown to save up to $2 million per year in some adult studies.[29] Financial support will also increase the capacity and potential impact of the program. Antimicrobials accounted for 17% of the pharmacy budget across 36 freestanding children's hospitals, with a few specific drugs accounting for a large proportion of the cost.[30] After an initial period of cost savings, eventually, cost decreases stabilize. ASPs need continued support as these programs mature, as improvements made quickly dissipate after support is withdrawn.[31]

Information technology resources are key to supporting the tracking and reporting of antibiotic use and other ASP outcomes. While some ASPs have dedicated data analysts, others receive support from hospital quality or infection prevention for data management.

Accountability and Drug Expertise

- *Stewardship Program Leader:* Identify a single leader who will be responsible for program outcomes. Physicians have been highly effective in this role.

- *Pharmacy Leader:* Identify a single pharmacy leader who will co-lead the program.

When possible, having both a physician and pharmacist is preferred. Additionally, representation from microbiology, information technology/data analysis, infection prevention, quality and patient safety, and hospital leadership should be included. Large facilities generally have full-time staff to manage their ASPs; however, smaller facilities have reported arrangements such as off-site expertise, part-time staff, physicians with interest in the topic that are not specifically infectious disease–trained. Hospitalists have become integral to ASPs, given their increasing popularity in inpatient medicine,[32,33] and pediatric hospitalists may be a natural fit to lead ASPs in facilities without pediatric infectious disease physician support. Special populations such as NICU, surgical, or immunocompromised patients may need specific ASP interventions. Sometimes these clinicians need assurance that the ASP team understands the unique problems associated with these patients. Identifying local champions with an interest in stewardship can be the key to success. These champions can be anyone on the care delivery team, including physicians, advanced practice practitioners, nurses, or pharmacists.

Other Key Support

- *Clinicians and Department Heads:* As the prescribers of antibiotics, it is vital that clinicians be fully engaged in and supportive of efforts to improve antibiotic use in hospitals.
- *Infection Preventionists and Hospital Epidemiologists*: These partners can readily bring their skills to auditing, analyzing, and reporting data. They can also assist with monitoring and reporting of resistance and *Clostridioides difficile* infection (CDI) trends, educating staff on the importance of appropriate antibiotic use, and implementing strategies to optimize the use of antibiotics.
- *Quality Improvement Staff:* Key partners, given that optimizing antibiotic use is a medical quality and patient safety issue.
- *Laboratory Staff:* Can guide the proper use of tests and the flow of results. They can also guide empiric therapy by creating and interpreting a facility cumulative antibiotic resistance report, known as an *antibiogram.* Lab and stewardship staff can work collaboratively to ensure that lab reports present data in a way that supports optimal antibiotic use. For facilities that have laboratory services

performed off-site, information provided should be useful to stewardship efforts, and contracts should be written to ensure this is the case.

- *Information Technology Staff*: These partners are critical to integrating stewardship protocols into existing workflow. Examples include embedding relevant information and protocols at the point of care (e.g., immediate access to facility-specific guidelines at point of prescribing), implementing clinical decision support for antibiotic use, creating prompts for action to review antibiotics in key situations, and facilitating the collection and reporting of antibiotic use data.
- *Clinical Nurses:* Nurses can ensure that cultures are performed before starting antibiotics. In addition, nurses review medications as part of their routine duties and can prompt discussions of antibiotic treatment (especially readiness to change to oral therapy if indicated), indication, and duration.

Action

Implement Policies and Interventions to Improve Antibiotic Use

Key Points

- Implement policies that support optimal antibiotic use.
- Utilize specific interventions that can be divided into three categories: broad, pharmacy-driven, and infection/syndrome-specific.
- Avoid implementing too many policies and interventions simultaneously; always prioritize interventions based on the needs of the hospital as defined by measures of overall use and other tracking and reporting metrics.

Policies That Support Optimal Antibiotic Use

From an institutional perspective, policy management can have a great impact on local antimicrobial prescribing. Simple strategies such as requiring documentation of the duration and indication for all courses of antibiotics help pharmacists and nurses check the appropriateness of the antibiotic order and ensure timely discontinuation of antibiotics when appropriate. Other facility-specific policies such as evidence-based care process models or treatment algorithms[10,13,34] for common conditions can be useful by providing clinicians with suggested antimicrobial regimens that consider available evidence, local susceptibility patterns, formulary, and/or culture results. Computerized decision support through electronic medical records can support optimization of prescribing. Condition- or population-specific antibiograms can also be very useful in identifying ASP targets.

Interventions to Improve Antibiotic Use

Choosing where to start is often difficult, as ASP leaders often want to implement many projects at once. Careful consideration of the facility, the culture, the most imminent risks or low-hanging fruit, and the availability of resources should guide ASP interventions. Many programs will pilot an intervention in a specific population or unit prior to disseminating it to the entire facility to identify any concerns. This section will discuss how to identify interventions and then classify the types of interventions as broad, pharmacy-driven, and infection- or syndrome-specific.

Identifying Interventions The CDC/IHI Antibiotic Stewardship Driver Diagram (Figure 13.1) and Change Package (http://www.cdc.gov/getsmart/healthcare/implementation.html)[5] are great tools to understand various processes that can lead to optimal antibiotic use. The Driver Diagram visually identifies various processes that can lead to appropriate antimicrobial use. The broad categories are labeled as Primary and Secondary Drivers. The Change Package includes lists of specific interventions believed to "drive" improved antibiotic use within each driver category. The goal is not to implement all Change Package interventions at once, but to provide ASPs with a list of options to help institutions identify and select specific interventions to drive optimal antibiotic use. The Driver Diagram also includes a measurement framework, which encourages selection of key metrics that may be helpful in evaluating the effectiveness of the intervention.

Speaking with clinical staff is also helpful for identifying potential concerns and gathering suggestions to facilitate implementation of interventions (Handout 13.2). Measures are suggested for each of the primary drivers. Measures such as the percentage of patients with cultures obtained prior to the first dose of antibiotics, and the percentage of patients sampled with indication documented at point of care, are suggested to evaluate timely antibiotic management.

Let's look at a hypothetical example of an ASP using the Driver Diagram to enact change. The ASP is concerned that children with urinary tract infections (UTIs) in the Emergency Department (ED) are receiving inappropriate antibiotics. The team evaluates the Driver Diagram,

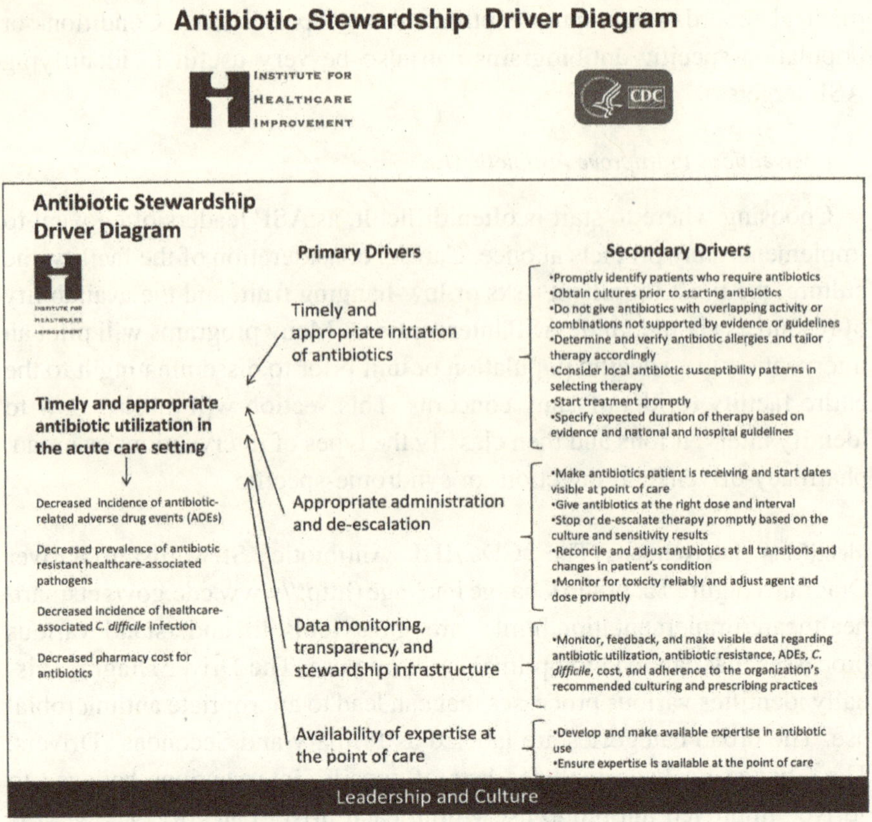

FIGURE 13.1 Institute for Healthcare Improvement Driver Diagram.

and identifies "Primary Driver 1: Timely and Appropriate Initiation of Antibiotics" as a target. The team reviews the secondary drivers to generate ideas for change. Amongst the secondary drivers, the team identifies two that they feel will lead to more appropriate initiation of antibiotics:

1. Obtain cultures prior to starting antibiotics.
2. Consider local susceptibility patterns in selecting therapy.

The team then reviews and selects interventions from the specific change ideas suggested for these secondary drivers. In this example, the team chooses to develop facility-specific guidance for diagnosing and treating community-acquired UTIs. The team uses the local susceptibilities of

Antibiotic Stewardship Measurement Framework

This document describes selected measures that could be used to measure the change concepts summarized in the Antibiotic Stewardship Drivers and Change Package. These measures are recommended, based on initial pilot testing across eight pilot testing hospitals (September 2011 – July 2012) and are not meant to reflect a complete set of measures. Because each concept can be measured in a variety of ways, those listed here are provided as a starting point to stimulate investigation. Each organization using these measures needs to provide further detail on specific operational definitions (numerator/ denominator) and data collection strategy. The availability of an electronic health record (EHR) and supporting software may be required for routine use of the process measures, although incorporating assessment into the process of care (rounding) has been demonstrated to be an effective approach. The utility of each measure for an organization will need to be assessed against the availability of data and the ease and frequency with which it can be collected.

Outcomes	Measure
Healthcare-associated *C. difficile* infections	• Rate of healthcare-associated *C. difficile* per 10,000 pt. days • When *C. diff* is a "rare event": days (or admissions) between *C. diff*-associated disease
Pharmacy cost for antibiotics	• Total pharmacy cost for antibiotics per month • When census is variable: Pharmacy cost for antibiotics per discharge per month
Antibiotic-related adverse drug events (ADEs)	Currently not feasible method
Antibiotic-resistant healthcare-associated pathogens	Percent of antibiotic-resistant healthcare-associated pathogens (prevalence) (Note: targeting pathogens based on local circumstances, i.e., MRSA, VRE, etc.)

Primary Driver	Measure
Timely antibiotic management	***Recommended measures, based on pilot testing:*** • Percentage of patients where cultures were obtained prior to first dose of antibiotics • Percentage of patients sampled where antibiotic start date was documented/visible at the point of care • Percentage of patients sampled where antibiotic stop date/duration was documented/visible at the point of care • Percentage of patients sampled where antibiotic indication was documented/visible at the point of care • **COMPOSITE MEASURE:** Percentage of patients sampled where antibiotic start date, stop date/duration, and indication were documented/visible at the point of care
Appropriate administration and de-escalation	
Data monitoring, transparency, and stewardship infrastructure	***Suggested measure for consideration:*** Percentage of clinicians responding positively to a survey on their receipt, or knowledge, of selected antibiotic information (e.g., antibiotic utilization, antibiotic resistance, *C. difficile* rate, cost associated with antibiotics, adherence to organization prescribing practices)
Availability of expertise at the point of care	***Suggested measures for consideration:*** • Percentage of providers who can state how to secure expertise on pharmacology and antimicrobial spectrum • Percentage of cases sampled where expertise was available at the point of care

urine cultures to select a preferred antimicrobial, and embeds this choice into the electronic health record order set. Measures such as the percentage of patients with cultures obtained prior to the first dose of antibiotics, the percentage of patients sampled with indication documented at point of care are recommended by the Measurement Framework. In order to determine if this specific intervention worked, the team identifies patients with urinalysis performed in the ED. They review the percentage diagnosed with UTI, the percentage receiving the recommended antibiotic regimen, and the percentage receiving urine culture prior to initiation of antibiotics, compared to their local facility-specific guidance.

Broad Interventions When resources are available, the core actions in any ASP are generally performed by the physician/pharmacist team when available and include one of three broad strategies.

Antibiotic "timeouts" are utilized to address the fact that clinicians often neglect to revisit an initial antibiotic prescription once it is ordered in hospitalized patients.[35] This is generally necessary when clinical and laboratory data become available to aid in decision-making for the patient. Timeouts should be performed at 48 hours after initiation of antibiotics, and should answer these four questions:

- Does this patient have an infection that will respond to antibiotics?
- If yes, is the patient on the right antibiotic(s), dose, and route of administration?
- Can a more targeted antibiotic be used to treat the infection (de-escalate)?
- How long should the patient receive the antibiotic(s)?

Prospective audit with feedback (PAF) is a strategy similar to the antibiotic timeout, with the exception that a physician or pharmacist with infectious diseases training, who is not on the clinical team, is reviewing the antibiotic use and provides direct interaction and feedback to the prescriber. Using PAF, the overall antibiotic use in one children's hospital decreased from 883 days of therapy (DOT)/1000 patient-days to 787 DOT/1000 patient-days, a decrease of 7%.[36] A greater impact was seen on the selected antimicrobials, with a decrease of 17% in DOT/1000 patient-days. Clinicians were compliant with agreed-upon ASP recommendations in 92% of patients. After incorporating antimicrobial-use indications as a mandatory field in the computerized order entry system and PAF, another hospital demonstrated that both targeted and non-targeted antimicrobial use declined by 21%.[37] Dose adjustment and modification of antibiotic therapy accounted for ~75% of those interactions

PAF requires access to expertise. Reviews are done after drug initiation; therefore the reviews can take place when that expertise is available. Some programs will have PAF available seven days a week, while others may review patients less often or on a case-by-case basis. Reviews can also be done remotely if pediatric expertise is not locally available.

Prior authorization (PA) is restriction of certain or all antimicrobials based on their spectrum of activity, toxicity profile, drug formulary, or cost. PA ensures the expert review of an antibiotic prior to initiation. As authorization is obtained prior to the dispensing of the drug, availability of ASP-trained team members is key. In pediatrics, this strategy has been shown to be effective, both in an internet-based restriction and approval program that was also linked to decision support, and in a PA program staffed by both pharmacists and pediatric infectious diseases fellows.[38,39]

Pharmacy-Driven Interventions There are several interventions that can be led by ASP or other hospital pharmacists that can impact overall antibiotic use. The CDC highlights the following:

- *Automatic changes from intravenous to oral antibiotic therapy* in appropriate situations and for antibiotics with good absorption (e.g., clindamycin, fluconazole, fluoroquinolones, trimethoprim-sulfamethoxazole, metronidazole, etc.), which improves patient safety by reducing the need for intravenous access.
- *Dose adjustments* in cases of organ dysfunction (e.g., renal adjustment).
- *Dose optimization,* including dose adjustments based on therapeutic drug monitoring, optimizing therapy for highly drug-resistant bacteria, achieving central nervous system penetration, extended-infusion administration of beta-lactams, etc.
- *Automatic alerts in situations where therapy might be unnecessarily duplicative,* including simultaneous use of multiple agents with overlapping spectra such as anaerobic activity, Gram-negative activity, and resistant Gram-positive activity.
- *Time-sensitive automatic stop orders* for specified antibiotic prescriptions, especially antibiotics administered for surgical prophylaxis.
- *Detection and prevention of antibiotic-related drug–drug interactions*—e.g., interactions between orally administered fluoroquinolone and certain vitamins or enteral feeds.

Additionally, collaborative practice agreements—which are formal agreements in which a licensed clinician makes a diagnosis, supervises patient care, and refers patients to a pharmacist for drug dosage adjustment and monitoring that allows the pharmacist to perform specific patient care functions[40]—may be useful in certain circumstances involving antibiotics with a need for therapeutic drug monitoring, such as vancomycin. Laws regarding collaborative practice agreements differ between states, so this should be considered.

Infection- and Syndrome-Specific Interventions Condition-specific guidance on common problems is another way to influence local antibiotic prescribing. Many programs issue guidance in the form of evidence-based care processes, guidelines, treatment algorithms, or computer decision support. A study looking at targets for stewardship in pediatrics showed that four clinical conditions accounted for 10% of the DOT, but only 1% of admitting diagnoses.[41] These included pneumonia, appendicitis, cystic fibrosis, and skin and soft tissue infections. Other common conditions or syndromes in pediatrics that are good targets (although this is in no way a comprehensive list) include: urinary tract infections, empiric methicillin-resistant *Staphylococcus aureus* (MRSA) coverage, CDIs, bloodstream infections, and febrile infants. NICU conditions such as early- and late-onset sepsis and necrotizing enterocolitis (NEC) may also be useful targets. The pediatric literature supports use of guidelines to improve antibiotic use. After implementation of a care process model for febrile infants, Intermountain Healthcare, an integrated healthcare system, improved both antibiotic selection and duration, while concomitantly improving identification and treatment of infants with known serious bacterial infection (SBI), and decreasing antibiotic exposure and hospital stay in those without SBI in their target facilities.[10] Another pediatric study at three centers showed that after national guidelines for pediatric pneumonia were disseminated, narrow-spectrum antibiotic choice increased among hospitalized children, and those changes were boosted in institutions with proactive dissemination of this guideline.[42]

Pediatric surgical patients are an important population to include in ASP activities, as 80% of surgical patients admitted to children's hospitals receive antibiotics.[41] Surgical prophylaxis is a common target for ASPs. One pediatric study looking at compliance with published recommendations in appendicitis showed that 52% of patients with non-perforated appendicitis and 62% of perforated appendicitis cases received antibiotics longer than recommended,[43] which correlates with the preceding stewardship target. Other surgical targets relate to large variations identified among surgical patients at 37 children's hospitals.[11] Among the top 10 conditions, which accounted for more than 50% of all antibiotic use, the adjusted use of postoperative and perioperative vancomycin had high variation among craniotomy and cardiothoracic surgery patients. High variation in anti-*Pseudomonas* agents in gastrointestinal surgery patients was also noted.

Tracking and Reporting

Improving antimicrobial prescribing requires measurement.[44] Measurement aids in identification of potential opportunities for improvement and evaluates program impact.

The goal of ASPs is to optimize patient outcomes while minimizing unintended consequences of antimicrobial use by using the right drug, dose, route, and duration.[4] A survey of pharmacists and physicians sought to understand the most important metrics of those commonly collected by ASPs.[45] The two most commonly used metrics were antimicrobial cost and antibiotic use, despite fewer than 20% of respondents identifying these outcomes as one of the top two most important. Infectious disease (ID) physicians felt that infection-related mortality was the most important outcome, yet few respondents' programs tracked this metric (7%). This study highlights the need for ASPs to measure more outcomes focusing on quality of care and minimizing negative patient outcomes in addition to process measures such as antibiotic cost and antibiotic use.[46]

Ideally, ASPs should evaluate process measures to understand antimicrobial use patterns, outcome measures to determine whether interventions are improving patient care, and balancing measures to determine whether processes are leading to negative outcomes in other parts of the system.

Antibiotic Use Measures

Measures of antimicrobial use quantify the aggregate amount of drug used at the level of the patient, hospital, or hospital unit. Commonly these metrics are reported as a rate, with patient days as a denominator to adjust antimicrobial use for census.

Defined daily dose (DDD) is a measurement that was developed in the 1970s and is promoted by the World Health Organization (WHO). It is a typical daily dose of an antibiotic for therapeutic purposes in an adult patient. The IDSA and SHEA stewardship guidelines advocated for DDDs/1000 patient days as a metric for hospital-based stewardship. DDD estimates antibiotic use by summing the total grams administered or purchased of each antibiotic, divided by the WHO-assigned DDD. However, the use of DDDs is not appropriate for children. Since the WHO-DDD is determined using average adult daily doses, the calculated DDD is highly influenced by the average size of the patient, limiting its utility in children.

Days of therapy (DOT) are the sum of the total days of a particular antimicrobial divided by patient days or number of admissions. This overcomes the limitation of one dose per drug of DDDs and provides more clinically relevant data to pediatric facilities. The Pediatric Health Information System's antimicrobial stewardship report uses this metric per 1000 patient days to help participating pediatric hospitals benchmark antimicrobial use. The National Healthcare Safety Network (NHSN) has developed an Antibiotic Use (AU) Option that collects and reports monthly DOT data per 1000 days present and per 100 admissions. Analysis can be performed in aggregate by facility, by patient care location, and by specific agents.

The CDC has also developed the Standardized Antimicrobial Administration Ration (SAAR) to report antimicrobial use in standardized form. It is calculated by dividing the observed antimicrobial use by the predicted antimicrobial use. The predicted antimicrobial use is derived using models developed by the CDC from the nationally aggregated AU data. The SAAR is generated for the following categories of antimicrobials: broad-spectrum antibacterials for treatment of multidrug-resistant infections, broad-spectrum antibacterials for treatment of community-acquired infections, anti-MRSA antibacterials, antibacterials used for surgical prophylaxis, and all antibacterial agents. Currently, all SAARs are available for pediatric medical wards. SAARS are also available for pediatric ICUs and surgical wards for surgical site infection prophylaxis and all antibacterial agents. As more data are obtained, the CDC will calculate SAARs for additional patient locations. SAARs above 1 that achieve statistical significance suggest there may be excessive antimicrobial use and should prompt evaluation by the ASP. Ensuring that the unit is correctly categorized is a first step in this analysis. (For more information, please see https://www.cdc.gov/nhsn/PDFs/pscManual/11pscAURcurrent.pdf.)

Both DDDs and DOTs are calculated by drug use, such that if a patient receives two antimicrobials for 10 days, the DOT is 20. If one is reporting only overall DOT, there may be an incentive to use broad-spectrum antimicrobials to decrease the overall DOT. To overcome this, most institutions evaluate both selected broad-spectrum antibiotic DOT per 1000 patient days and overall DOT per 1000 patient days.

In addition to overall hospital use, ASPs should evaluate specific antibiotics and locations where stewardship efforts are implemented.

A Structured Taskforce of Experts Working at Reliable Standards for Stewardship (STEWARDS) panel evaluated ASP metrics for usefulness and feasibility. The panel recommends that DOT per admission and DOT per patient-days be measured to track antimicrobial utilization.[47]

Antimicrobial Cost

Antimicrobial costs are often collected to justify ASP programs. Although cost reduction is not the primary goal of ASPs, programs are generally cost-effective and pay for themselves. For many institutions, this may be the easiest variable to track. Since cost of antimicrobials is contract-dependent, this variable cannot be used as a benchmark. One caveat: collecting cost information from purchasing can be misleading, as savvy buyers often purchase products in large quantities at low prices, and it may remain in inventory for long periods of time. It is more accurate to correlate antimicrobial cost savings with antimicrobial dispensing or charting. The IDSA guidelines recommend measuring costs based on antimicrobial administration or prescriptions instead of purchasing data. When considering cost, it is also important to monitor the slope of rising costs before and after ASP initiation, with the realization that costs often stabilize over time. Calculating antimicrobial acquisition cost for pediatric patients poses some difficulty.

As doses are dependent on weight of the patient, cost per dose for the same antimicrobial may be different for each patient. Estimating cost savings by calculating an average dose and cost per dose, then multiplying the average cost per dose by the reduction in DOT, may be the most pragmatic method in a pediatric facility of determining antimicrobial cost reductions. The difficulty of this metric is highlighted by the lower number of pediatric studies assessing antimicrobial cost compared to adult facilities in the stewardship literature.

Recently, experts have suggested that ASPs abandon drug cost as a measure of process and outcome. Since the goal of ASPs is to improve the quality of care, estimating overall cost of care may be a better measure.[46] Length of stay is the primary driver of cost, and some ASPs have found interventions that can help drive down that cost. In pediatrics, standardization of care of patients with appendicitis and of febrile infants was shown to decrease length of stay (and therefore cost).[10,48]

Antimicrobial Appropriateness

Improving the use of antimicrobials is a key goal of ASP. Although aggregate data are the most readily available, they do not adequately account for clinical indications.[49] Ensuring that appropriate diagnostic criteria are applied, that appropriate cultures are obtained, and that antimicrobial selection is appropriate may require manual review. The CDC has standardized tools for drug use evaluations or antibiotic audit forms that are available to assist ASPs. (See the Centers for Disease Control and Prevention, Antibiotic audit forms, 2013; http://www.cdc.gov/getsmart/healthcare/implementation.html; Handout 13.3.) These data collection forms allow ASPs to evaluate the quality of antimicrobial use through chart review by answering questions such as, "Were cultures collected prior to antibiotic administration?" "What was the indication for the antimicrobial regimen?" "Was the duration appropriate?" etc. These tools can be modified as seen fit by the ASP to collect pertinent information regarding a specific intervention.

When evaluating for appropriateness, disease-based evaluation may allow for a more evidence-based review of appropriateness and may identify opportunities to evaluate the adherence to institutional or national guidelines. The following metrics may be considered when performing these reviews: appropriate antimicrobial, dose, route, frequency, documentation of indication for use, length of therapy, adherence to clinical pathway or guidelines, and appropriate de-escalation, if applicable.[46] Assessing appropriateness is a labor-intensive process. Using a sample from a specific population (e.g., patients with pneumonia) or using a point-prevalence methodology may make this goal more feasible.[49] During a point-prevalence study, assessment of an institution's antimicrobial use on a specific day is used to sample the antimicrobial appropriateness of an institution. This information can be used to identify and evaluate ASP interventions.

Number of Interventions

Many ASPs measure and report the number of recommendations made to clinicians. Experts have called this practice into question, since the recommendations themselves provide no information on desired outcomes.[46] As the goal of the ASP is to optimize antimicrobial use and not to maximize the number of times the ASP intervenes, evaluating a program by the number of recommendations made is unlikely to be important.

Clinical Outcomes

Clinical outcomes are reported in a minority of ASPs. Infection-related mortality, infection-related length of stay, cure, and infection-related readmission have been proposed as outcome measures. However,

Assessment of Appropriateness of Inpatient Antibiotics

1. Date: ______________________________

   Gender: Male: Female

   Age: ___________________________

   Service: _______________________

   Antibiotic: _____________________

2. Was an indication for antibiotic use documented? Yes No

   A. If **Yes**, please document the indication below:

   ____

3. Were cultures collected? Yes No

   A. If **Yes**, please document what site(s) or body fluid(s) were cultured.

   ____

   B. If **Yes**, were antibiotics administered before collection of cultures?

   Yes No

   C. If **Yes** (cultures were collected), was an organism isolated by culture within 72 hours of the first dose of antibiotics? (If **Yes**, skip to question #5):

   Yes No

4. If no organism was isolated with 72 hours of the first dose of antibiotics, were antibiotics prescribed? Yes No

   A. If No, was a reason for continuation documented? (Please document reason below):

   ____

5. If an organism was isolated by culture, was it susceptible to the prescribed antibiotic? **(PRINT ANTIOBIOTIC SUSCEPTIBILITY REPORT)**

   Yes No

6. If an organism was isolated by culture, were antibiotics changed or stopped after culture results were available? Yes No

   A. If **Yes**, please document antibiotic change or check box below if stopped:

   ____

   __________Antibiotics Stopped

7. Was the patient initially prescribed an intravenous (IV) antibiotic with good oral bioavailability? (See Appendix A): Yes No

   A. If **Yes**, was the antibiotic changed to an oral formulation (PO), within 24 hours of being eligible for oral medications? (See Appendix B for criteria):

   Yes No

8. Total duration of antibiotic therapy while an inpatient for the above indication? ____ Days

Assessment of Appropriateness of Inpatient Antibiotics

Appendix A

Amoxicillin

Amoxicillin/Clavulanate

Azithromycin

Cefpodoxime

Ciprofloxacin

Clindamycin

Doxycycline

Levofloxacin

Linezolid

Moxifloxacin

Trimethoprim/Sulfamethoxazole

Appendix B

1. Patients must meet the following criteria:
    A. Receiving oral or gastric tube intake
    B. Taking other oral medications
2. Patients are considered inappropriate for IV to PO conversion if any of the following are present:
    A. Mucositis
    B. Malabsorption syndrome or gastrointestinal motility disorder
    C. Severe nausea, vomiting, or diarrhea
    D. Continuous nasogastric suctioning
    E. Continuous enteral feeds are contraindicated with oral ciprofloxacin, levofloxacin, or moxifloxacin

multiple confounders in addition to antimicrobial selection affect these outcomes, such as other improvements in care, diagnosis distribution, and secular trends emphasizing early discharge.[49] Improving antibiotic use can have significant impact on the rates of hospital-onset CDI; however, this is also confounded in that most infection prevention programs also prioritize interventions to decrease CDI, and ASP interventions are therefore part of a bundled approach. An expert panel evaluating ASP metrics determined that, in their opinion, no clinical outcome was ready for immediate use and tracking under the current healthcare system, although readmission due to infectious diagnosis was identified as an area for future study.[47]

Intervention-Specific Metrics

When considering implementation of a specific intervention, such as a care process model, ASPs should consider the metrics necessary to determine whether the change is positive. Process measures, outcome measures, and balancing measures should be specific to the intervention. The Driver Diagram can be helpful to determine appropriate metrics for the intervention.

Plotting Data over Time

Evaluating metrics over time is a helpful quality improvement tool.[50] The use of run charts and control charts allows ASPs to annotate interventions and visualize the change in the metric over time. Interrupted-time series (ITS) analysis is a powerful tool to evaluate the impact of an intervention. ITS controls for trends in the data before implementation and after implementation of the intervention. This method estimates the immediate change after an intervention and the trend of a segment of time prior to and after the intervention.[51]

Education

Education is a critical element to a successful ASP, although education alone has not been shown to be a sustainable strategy for improvement in hospitals.[52] Education is most effective when paired with other interventions.[4] ASPs should educate hospital leadership and other interested parties regarding the data on antimicrobial prescribing, antimicrobial resistance, adherence to ASP recommendations, and status of other interventions. The ASP team should educate frontline healthcare personnel (HCP) about bacterial resistance, antibiotics, proper diagnosis and principles of infection management, and infection prevention.[53] The goal of education is to change the clinicians' attitude toward infection management as well as their prescribing behavior.[53] This can be accomplished in many formats, including didactic presentations, flyers and posters, computer screen savers, or through other electronic communication. Tools used in decision support can also be educational. Even more importantly, education must be provided when making audit and feedback recommendations associated with specific patients.

Approach to the Clinical Scenario

As defined by the CDC, the most important elements of a successful ASP are:

- *Leadership Commitment*: Dedicating necessary human, financial, and information technology resources.
- *Accountability*: Appointing a single leader responsible for program outcomes. Experience with successful programs shows that a physician leader is effective.
- *Drug Expertise*: Appointing a single pharmacist leader responsible for working to improve antibiotic use.
- *Action*: Implementing at least one recommended action, such as systemic evaluation of ongoing treatment need after a set period of initial treatment (i.e., "antibiotic timeout" after 48 hours).
- *Tracking*: Monitoring antibiotic prescribing and resistance patterns.
- *Reporting*: Regular reporting information on antibiotic use and resistance to doctors, nurses, and relevant staff.
- *Education*: Educating clinicians about resistance and optimal prescribing.

The hospital pharmacist in the clinical scenario should consider these elements when when developing an ASP to address broad-spectrum antibiotic use in pediatric inpatient units. Objective metrics to gauge success of the program include:

- Overall, drug-specific, and population-specific antibiotic use
- Appropriateness of prescribing
- Clinical outcomes if measureable
- Cost

Unresolved Issues

There are many unresolved issued in the area of antimicrobial stewardship, especially in the pediatric population. The evolution of diagnostic testing is an exciting area for evaluation and research, and ASPs have been key in assessing the need for and success of these tests. Rapid diagnostic testing with biomarkers and molecular techniques can be very useful for ASPs, as more narrow or definitive therapy can be prescribed sooner. There are limited cost and outcome studies in pediatrics regarding rapid diagnostic testing. Several single-center studies have shown positive impact of pediatric ASPs, but there are no multi-center pediatric studies to evaluate which strategies are the most optimal to improve outcomes. Resource allocation for ASP may not include pediatrics, as the regulatory requirements do not mention pediatrics specifically. Therefore pediatric-specific recommendations may be overlooked without a champion in place. Alternatively, ASP guidance from a children's hospital may not be appropriate to implement in community hospitals or other tertiary care centers with children's units. There are also educational shortcomings, as curricula around antimicrobial prescribing, antibiotic resistance, and principles of antimicrobial stewardship are not standard in training programs.

References

1. Federal Register. Executive Order combating antibiotic resistant bacteria 2014. Available from: https://www.federalregister.gov/documents/2014/09/23/2014-22805/combating-antibiotic-resistant-bacteria. Accessed October 28, 2018.
2. Federal Register. Meeting of the Presidential Advisory Council on combating antibiotic-resistant bacteria 2015. Available from: https://www.federalregister.gov/documents/2015/09/11/2015-22920/meeting-of-the-presidential-advisory-council-on-combating-antibiotic-resistant-bacteria. Accessed October 28, 2018.
3. Siegel JD, Rhinehart E, Jackson M, Chiarello L. Healthcare Infection Control Practices Advisory Committee. Management of multidrug-resistant organisms in healthcare settings, 2006. *Am J Infect Control.* 2007;35(10 Suppl 2):S165–S193.
4. Dellit TH, Owens RC, McGowan JE, et al. Infectious Diseases Society of America and the Society for Healthcare Epidemiology of America guidelines for developing an institutional program to enhance antimicrobial stewardship. *Clin Infect Dis.* 2007;44(2):159–177.
5. Centers for Disease Control and Prevention. Get Smart for Healthcare: implementation resources 2012. Available from: http://www.cdc.gov/getsmart/healthcare/implementation.html. Accessed October 28, 2018,
6. Fishman N. Policy statement on antimicrobial stewardship by the Society for Healthcare Epidemiology of America (SHEA), the Infectious Diseases Society of America (IDSA), and the Pediatric Infectious Diseases Society (PIDS). *Infect Control Hosp Epidemiol.* 2012;33(4):322–327.
7. Centers for Disease Control and Prevention. Core elements of hospital antibiotic stewardship programs. 2014. Available from: http://www.cdc.gov/getsmart/healthcare/implementation/core-elements.html. Accessed October 28, 2018.
8. Barlam TF, Cosgrove SE, Abbo LM, et al. Implementing an antibiotic stewardship program: guidelines by the Infectious Diseases Society of America and the Society for Healthcare Epidemiology of America. *Clin Infect Dis.* 2016;62(10):e51–e77.

9. Olmstead MG, Geisen E, Powell R, Murphy J, Bell D, Stanley M. *U.S. News & World Report*, Methodology: *U.S. News & World* Report best children's hospitals 2016–17. 2016. http://static.usnews.com/documents/health/best-hospitals/BCH_Methodology_2016-17.pdf. Accessed October 26, 2018.
10. Byington CL, Reynolds CC, Korgenski K, et al. Costs and infant outcomes after implementation of a care process model for febrile infants. *Pediatrics*. 2012;130(1):e16–e24.
11. Kronman MP, Hersh AL, Gerber JS, et al. Identifying antimicrobial stewardship targets for pediatric surgical patients. *J Pediatr Infect Dis Soc*. 2015;4(4):e100–8.
12. Gerber JS, Newland JG, Coffin SE, et al. Variability in antibiotic use at children's hospitals. *Pediatrics*. 2010;126(6):1067–1073.
13. Skarda DE, Schall K, Rollins M, et al. A dynamic postoperative protocol provides efficient care for pediatric patients with non-ruptured appendicitis. *J Pediatr Surg*. 2015;50(1):149–152.
14. Saari A, Virta LJ, Sankilampi U, Dunkel L, Saxen H. Antibiotic exposure in infancy and risk of being overweight in the first 24 months of life. *Pediatrics*. 2015;135(4):617–626.
15. Kronman MP, Zaoutis TE, Haynes K, Feng R, Coffin SE. Antibiotic exposure and IBD development among children: a population-based cohort study. *Pediatrics*. 2012;130(4):e794–803.
16. Horton DB, Scott FI, Haynes K, et al. Antibiotic exposure and juvenile idiopathic arthritis: a case–control study. *Pediatrics*. 2015;136(2):e333–e343.
17. Shehab N, Lovegrove MC, Geller AI, Rose KO, Weidle NJ, Budnitz DS. US emergency department visits for outpatient adverse drug events, 2013–2014. *JAMA*. 2016;316(20):2115–2125.
18. Grohskopf LA, Huskins WC, Sinkowitz-Cochran RL, Levine GL, Goldmann DA, Jarvis WR. Use of antimicrobial agents in United States neonatal and pediatric intensive care patients. *Pediatr Infect Dis J*. 2005;24(9):766–773.
19. Singh N, Patel KM, Leger MM, et al. Risk of resistant infections with *Enterobacteriaceae* in hospitalized neonates. *Pediatr Infect Dis J*. 2002;21(11):1029–1033.
20. Benjamin DK Jr, Stoll BJ, Gantz MG, et al. Neonatal candidiasis: epidemiology, risk factors, and clinical judgment. *Pediatrics*. 2010;126(4):e865–e873.
21. Patel SJ, Saiman L. Principles and strategies of antimicrobial stewardship in the neonatal intensive care unit. *Semin Perinatol*. 2012;36(6):431–436.
22. Schulman J, Dimand RJ, Lee HC, Duenas GV, Bennett MV, Gould JB. Neonatal intensive care unit antibiotic use. *Pediatrics*. 2015;135(5):826–833.
23. Cotten CM, Taylor S, Stoll B, et al. Prolonged duration of initial empirical antibiotic treatment is associated with increased rates of necrotizing enterocolitis and death for extremely low birth weight infants. *Pediatrics*. 2009;123(1):58–66.
24. Lortholary O, Desnos-Ollivier M, Sitbon K, et al. Recent exposure to caspofungin or fluconazole influences the epidemiology of candidemia: a prospective multicenter study involving 2,441 patients. *Antimicrob Agents Chemother*. 2011;55(2):532–538.
25. Shah DN, Yau R, Lasco TM, et al. Impact of prior inappropriate fluconazole dosing on isolation of fluconazole-nonsusceptible *Candida* species in hospitalized patients with candidemia. *Antimicrob Agents Chemother*. 2012;56(6):3239–3243.

26.. Wolf J, Sun Y, Tang L, et al. Antimicrobial stewardship barriers and goals in pediatric oncology and bone marrow transplantation: a survey of antimicrobial stewardship practitioners. *Infect Control Hosp Epidemiol.* 2016;37(3):343–347.
27. Newland JG, Gerber JS, Weissman SJ, et al. Prevalence and characteristics of antimicrobial stewardship programs at freestanding children's hospitals in the United States. *Infect Control Hosp Epidemiol.* 2014;35(3):265–271.
28. Hersh AL, De Lurgio SA, Thurm C, et al. Antimicrobial stewardship programs in freestanding children's hospitals. *Pediatrics.* 2015;135(1):33–39.
29. Beardsley JR, Williamson JC, Johnson JW, Luther VP, Wrenn RH, Ohl CC. Show me the money: long-term financial impact of an antimicrobial stewardship program. *Infect Control Hosp Epidemiol.* 2012;33(4):398–400.
30. Ross RK, Hersh AL, Kronman MP, Newland JG, Gerber JS. Cost of antimicrobial therapy across US children's hospitals. *Infect Control Hosp Epidemiol.* 2015;36(10):1242–1244.
31. Standiford HC, Chan S, Tripoli M, Weekes E, Forrest GN. Antimicrobial stewardship at a large tertiary care academic medical center: cost analysis before, during, and after a 7-year program. *Infect Control Hosp Epidemiol.* 2012;33(4):338–345.
32. Srinivasan A. Engaging hospitalists in antimicrobial stewardship: the CDC perspective. *J Hosp Med.* 2011;6(Suppl 1):S31–S33.
33. Rohde JM, Jacobsen D, Rosenberg DJ. Role of the hospitalist in antimicrobial stewardship: a review of work completed and description of a multisite collaborative. *Clin Ther.* 2013;35(6):751–757.
34. Newman RE, Hedican EB, Herigon JC, Williams DD, Williams AR, Newland JG. Impact of a guideline on management of children hospitalized with community-acquired pneumonia. *Pediatrics.* 2012;129(3):e597–e604.
35. Kaye KS. Antimicrobial de-escalation strategies in hospitalized patients with pneumonia, intra-abdominal infections, and bacteremia. *J Hosp Med.* 2012;7(Suppl 1):S13–S21.
36. Newland JG, Stach LM, De Lurgio SA, et al. Impact of a prospective-audit-with-feedback antimicrobial stewardship program at a children's hospital. *J Pediatr Infect Dis Soc.* 2012;1(3):179–186.
37. Di Pentima MC, Chan S, Hossain J. Benefits of a pediatric antimicrobial stewardship program at a children's hospital. *Pediatrics.* 2011;128(6):1062–1070.
38. Agwu AL, Lee CK, Jain SK, et al. A World Wide Web-based antimicrobial stewardship program improves efficiency, communication, and user satisfaction and reduces cost in a tertiary care pediatric medical center. *Clin Infect Dis.* 2008;47(6):747–753.
39. Metjian TA, Prasad PA, Kogon A, Coffin SE, Zaoutis TE. Evaluation of an antimicrobial stewardship program at a pediatric teaching hospital. *Pediatr Infect Dis J.* 2008;27(2):106–111.
40. Centers for Disease Control and Prevention. Collaborative practice agreements and pharmacists' patient care services. A resource for pharmacists. 2013. Available from: https://www.cdc.gov/dhdsp/pubs/docs/Translational_Tools_Pharmacists.pdf.
41. Gerber JS, Kronman MP, Ross RK, et al. Identifying targets for antimicrobial stewardship in children's hospitals. *Infect Control Hosp Epidemiol.* 2013;34(12):1252–1258.
42. Williams DJ, Edwards KM, Self WH, et al. Antibiotic choice for children hospitalized with pneumonia and adherence to national guidelines. *Pediatrics.* 2015;136(1):44–52.

43. Shawyer AC, Hatchell AC, Pemberton J, Flageole H. Compliance with published recommendations for postoperative antibiotic management of children with appendicitis: a chart audit. *J Pediatr Surg*. 2015;50(5):783–785.
44. Berrington A. Antimicrobial prescribing in hospitals: be careful what you measure. *J Antimicrob Chemother*. 2010;65(1):163–168.
45. Bumpass JB, McDaneld PM, DePestel DD, et al. Outcomes and metrics for antimicrobial stewardship: survey of physicians and pharmacists. *Clin Infect Dis*. 2014;59(Suppl 3):S108–S111.
46. Dodds Ashley ES, Kaye KS, DePestel DD, Hermsen ED. Antimicrobial stewardship: philosophy versus practice. *Clin Infect Dis*. 2014;59(Suppl 3):S112–S121.
47. Moehring RW, Anderson DJ, Cochran RL, et al. Expert consensus on metrics to assess the impact of patient-level antimicrobial stewardship interventions in acute-care settings. *Clin Infect Dis*. 2017;64(3):377–383.
48. Skarda DE, Schall K, Rollins M, et al. Response-based therapy for ruptured appendicitis reduces resource utilization. *J Pediatr Surg*. 2014;49(12):1726–1729.
49. Morris AM. Antimicrobial stewardship programs: appropriate measures and metrics to study their impact. *Curr Treat Options Infect Dis*. 2014;6(2):101–112.
50. Institute for Helathcare Improvement. Science of improvement: establishing measures. Available from: http://www.ihi.org/resources/Pages/HowtoImprove/ScienceofImprovementEstablishingMeasures.aspx. Accessed October 26, 2018.
51. Penfold RB, Zhang F. Use of interrupted time series analysis in evaluating health care quality improvements. *Acad Pediatr*. 2013;13(6 Suppl):S38–S44.
52. Belongia EA, Knobloch MJ, Kieke BA, Davis JP, Janette C, Besser RE. Impact of statewide program to promote appropriate antimicrobial drug use. *Emerg Infect Dis*. 2005;11(6):912–920.
53. Ohl CA, Luther VP. Health care provider education as a tool to enhance antibiotic stewardship practices. *Infect Dis Clin North Am*. 2014;28(2):177–193.

APPENDIX | Overview of Transmission-Based Precautions and Personal Protective Equipment

Personal Protective Equipment (PPE)

Personal protective equipment (PPE) refers to the various barriers used alone or in combination to protect healthcare personnel (HCP) from contact with infectious microorganisms. PPE includes gloves, isolation gowns, masks, goggles, and face shields. Precautions to prevent transmission of infectious pathogens include standard, contact, droplet, or airborne precautions (Table A.1). In some situations, a combination of precaution categories is required (e.g., contact plus droplet precautions for adenovirus bronchiolitis).

Standard Precautions

Standard precautions should be followed with every single patient encounter; HCP should assume that all patients are potentially infected or colonized with pathogens that may be transmitted in the healthcare setting. Thus, HCP should wear the appropriate PPE to prevent potential occupational exposures.

PPE recommendations may differ based on the anticipated extent of exposure (e.g., wearing gloves while changing a wound dressing, regardless of culture results) and the potential (or known) pathogens with which the patient is colonized or infected (e.g., wearing a mask when entering the room of a coughing infant who has possible pertussis). When the etiological agent of an individual's infection is unknown, HCP should choose PPE based on the differential diagnosis of possible pathogens, until diagnostic test results are available.

TABLE A.1 Transmission-Based Precautions

TRANSMISSION PRECAUTIONS	DEFINITION	PPE COMPONENTS	EXAMPLE
Standard Precautions	Prevents potential transmission of pathogens in various situations, dependent on the HCP–patient interaction. Before every patient encounter, the HCP should consider what potential exposure may occur.	Dependent on anticipated exposure(s) during patient care	HCP wearing goggles and mask during aerosol-generating procedure, or HCP wearing disposable gloves when handling blood and body fluids
Contact Precautions	Prevents transmission of pathogens that are spread by direct or indirect contact with the patient or his/her environment.	Disposable gloves and gown	Draining open wounds, *Herpes simplex* skin lesions, respiratory syncytial virus, multi-drug-resistant organisms (e.g., carbapenem-resistant *Enterobacteriaceae*)
Droplet Precautions	Prevents transmission of pathogens spread via close contact with respiratory secretions within short distance (<3 feet).	Disposable mask	Pertussis
Airborne Precautions	Prevents transmission of pathogens that are capable of travel over long distances when suspended in air.	Fit-tested N95 respirator or powered air-purifying respirator (PAPR)	Measles, varicella, active pulmonary tuberculosis
Combination: Contact + Droplet Precautions	See above.	Disposable gloves, gown, mask	Adenovirus bronchiolitis in an infant

Vertical vs. Horizontal Strategies in Infection Prevention

Infection prevention approaches can be broadly categorized as "vertical" or "horizontal."

Vertical Approach

The vertical approach is pathogen-specific; the goal is the reduce one pathogen. Examples of vertical approach include *active surveillance* for an MDRO (e.g., screening every ICU admission for MRSA colonization), *contact precautions* for patients with VRE colonization or infection, and *pathogen-specific decolonization* (e.g., nasal mupirocin to eradicate anterior nares colonization of *Staphylococcus aureus*).

Horizontal Approach

A horizontal approach to decrease MDRO transmission widens the scope to reduce *all* infections and/or transmission. Examples of horizontal approaches include *standard precautions* (general interventions to decrease risk of MDRO transmission, including syndromic PPE use, hand hygiene, and respiratory etiquette), *chlorhexidine gluconate (CHG) skin bathing* to decrease the bioburden of MDRO skin colonization, and *prevention care bundles* (e.g., central line–associated bloodstream infection [CLABSI] prevention bundle).

INDEX

Page numbers followed by *f*, and *t* refer to figures, and tables, respectively.